Contributors

Paolo Campisi, MSc, MD, FRCSC, FAAP
Assistant Professor
Department of Otolaryngology—Head
& Neck Surgery
University of Toronto
Toronto, Ontario
Canada

Adam Cheng, MD, FRCPC (Ped EM), FAAP
Fellowship Director and Staff Physician
Division of Pediatric Emergency Medicine
British Columbia Children's Hospital
Clinical Assistant Professor,
University of British Columbia
British Columbia, Vancouver, Canada

Priscilla Chiu, MD, PhD, FRCSC
Assistant Professor and Associate
Pediatric Surgeon
Division of General Surgery
The Hospital for Sick Children
University of Toronto
Toronto, Ontario
Canada

Howard Clarke, MD, PhD, FRCS,
FAAP, FACS
Medical Director, Burn Unit
Division of Plastic Surgery
The Hospital for Sick Children;
Professor
Department of Surgery
University of Toronto
Toronto, Ontario
Canada

Sandrine de Ribaupierre, MD, FRCSC
Fellow, Pediatric Neurosurgery
The Hospital for Sick Children
Toronto, Ontario
Canada

Peter Dirks, MD, PhD, FRCSC
Staff Neurosurgeon
Division of Neurosurgery
The Hospital for Sick Children;

Assistant Professor
Department of Surgery
University of Toronto
Toronto, Ontario
Canada

James M. Drake, BSE, MBBCh, iMSc,
FRCSC, FACS
Division Head
Department of Surgery Division
of Neurosurgery
The Hospital for Sick Children
University of Toronto Faculty of Medicine
Toronto, Ontario
Canada

Christopher R. Forrest, MD, MSc,
FRCSC, FACS
Chief, Division of Plastic Surgery
Medical Director, HSC Centre for
Craniofacial Care and Research
Professor
Division of Plastic Surgery
Department of Surgery
University of Toronto
Toronto, Ontario
Canada

Anne-Marie Guerguerian, MD,
FAAP, FRCPC
Staff Physician, Department of Critical
Care Medicine
Hospital for Sick Children
Assistant Professor, Pediatrics
and Critical Care
Faculty of Medicine
University of Toronto
Toronto, Ontario
Canada

Patricio Herrera, MD
Cirugía Pediátrica
Hospital Padre Hurtado —Clínica Alemana
de Santiago
Santiago
Chile

Andrew Howard, MD, MSc, FRCS(C)
Staff Orthopaedic Surgeon
Division of Orthopaedic Surgery
Director, Trauma Program
The Hospital for Sick Children
University of Toronto
Toronto, Ontario
Canada

James Hutchison, MD, FRCPC, FAAP
Staff Physician, Department of Critical Care
The Hospital for Sick Children;
Associate Professor, Pediatrics
and Critical Care
Faculty of Medicine
University of Toronto
Toronto, Ontario
Canada

Shauna Jain, MD, FRCPC
Staff Emergency Physician
Hospital for Sick Children;
Assistant Professor of Pediatrics
University of Toronto
Toronto, Ontario
Canada

Andrew Jea, MD
Chief Fellow
Department of Surgery
Division of Neurosurgery
Hospital for Sick Children;
Faculty of Medicine
University of Toronto
Toronto, Ontario
Canada

Cengiz Karsli, BSc, MD, FRCPC
Assistant Professor
The Hospital for Sick Children
University of Toronto
Toronto, Ontario
Canada

Amina Lalani, MD, FRCPC
Staff Emergency Physician
The Hospital for Sick Children
Assistant Professor of Pediatrics
The University of Toronto
Toronto, Ontario
Canada

Jacob C. Langer, MD, FRCPC
Professor
Department of Surgery
University of Toronto;
Chief, Division of Pediatric General Surgery
The Hospital for Sick Children
Toronto, Ontario
Canada

Sanjay V. Mehta, MD, MEd, FRCPC,
FAAP, FACEP
Assistant Professor
Division of Pediatric Emergency Medicine
Department of Pediatrics
University of Toronto
Toronto, Ontario
Canada

Angelo Mikrogianakis, MD, FRCPC
Emergency Physician and Trauma
Team Leader
Division of Emergency Medicine
and Critical Care
The Hospital for Sick Children
Assistant Professor of Pediatrics
University of Toronto
Toronto, Ontario
Canada

Stephen F. Miller, MD, FRCPC
Assistant Professor
Department of Medical Imaging
University of Toronto;
Staff Pediatric Radiologist
The Hospital for Sick Children
Toronto, Ontario
Canada

Michelle Shouldice, MD, FRCPC
Director, Suspected Child Abuse
and Neglect (SCAN) Program
Division of Pediatric Medicine
The Hospital for Sick Children;
Assistant Professor, University of Toronto
Toronto, Ontario
Canada

Laura Snell, MD
Resident
Department of Plastic Surgery
University of Toronto
Toronto, Ontario
Canada

Rahim Valani, MD, CCFP-EM, FRCPC,
PG Dip Med Ed
Division of Pediatric Emergency Medicine
Hospital for Sick Children
Toronto, Ontario
Canada

THE HOSPITAL FOR SICK CHILDREN
MANUAL OF
PEDIATRIC TRAUMA

THE HOSPITAL FOR SICK CHILDREN
MANUAL OF
PEDIATRIC TRAUMA

Angelo Mikrogianakis, MD, FRCPC
Emergency Physician and Trauma Team Leader
Division of Emergency Medicine and Critical Care
The Hospital for Sick Children
Assistant Professor of Pediatrics
University of Toronto
Toronto, Ontario
Canada

**Rahim Valani, MD, CCFP-EM, FRCPC,
PG Dip Med Ed**
Division of Pediatric Emergency Medicine
The Hospital for Sick Children
University of Toronto
Sunnybrook Health Sciences Centre
Division of Emergency Medicine
Toronto, Ontario
Canada

Adam Cheng, MD, FRCPC, FAAP
Fellowship Director and Staff Physician
Division of Pediatric Emergency Medicine
British Columbia Children's Hospital
Clinical Assistant Professor,
University of British Columbia
British Columbia,Vancouver, Canada

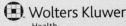 Wolters Kluwer | Lippincott Williams & Wilkins
Health
Philadelphia • Baltimore • New York • London
Buenos Aires • Hong Kong • Sydney • Tokyo

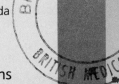

Acquisitions Editor: Frances R. DeStefano
Managing Editor: Michelle LaPlante
Project Manager: Bridgett Dougherty
Manufacturing Manager: Kathleen Brown
Marketing Manager: Angela Panetta
Design Coordinator: Teresa Mallon
Production Services: International Typesetting and Composition

© 2008 The Hospital for Sick Children
530 Walnut Street
Philadelphia, PA 19106
LWW.com

Printed in the USA

Library of Congress Cataloging-in-Publication Data

The Hospital for Sick Children manual of pediatric trauma / [edited by] Angelo Mikrogianakis, Rahim Valani, Adam Cheng.—1st ed.
    p. ; cm.
  Includes bibliographical references and index.
  ISBN-13: 978-0-7817-7816-9
  ISBN-10: 0-7817-7816-6
  1. Children—Wounds and injuries—Treatment—Handbooks, manuals, etc.   I. Mikrogianakis, Angelo.   II. Valani, Rahim.   III. Cheng, Adam.   IV. Hospital for Sick Children.   V. Title: Manual of pediatric trauma.
  [DNLM: 1. Wounds and Injuries—Handbooks.   2. Wounds and Injuries—therapy—Handbooks.   3. Child.   4. Infant. WO 39 H828 2008]
  RD93.5.C4H67 2008
  617.10083—dc22

                                                          2007025181

Care has been taken to confirm the accuracy of the information presented and to describe generally accepted practices. However, the authors, editors, and publisher are not responsible for errors or omissions or for any consequences from application of the information in this book and make no warranty, expressed or implied, with respect to the currency, completeness, or accuracy of the contents of the publication. Application of this information in a particular situation remains the professional responsibility of the practitioner.

The authors, editors, and publisher have exerted every effort to ensure that drug selection and dosage set forth in this text are in accordance with current recommendations and practice at the time of publication. However, in view of ongoing research, changes in government regulations, and the constant flow of information relating to drug therapy and drug reactions, the reader is urged to check the package insert for each drug for any change in indications and dosage and for added warnings and precautions. This is particularly important when the recommended agent is a new or infrequently employed drug.

Some drugs and medical devices presented in this publication have Food and Drug Administration (FDA) clearance for limited use in restricted research settings. It is the responsibility of the health care provider to ascertain the FDA status of each drug or device planned for use in their clinical practice.

To purchase additional copies of this book, call our customer service department at (800) 638-3030 or fax orders to (301) 223-2320. International customers should call (301) 223-2300.

Visit Lippincott Williams & Wilkins on the Internet: at LWW.com. Lippincott Williams & Wilkins customer service representatives are available from 8:30 am to 6pm, EST.

10 9 8 7 6 5 4 3 2 1

Dedication

Thank you to my parents and sister who have always guided me with wisdom, support and love. Above all, dedicated to my dearest wife and three little darlings, Payton, Felicia and Nicholas. You are my inspiration, motivation and joy.

—Angelo Mikrogianakis

To my parents and brothers for being a source of inspiration for me over the years, and supporting my ideas; my mentors and teachers who have taught me the ropes; and to my friends and colleagues for their understanding and support. A special thanks to Serena for your support and encouragement to make it through.

—Rahim Valani

Special thanks to my parents, Jane and Smiley, for providing the guiding light throughout my life; my sister Aisha for being a constant support and friend; my fiancé Natalie for making me happier than I've ever been; and to my friends for remaining by my side through the thick and the thin!

—Adam Cheng

Preface

Every child who suffers a traumatic injury deserves the best care to ensure a successful recovery. We wish to share what we know and what we have learned, to ensure that all children, no matter where they present, receive excellent and knowledgeable care.

Welcome to the Hospital for Sick Children Manual of Pediatric Trauma. This book was inspired by:

- Our perceived need for further education regarding pediatric trauma patients.
- Knowledge translation, which is imperative in the pursuit of medical excellence.
- The SickKids core values, which encourage the continued pursuit of:
  - Excellence
  - Collaboration
  - Innovation
  - Integrity

—*Angelo Mikrogianakis*
—*Rahim Valani*
—*Adam Cheng*

Paul W. Wales, MD, MSc, FRCSC, FACS
Staff Surgeon
Division of General Surgery
Clinical Director
Trauma Program
The Hospital for Sick Children;
Assistant Professor
Department of Surgery
University of Toronto
Toronto, Ontario
Canada

Mohammed Zamakhshary, MD,
MEd, FRCSC
Fellow, Pediatric General Surgery
The Hospital for Sick Children
University of Toronto
Toronto, Ontario
Canada

Acknowledgments

Special thanks to the Sick Kids Trauma Program Management Team; our colleagues in the Division of Emergency Medicine, Department of Critical Care Medicine, and Department of Surgery at The Hospital for Sick Children; all our contributing authors; Heidi Falckh and Susana Andres from the Office of Corporate Ventures; Agnes Bellegris for her superior editorial skills; and Lippincott Williams & Wilkins for seeing the value in this project and helping to make our dream real.

—*Angelo Mikrogianakis*
—*Rahim Valani*
—*Adam Cheng*

Table of Contents

CHAPTER 1

Introduction

Angelo Mikrogianakis, MD, FRCPC

EPIDEMIOLOGY OF PEDIATRIC TRAUMATIC INJURY[1]
- Traumatic injury is the leading preventable health problem in children.
- Trauma is the leading cause of death in children after infancy.
- Most common causes of injury-related deaths are:
  - Motor vehicle crashes.
  - Submersion injury.
  - Homicide.
  - Suicide.
  - Fires.
- In 2003 there were 11,090 injury-related deaths in the United States in those less than 20 years old.[2]
- 10 million ED visits in those under 20 and >10 million primary care office visits yearly.[3]
- Traumatic injury is the leading cause of childhood hospitalization.
  - 300,000 hospitalizations yearly in the United States.[4]
- Injury in children aged 5 to 14 is the leading cause of medical spending in the United States.
- Billions of dollars are spent on direct and indirect expenses related to injury annually.
  - Annual lifetime cost of injuries to children under 15: $254 billion in 1992.
  - Medical care: $11 billion.[4]

TRAUMA IS NOT RANDOM
- Injuries commonly referred to as "accidents."
  - But injuries are not random, unpredictable tragedies.[5,6]
- Trauma has patterns, defined risk factors, and distinct preventative interventions.
- Can identify high-risk populations and target interventions.[7]
- Emergency physicians can engage in both improved acute care and prevention efforts of the severely injured child.

AGE
- Bimodal distribution in injury death rates for children and teenagers.
  - Reflects developmental and activity-related differences.
- Infants at higher risk of inflicted trauma.
  - Small size.
  - Inability to protect themselves.
- Teenagers
  - Risks amplified from increased exposure to hazards (e.g., automobile travel).
  - Increase in risk-taking behaviors (e.g., alcohol and drug use).[8]

SEX
- Males at higher death risk from all types of injury.
- Ratio of male-to-female deaths varies by injury mechanism.

- Death rate from motorcycles crashes, firearms, and falls in teenage boys approximately tenfold greater than girls.
- Pedestrian deaths only slightly higher in boys compared with girls.[8]

SOCIOECONOMIC STATUS AND RACE
- Minority and low-income children have higher rates of fatal and nonfatal traumatic injury. [9–11]
- Higher injuries in low-income neighborhoods related to educational and environmental factors.[9]

GEOGRAPHY
- Injuries not randomly or equally distributed geographically.
- Certain injuries more common in particular geographic locations due to differences in exposure to injury-associated natural features or hazards.[12,13]

TRAUMA TRIAGE SCORES[14]
- Aid prehospital personnel to determine which patients require trauma center care.
- Assist emergency physicians to determine level of trauma triage.
- Should be easy to use and reliable.
- Must accurately identify all patients requiring trauma center services.
- Should reduce overtriage of minor trauma and minimize undertriage of major trauma.[15]
- Trauma scores should not be used as sole determinant of injury triage.[16]

Revised Trauma Score (RTS) (Table 1-1)
- Trauma triage scoring system.[17]
- Elements of score are considered reliable:
  - Respiratory rate (RR) (score 0–4).
  - Systolic blood pressure (SBP) (score 0–4).
  - Glasgow Coma Scale (GCS) (score 0–4).
- Triage RTS used as prehospital triage score.
  - The integer sum of the score's three components.
    - Triage RTS has been incorporated into EMS trauma triage algorithms.[18,19]
    - Trauma patients with Triage RTS ≤11 should be taken to a trauma center.[20]
  - RTS calculated by multiplying each of the component scores by weighted coefficients:
    - RTS = 0.9368 (GCS value) + 0.7326 (SBP value) + 0.2908 (RR value).
  - RTS
    - Ranges from 0 to 7.84.
    - Correlates well with survival.
    - Higher values more predictive of survival.
  - RTS should NOT be used as sole predictor of mortality.[20,21]

Pediatric Trauma Score (PTS) (Table 1-2)
- Designed explicitly to triage pediatric trauma patients.
- Calculated from six clinical variables:
  1. Weight (kg).
  2. Airway.
  3. Systolic blood pressure.
  4. Central nervous system.
  5. Open wound.
  6. Skeletal.
- Accounts for pediatric trauma patients' frequent cerebral and cardiopulmonary instability.
- A PTS ≤8 requires triage to designated trauma center.
  - Correlates well with risk of severe injury and mortality.[22]
- Using pediatric scores makes sense but some studies have failed to demonstrate significant advantage of the PTS over RTS or clinical judgment. [20,23–26]

TABLE 1-1

Revised Trauma Score[17]

Clinical Parameter	Parameter Category	Score
Respiratory Rate (breaths/min)	10–24	4
	25–35	3
	>35	2
	<10	1
	0	0
Systolic Blood Pressure	>90	4
	70–89	3
	50–69	2
	<50	1
	0	0
Glasgow Coma Scale	14–15	4
	11–13	3
	8–10	2
	5–7	1
	3–4	0

SEVERITY OF ILLNESS (SOI) MEASURES

- Used to predict mortality risk.
- Calculated retrospectively on a group of trauma patients.
- Estimate the average SOI or expected population mortality rate.
- Can be complex and use variables that may not be available at time of injury.

TABLE 1-2

Pediatric Trauma Score[27,28]

Clinical Parameter	Parameter Category	Score Value
Weight (kg)	≥20	2
	10–19	1
	<10	−1
Airway	Normal	2
	Maintainable	1
	Unmaintainable	−1
Systolic Blood Pressure	>90	2
	50–89	1
	<50	−1
Central Nervous System	Awake	2
	Obtunded or LOC	1
	Coma or decerebrate	−1
Open Wound	None	2
	Minor	1
	Major	−1
Skeletal	None	2
	Closed fracture	1
	Open or multiple fractures	−1

- Accuracy important with SOI because used in quality-of-care assessments, institutional benchmarking, and health services research.
- Data composed of demographics, anatomic injuries, diagnostic, or physiologic.
- Lack of accuracy in medical coding is a limitation of SOI and mortality prediction models that use hospital discharge databases as measure of outcome.[29,30]

INJURY SEVERITY SCORE (ISS)

- Provides overall score for patients with multiple injuries.[31,32]
- Each injury assigned Abbreviated Injury Scale (AIS) score and is allocated to one of six body regions:
  1. Head.
  2. Face.
  3. Chest.
  4. Abdominal and pelvic contents.
  5. Extremities or pelvic girdle.
  6. External injuries.
- Only highest score in each body region is used.
- ISS calculated by adding together the squares of the 3 most severely injured body regions.
- **ISS = (AIS-body region 1)^2 + (AIS-body region 2)^2 + (AIS-body region 3)^2.**
- ISS values range from 0 to 75.

Limitations of ISS[14]

- Includes only highest value for a given body region used.
- Cannot adjust for cumulative effects of more than one injury in a body region.
- Not a continuous interval scale.
- Does not allow some integer values; therefore not linearly related to risk of mortality.
- Different injury patterns can result in similar scores even if the injuries differ significantly in their mortality risk.
  - For example, ISS of 16 from a single system injury may be associated with a higher risk of mortality than an ISS of 18 from multiple injuries.
- Similarly, one may have very different risks of mortality with the same score from a single severe injury or two smaller injuries.
- Precision and validity rely on accuracy of medical coding.

TRAUMA SYSTEMS[33]

- Trauma systems arose out of the lessons learned from casualty evacuation and injury management in the military.[34–37]
- Pediatric trauma systems originally developed using adult scenarios.
- Continued system development, assessment, and educational efforts about how childhood injuries are different are essential to combat this leading killer of children. [34–37]

Sentinel Paper

- *Accidental Death and Disability: The Neglected Disease of Modern Society*[38] published by the National Academy of Sciences of the National Research Council.
- 1966 report described magnitude of trauma in the United States.
- Examined prehospital care and hospital staffing, and made recommendations for improving trauma patient care.
- Likened trauma to infectious epidemics of the past, leading to countless preventable deaths.
- Report led to recommendations for:
  - Ambulance design.
  - Prehospital care.
  - Communications between prehospital care providers and the hospital.
  - Trauma center development.
- Emphasized research into effectiveness of these systems and recommended development of National Institute of Trauma and the National Institute of Health.
- American College of Surgeons (ACS) designated trauma committee in 1976, published *Optimal Hospital Resources for Care of the Seriously Injured*. ACS also developed Advanced Trauma Life Support (ATLS) in 1979.[36,37,39–41]

Organization of Trauma Systems

- Ranges from injury prevention programs to prehospital care:
  - Dispatch.
  - Hospital communication.
  - Medial care en route to hospital.
  - Acute hospital care.
  - Rehabilitation.
  - Quality assurance endeavors.
  - Research to assess effectiveness and guide improvements in the above.
- An effective multidisciplinary acute-care team includes:
  - Trauma surgeons.
  - Emergency medicine specialists.
  - Intensivists.
  - Pediatricians.
  - Prehospital personnel.
  - Nursing.
  - Emergency department and operating room technical staff.
  - Radiologists and radiology technicians.
  - Consulting surgical subspecialists.
  - Social workers.
  - Clergy.
  - Blood bank expertise.

Pediatric Systems

- 25% of traumatic injuries occur in children.[42]
- Trauma has been leading cause of death for children aged 1 to 14 years for decades.[1,2,3,4]
- First pediatric-specific trauma centers developed in the early 1970s in Boston, Ann Arbor, Baltimore, Washington DC, Toronto, and Brooklyn.[34,43,44]
- 15 level I and II pediatric trauma centers have been verified by the ACS.
- 1983 ATLS course included a chapter for pediatric trauma care.
- National Pediatric Trauma Registry developed in 1985 collecting data up to 2001.[45]
- ACS exploring possibility of adding a pediatric registry to the National Trauma Data Bank—currently only collects data on adults.

EVALUATING TRAUMA CARE

- In pediatric trauma most deaths occur before arrival to hospital.
- Trauma systems may be costly and administratively difficult to implement, but long-term benefits to society and families are immeasurable.
- Children treated at pediatric trauma centers have better outcomes than predicted by Trauma Injury Severity Score (TRISS).[46]
- Recent study of outcomes for children treated at pediatric trauma centers versus adult trauma centers shows that children have lower mortality at pediatric trauma centers.
  - Particularly for those with liver, spleen, and traumatic brain injuries.[47]
  - Patients at pediatric trauma centers had fewer splenectomies but a higher rate of neurosurgical procedures.
- Nathens and associates[37] suggest that the greatest decrease in mortality in states with trauma systems was in the pediatric population.
- Children admitted to adult centers undergo more unnecessary procedures than those at pediatric centers.[48,49]
- Invasive procedures performed by adult surgeons are showing a decline as well.[50]
- Need to develop better methods for predicting survival and identifying excess mortality among pediatric patients. Telecommunications advances can help, allowing for pediatric-specific expertise to reach the patient.

IMPORTANT ASPECTS OF PEDIATRIC TRAUMA SYSTEMS

- Sustained educational efforts about childhood injury prevention and vehicle restraints.
- Must include educational programs.
- Organized transport system.
- Focused rehabilitation.

REFERENCES

1. Down DM, Keenan HT, Bratton SL. Epidemiology and prevention of childhood injuries. *Crit Care Med* 2002;30 No. 11:S385–S392.
2. National Center for Injury Prevention and Control. Available at "http://www.cdc.gov/ncipc/wisqars/".
3. Hambridge SJ, Davidson AJ, Gonzales R, et al. Epidemiology of pediatric injury-related primary care offices visits in the United Stated. *Pediatrics* 2002;109:559–565. Available at "http://www.cdc.gov/ncipc/wisqars/".
4. CSN. 1996 Children's Safety Network Economics and Insurance Resource Center.
5. Runyan CW. Using the Haddon matrix: Introducing the third dimension. *Injury Prev* 1998:4:302–301.
6. Davis RM, Pless IB. BMJ bans "accidents." *BMJ* 2001;332:1320–1321.
7. Scholer SJ, Hickson GB, Rjay WA. Sociodemographic factors identify U.S. infants at high risk of injury mortality. *Pediatrics* 1999;102:1183–1188.
8. Baker SP, O'Neill B, Ginsberg MJ, et al. (Eds.) Unintentional injury. In: *The Injury Fact Book*. 2nd ed. New York: Oxford University Press; 1992:39–77.
9. Pomerantz WJ, Dowd MD, Buncher CR. Relationship between socioeconomic factors and severe childhood injuries. *J Urban Health* 2001;78:141–151.
10. Durkin MS, Davidson LL, Kuhn, et al. Low-income neighborhoods and the risk of sever pediatric injury: A small area analysis of northern Manhattan. *Am J Public Health* 1994;84:587–592.
11. Slater SJ, Slater H, Goldfarb W. Burned children: a socioeconomic profile for focused prevention programs. *J Burn Care Rehabil* 1987;8:566–567.
12. Brenner RA, Trumble AC, Smith GS, et al. Where children drown, United States 1995. *Pediatrics* 2001;85:1115–1118.
13. Vane DW, Shackford SR. Epidemiology of rural traumatic death in children: a population-based study. *J Trauma Injury Infect Crit Care* 1995;38:867–870.
14. Marcin JP, Pollack MM. Triage scoring systems, severity of illness measures, and mortality prediction models in pediatric trauma. *Crit Care Med* 2002;30:S457–S467.
15. Maslanka AM. Scoring systems and triage from the field. *Emerg Med Clin North Am* 1993;11:15–27.
16. Baxt WG, Berry CC, Epperson MD, et al. The failure of prehospital trauma prediction rules to classify trauma patients accurately. *Ann Emerg Med* 1989;18:1–8.
17. Champion HR, Sacco WJ, Copes WS, et al. A revision of the trauma score. *J Trauma* 1989;29:623–629.
18. Spaite D, Benoit R, Brown D, et al. uniform prehospital data elements and definitions: a report from the uniform prehospital emergency medical services data conference. *Ann Emerg Med* 1995;25:525–534.
19. Committee on Trauma, ACoS. *Resources for Optimal Care of the Injured Patient*. Chicago: American College of Surgeons; 1998.
20. Champion HR, Copes WS, Sacco WJ, et al. The major trauma outcome study: establishing national norms for trauma care. *J Trauma* 1990;30:1356–1365.
21. Roorda J, van Beeck EF, Stapert JW, et al. Evaluating performance of the revised trauma score as a triage instrument in the prehospital setting. *Injury* 1996;27:163–167.
22. Aprahamian C, Cattey RP, Walker AP, et al. Pediatric trauma score: predictor of hospital resource use? *Arch Surg* 1990;125:1128–1131.
23. Eichelberger MR, Gotschall CS, Sacco WJ, et al. A comparison of the trauma score, the revised trauma score, and the pediatric trauma score. *Ann Emerg Med* 1989;18:1053–1058.
24. Kaufmann CR, Maier RV, Rivara FP, et al. Evaluation of the pediatric trauma score. *JAMA* 1990;263:69–72.
25. Ott R, Kramer R, Martus P, Bussenius-Kammerer M, et al. Prognostic value of trauma scores in pediatric patients with multiple injuries. *J Trauma* 2000;49:729–736.
26. Nayduch DA, Moylan J, Rutledge R, et al. Comparison of the ability of adult and pediatric outcome following major trauma. *J Trauma* 1991;31:452–457.
27. Tepas JJ III, Mollitt DL, Talbert JL, et al. The pediatric trauma score as a predictor of injury severity in the injured child. *J Pediatr Surg* 1987;22:14–18.
28. Tepas JJ III, Ramenofsky ML, Mollitt DL, et al. The pediatric trauma score as a predictor of injury severity: an objective assessment. *J Trauma* 1988;28:425–429.
29. Mullins RJ, Mann NC. Population-based research assessing the effectiveness of trauma systems. *J Trauma* 1999; 47(suppl):S59–S66.
30. Hunt JP, Baker CC, Fakhry SM, et al. Accuracy of administrative data in trauma. *Surgery* 1999;126: 191–197.
31. Baker SP, O'Neill B. The injury severity score: an update. *J Trauma* 1976;16:882–885.
32. Baker SP, O'Neill B, Haddon W Jr, et al. The injury severity score: a method for describing patients with multiple injuries and evaluating emergency care. *J Trauma* 1974;14:187–196.
33. Morrison W, Wright JL, Paidas CN. Pediatric trauma systems. *Crit Care Med* 2002;11(suppl):S448–S456.

34. Haller JA Jr. Life-threatening injuries in children: what have we learned and what are the challenges? *Bull Am Coll Surg* 1995;80:8–18,43.
35. Howard JM. Historical background to accidental death and disability: The neglected disease of modern society. *Prehospital Emerg Care* 2000;4:285–289.
36. Mullins RJ. A historical perspective of trauma systems developed in the United States. *J Trauma* 1999; 47(suppl):S8–S14.
37. Nathens AB, Jurkovich GJ, Rivara FP, et al. Effectiveness of state trauma systems in reducing injury-related mortality: a national evaluation. *J Trauma* 2000;48:25–30.
38. *Accidental death and disability: the neglected disease of modern society.* Washington, DC: National Committee of Trauma and Committee of Shock National Academy of Sciences/National Research Council; 1966.
39. Mullins RJ, Mann NC. Introduction to the academic symposium to evaluate evidence regarding the efficacy of trauma systems. *J Trauma* 1999;47(suppl):S3–S7.
40. Wright J, Klein B. Regionalized pediatric trauma systems. *Clin Pediatr Emerg Med* 2001;2:3–12.
41. ACoSCoT. Optimal hospital resources for care of the seriously injured. *Bull Am Coll Surgeons* 1976;61: 15–22.
42. *Resources for optimal care of the injured patient.* Chicago: American College of Surgeons, Committee on Trauma; 1998:39–42.
43. Colombani PN, Buck JR, Dudgeon DL, et al. One-year experience in a regional pediatric trauma center. *J Pediatr Surg* 1985;20:8–13.
44. Harris BH, Latchaw LA, Murphy RE, et al. A protocol for pediatric trauma receiving units. *J Pediatr Surg* 1989;24:419–422.
45. Tepas JJ III, Romenofsky ML, Barlow B, et al. National pediatric trauma registry. *J Pediatr Surg* 1989;24:156–158.
46. Hall JR, Reyes HM, Meller JL, et al. The outcome for children with blunt trauma is best at a pediatric trauma center. *J Pediatr Surg* 1996;31:72–76.
47. Potoka DA, Schall LC, Gardner MJ, et al. Impact of pediatric trauma centers on mortality in a statewide system. *J Trauma* 2000;49:237–245.
48. Sanchez JL, Lucas J, Feustel PJ. Outcome of adolescent trauma admitted to an adult surgical intensive care unit versus a pediatric intensive care unit. *J Trauma* 2001;51:478–480.
49. Keller MS, Vane DW. Management of pediatric blunt splenic injury: comparison of pediatric and adult trauma surgeons. *J Pediatr Surg* 1995;30:221–224.
50. Patric DA, Moore EE, Bensard DD, et al. Operative management of injured children at an adult level I trauma center. *J Trauma* 2000;48:894–901.

CHAPTER 2

Primary Survey, Secondary Survey, and Adjuncts

Priscilla Chiu, MD, PhD, FRCSC

EPIDEMIOLOGY
- Trauma is the leading cause of death in children age 16 and under.[4]
- Blunt trauma is the most common mechanism of injury in children due to[5]:
  - Falls.
  - Motor vehicle accidents: passenger, pedestrian, bicycle.
- Most common injuries: fractures, intracranial, internal.
- Neurologic injury is the leading cause of long-term morbidity.[6,7]
- Young children have better outcomes when treated at pediatric trauma centers.[8]
- Children have better outcomes than adults following traumatic injuries.[3]
- Traumatic injuries suspicious for abuse must be documented, investigated, and reported as per local practice patterns (such as Children's Aid Society in Ontario).
- Penetrating trauma incidence is increasing in some large urban centers.[9]

DEFINITIONS[10]
Primary Survey
- Quick, initial patient assessment to identify life-threatening injuries.
- Occurs simultaneously with active resuscitation (securing airway, establishing IV, fluid resuscitation, control of bleeding).
- Happens in a systematic and logical sequence.

Secondary Survey
- More detailed assessment of injuries.
- Reevaluation of the interventions with the transition toward definitive care.

PRIMARY SURVEY
Pediatric Primary Survey: ABCDEs (Fig. 2-1)
- Every trauma patient should arrive on a board with C-spine immobilization.
  - Collar on for school-age and adolescent children.
  - Rolls and tape for infants and toddlers.
- Immediately check vital signs and temperature.
- The initial management is always the ABCs, described next.

A: Airway with Cervical Spine Protection
- Clear secretions, assess patency and need for intubation.
- Look for foreign bodies.
- Be cautious when small children have associated neurologic or craniofacial injuries—intubate early.

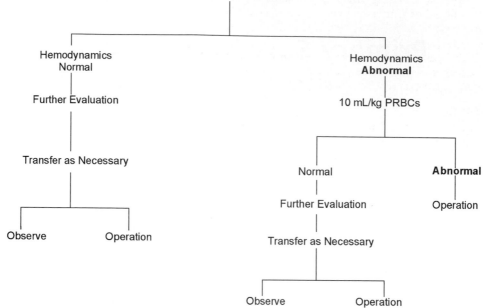

FIGURE 2-1 ● Algorithm for the hemodynamic resuscitation of the pediatric trauma patient. (From American College of Surgeons' Committee on Trauma. *Advanced Trauma Life Support for Doctors (ATLS) Student Manual.* 7th ed. Chicago: American College of Surgeons; 2004, with permission.)

- Significant airway burns or inhalation injury (based on mechanism, length of time of rescue, initial saturations) will require early intubation.
- Ensure adequate C-spine protection, particularly when moving the patient.
- See Chapter 9 on C-spine Management for details.

B: Breathing
- Assess adequacy of respirations (effort, efficacy, breath sounds, and oxygenation).
- Apply oxygen in the tachypneic patient or if oxygen saturations <93% on room air or based on mechanism (smoke/carbon monoxide inhalation).
  - Via face mask in the older patient.
  - Via blow-by or hood in infants.
- Low threshold to intubate if poor oxygenation and poor respiratory effort.
  - See Chapter 3 on Airway Management for details.
- If intubated in the field, always reassess respirations bilaterally and confirm ETT position.
  - Common to find right mainstem intubations in children.
  - Monitor end-tidal CO_2 continuously.
  - Obtain CXR.

C: Circulation with Control of External Hemorrhage
- Most common cause of shock in pediatric trauma patients is hypovolemia.
- Total blood volume in child = 80 mL/kg.
- Start IVs and draw blood work while the ABCs are being assessed.
  - Order cross-match or type and screen.
- Start IV: 20 mL/kg crystalloid bolus over 15–30 minutes.
- Use warmed solutions if patient hypothermic.

- Assess for and control obvious sources of bleeding.
  - Look for blood-soaked clothing or scalp laceration—apply direct pressure.
  - Internal bleeding (bulging abdomen, hemothorax) requires aggressive resuscitation toward definitive management and possible OR.
  - Wrap or splint unstable pelvic fracture to decrease bleeding in pelvic/retroperitoneal space.
- Stable patients are apparent in the primary survey because a talking or crying child has a **patent airway,** is **breathing spontaneously,** and has **sufficient blood pressure** to maintain cerebral perfusion.

D: Disability

- Brief musculoskeletal/neurologic examination for obvious limb deformities, check neurologic and pupillary responses:
  - Spontaneous movement.
  - Sensation or complaints of pain.
  - Responsiveness to voice.
  - Assess with modified GCS or Verbal Score (see below).

E: Expose Patient

- Assess all surface areas (including diaper).
- Prevent hypothermia.
  - Keep trauma room warm.
  - Cover patient with warm blankets after assessment.
  - Use overhead warmer for infants.
- Burns should be calculated based on patient's palmar surface = 1% BSA.
  - Quickly cover burns with moist, warm dressings.
  - See Chapter 14 on Thermal Injuries for details.

History

- If patient can communicate, obtain details leading to injury and relevant medical history.
- If patient cannot communicate, obtain history from EMS crew, witnesses at the scene, friends, family members, and authorities.
- Important details of history requiring special attention:
  - Mechanism of injury (e.g., vehicle speed, distance thrown, fall from height, landing surface, farm accident).
  - Use of protective devices (e.g., child seat, seatbelt, helmet).
  - Patient's initial exam at scene (e.g., initial responsiveness, any loss or changes in level of consciousness, any seizure activity, any evidence of bleeding and quantity at scene).
  - Initial vitals (*Note:* <u>Not</u> unusual to have tachycardia in frightened child, but important as a baseline).
- Be sure to obtain pertinent AMPLE history:
  - **A:** Allergies.
  - **M:** Medications currently taking.
  - **P:** Past medical history/illnesses.
  - **L:** Last meal.
  - **E:** Events relating to injury.
- Obtain immunization history from patient or family, especially last tetanus booster.

Specific Life-Threatening Injuries to Be Identified and Treated in the Primary Survey

- Children are less likely to demonstrate changes in vital signs from hypovolemia until they can no longer compensate, at which point they may arrest.
  - The earliest sign of hypovolemia is tachycardia (Table 2-1).
  - Greatest risk is tension pneumothorax due to a mobile mediastinum.
    - Maintain a high index of suspicion!
- Physical examination during primary survey must rule out presence of these life-threatening conditions that require immediate intervention:

TABLE 2-1

Systemic Responses to Blood Loss in the Pediatric Patient

System	Mild Blood Volume Loss (<30%)	Moderate Blood Volume Loss (30–45%)	Severe Blood Volume Loss (>45%)
Cardiovascular	↑ Heart rate; weak, thready peripheral pulses	Low normal blood pressure, narrowed pulse pressure, markedly ↑ heart rate; absent peripheral pulses with weak, thready central pulses	Hypotension; tachycardia then bradycardia
Central Nervous System	Anxious, irritable, confused	Lethargic, dulled response to pain[a]	Comatose
Skin	Cool, mottled; prolonged capillary refill	Cyanotic; markedly prolonged capillary refill	Pale, cold
Urinary Output	Minimal ↓	Minimal	None

[a]Child's dulled response to pain with this degree of blood loss (30–45%) is often indicated by the decreased response noted when an IV catheter is inserted.
(From American College of Surgeons' Committee on Trauma. *Advanced Trauma Life Support for Doctors (ATLS) Student Manual.* 7th ed. Chicago: American College of Surgeons; 2004, with Permission).

- Tension hemopneumothorax—more common in older children with rib fractures (Figure 2.2).
  - Hemodynamic instability, decreased breath sounds, uneven chest contours, tracheal deviation.
  - Difficult to check neck veins in small children with short necks.
  - Don't wait for chest x-ray if patient unstable and clinical signs are present.
  - Needle decompression: 18-gauge angiocath at mid-clavicular line in 2nd intercostal space. Follow with chest tube insertion. See Chapter 21 on Procedures for details.
- Cardiac tamponade—rare.
  - Low-amplitude QRS complex on ECG suggestive.
  - Continue to resuscitate with IV fluids.
  - Consider pericardiocentesis: 20-gauge needle through subxiphoid if emergent intervention required. See Chapter 21 on Procedures for details.
  - Early thoracotomy or pericardial window best treatment.

Need for Reassessment

- Reassess:
  - Patient's vital signs.
  - Volume of fluids given and clinical response.
  - Determine whether antibiotic and tetanus prophylaxis are warranted.
- If vital signs have normalized after initial bolus, one can leave IV fluids at maintenance rate and proceed with imaging studies.
- If patient remains unstable, continue with resuscitation and reassess to determine if any injuries have been missed.
  - Give second or third bolus of 20 mL/kg warmed crystalloid IV if vitals unresponsive.
  - Increase venous access if current access not sufficient.
  - Administer warmed type-specific or O-negative PRBCs 10 mL/kg IV if third crystalloid bolus is required.

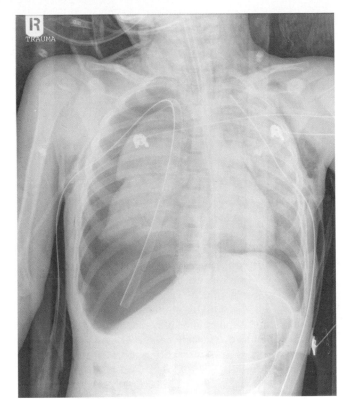

FIGURE 2-2 ● Right tension pneumothorax despite chest tube insertion. A right chest tube had been inserted for a right pneumothorax prior to patient transfer. The patient arrived at the trauma center hypotensive with high airway pressures. Breath sounds and chest movement were decreased on the right side. A second chest tube was subsequently inserted with complete decompression of the tension pneumothorax.

- Assess for ongoing blood loss or restrictive cardiac output (tension pneumothorax, pericardial tamponade).
- Involve surgical colleagues early.
- Consider need to stabilize for early transfer.
- NEVER transfer an unstable patient or send for lengthy radiologic imaging unaccompanied.

Adjuncts to the Primary Survey
- Vascular access should be established early.
  - One 22-gauge IV at minimum.
  - An unstable pediatric patient should have at least two IVs.
- Options for venous access if IV is unsuccessful:
  - Intraosseous (IO) access.
  - Central venous access (femoral preferable).
  - Venous cut-down (e.g., saphenous vein).
- The minimal monitoring requirements are:
  - Cardiorespiratory.
  - Pulse oximetry.
  - Cycling external BP cuff (properly sized).
- Unstable patients warrant the following additional monitors:
  - End-tidal carbon dioxide monitor if intubated.
  - Nasogastric/orogastric tube.
    - Choose appropriate size NG/OG to adequately decompress stomach.
    - Insert orogastric tube if child is unconscious and unable to protect airway.
    - DO NOT insert nasogastric tube if suspicion of basal skull fracture (persistent rhinorrhea, blood behind tympanic membranes).

- Urinary catheter.
  - DO NOT insert Foley catheter if:
    - Blood at the urethral meatus.
    - Bruising in the perineum or scrotum.
    - High-riding prostate on rectal exam.
    - In the presence of an unstable pelvic fracture.
  - Choose appropriate size to avoid drainage of urine around catheter.

Trauma Blood Work

- CBC, electrolytes, blood gas, creatinine and BUN, PT/PTT, cross-match, all liver function studies, amylase.
- β-hCG screen if female trauma patient of child-bearing age.
- Toxicology screen, cardiac enzymes if history and mechanism suggestive.

Interventions During Primary Survey

- Surgical airway (see Chapter 21 on Procedures for details).
  - Cricothyroidotomy should only be used in adolescents.
  - DO NOT perform cricothyroidotomy in pre-adolescent children as risk of future airway obstruction.
  - Use needle cricothyroidotomy with 16-gauge to 18-gauge angiocath in pre-adolescents.
  - Maintain C-spine immobilization.
- Chest tube insertion (see Chapter 21 on Procedures for details).
  - Chest tube output warranting thoracotomy (guidelines only):
    - Infant/toddler—initial drainage >2–3 mL/kg/hr or 20–30% of blood volume.
    - Older child >200 mL/hr output.
    - Adolescent >1,500 mL initial drainage.
- Thoracotomy
  - Should only be performed for witnessed arrest in the ER by the most experienced team member.
- Pericardiotomy/pericardial window.
  - Safest via left thoracotomy in children.
  - Poor outcomes as in adults.
- Diagnostic Peritoneal Lavage (DPL)—rarely performed in children because of the accuracy of CT imaging and the extensive use of nonoperative treatment for solid organ injuries.

Imaging Needed Prior to Secondary Survey

- X-rays:
  - Chest x-ray (AP only).
  - Pelvis (AP only).
  - C-spine—lateral (AP, and odontoid views if patient cooperative).
    - Controversial for infants and young children who are unable to cooperate and who will require head CT in the context of their injury.

FAST Ultrasound—Role in Pediatric Trauma Management

- Currently **no** studies validate FAST's role in abdominal pediatric trauma assessment.
- Potentially useful in early detection of diaphragmatic rupture, hemopneumothorax, cardiac tamponade as in adults, but depends on expertise of individual operator.
- See Chapter 4 on Diagnostic Imaging for details.

Role of Trauma Severity Scoring

- Acute injury scores (e.g., TRISS, ISS, PTS) are not useful in initial patient assessment during primary survey.
- Helpful in predicting outcomes and need for transfer to pediatric trauma center.
- See Chapter 1 on Introduction for details.

SECONDARY SURVEY: EXAMINATION AND HISTORY
Pediatric Anatomy/Pathophysiology
- The *anatomic proportions* of infants and young children differ significantly from adults.
- The larger **head to body mass ratio** decreases with age.
- Deceleration mechanisms (e.g., MVA) can cause massive and fatal C-spine injuries in improperly restrained infants.
- However, C-spine injuries are less common in children compared to adults.
- Formulas that calculate fluid resuscitation requirements for burns in children will have increased percentages of body surface area assigned to the head relative to trunk compared with adults.
- The **body surface area to body mass ratio** is high in infants and decreases with age.
- Core body temperature drops quickly with exposure in infants and pre-school-age children.
- Infants and young children have soft and pliable skull, rib cage, and bones.
- Injuries to deep soft tissues (e.g., brain, lung, abdomen, and pelvis) may be very significant even in the absence of bony fractures.
- Be suspicious for internal injuries based on mechanism of trauma rather than presence or absence of physical markings alone.

ABCDE of the Secondary Survey
- Secondary survey is a systematic head-to-toe examination of the patient.
  - Objective: determine extent of injuries and management plan.
- Abnormal findings interpreted based on need for additional investigations, interventions, and patient management/transfer.

Secondary Survey Essentially Same As in Adults with the Following Differences and Caveats
Head and Skull
- The head size and surface area relative to body size are disproportionately large in infants—heat loss significant, intracranial injuries common.
- Scalp lacerations → significant source of bleeding → clean, debride, and close as early as possible.
- Open fontanelles allow some decompression with raised ICP.
- Check fontanelles.
  - Depressed: under-resuscitated.
  - Bulging: intracranial injuries.
- Skull is soft and malleable in infants and young children.
- Unusual to have skull fractures but may have significant, life-threatening intracranial injuries.
- See Chapter 5 and 6 on Head Injuries for details.

Maxillofacial and Intra-oral
- Always recheck nasal and oral patency in the non-intubated patient.
  - Edema may develop following fluid resuscitation.
  - May contribute to upper airway obstruction if craniofacial trauma.
  - See Chapter 7 on Craniofacial Injuries or Chapter 8 on Neck and Airway Injuries for details.
- LOW threshold for early intubation if significant maxillofacial trauma.
- Blood in the oral cavity must be thoroughly examined.
  - Evidence of basal skull fracture.
  - Nasal or oral trauma, tongue laceration, loose or lost teeth.
  - Need to investigate for possible airway risk from missing teeth.
- Facial lacerations.
  - Remove any embedded foreign bodies.
  - Thoroughly irrigate, then cover with dressing before closure.
  - Consider need for antibiotics (infections rare).
- Keep any loose or avulsed teeth for possible reimplantation.
- Maxillofacial, orbital trauma, or trauma to the globe or extra-ocular muscles requires early plastic surgery and ophthalmology consultation.

Neck

- Short necks in infants and toddlers difficult to assess.
- May be difficult to clear C-spine clinically (uncooperative patient) or radiologically (unconscious or infant patient).
- Safest approach in unconscious patient is to keep C-spine immobilized for reassessment and possible neurosurgical consultation.
- An actively kicking and wiggling child is unlikely to have C-spine injury.
- Leave additional imaging to neurosurgical discretion.
- See Chapter 9 on Cervical Spine Injuries for details.

Chest

- Early CXR may not reveal extent of contusion.
- Rib fractures and flail segments are uncommon in young children.[11]
- Mechanism of injury predictive of significant lung contusion in children including motor vehicle accidents, crush injuries, falls.[11]
- Small chest size means penetrating trauma has high risk of injury to vital mediastinal structures.
- See Chapter 10 on Thoracic Trauma for details.

Abdomen/Pelvis (Including Spine)

- Frequent assessments for evidence of distension, peritonitis, and signs of trauma (e.g., seatbelt sign, penetrating trauma).
- Diffuse peritonitis—cross-table lateral x-ray may be helpful in detecting free air in lieu of CT imaging in children.
- Log-roll patient to assess and palpate spine and flanks.
- Presence of spinal injury should raise index of suspicion for associated chest and abdominal injuries.
- Shoulder tip and abdominal pain increase index of suspicion for splenic (most common) and liver (second most common) injuries.[12]
- Tender abdomen and associated spinal tenderness in child raises index of suspicion for Chance fracture and pancreatic injury (more common in children).
- Hemodynamically significant pelvic fractures less common in children compared to adults due to pliable pelvic bones.[13]
- Significant genitourinary trauma less common in children compared to adults but be suspicious if any blood present in urine.[13]
- See Chapter 11 on Abdominal and Pelvic Trauma for details.
- See Chapter 12 on Orthopedic Trauma for details.
- See Chapter 13 on Thoracic and Lumbar Spine Injuries for details.

Perineum/Rectum/Vagina

- Inspection of perineum/scrotum/vaginal orifice important because pelvic trauma more common in children than adults.
- No role for speculum examination of the vagina in prepubertal females unless blood is found in the perineum or on rectal exam.
- Rectal exam important but may not be useful for assessing rectal tone in small children.
- Blood on rectal exam or in perineum/vaginal orifice warrants examination under anesthesia to assess for rectal/vaginal injuries.

Musculoskeletal

- Splinted long bone fractures should be reassessed.
- Any vascular or neurologic compromise associated with long bone injuries or signs of compartment syndrome not responsive to closed reduction, or open/complex fractures warrant early orthopedic consultation.
- Open fractures should be cleaned with warm saline irrigation and covered with dressing and IV antibiotics given before definitive management.
- See Chapter 12 on Orthopedic Trauma for details.
- Unusual fractures (humerus, ribs, lower limbs in infants) not in keeping with mechanism of injury should raise suspicions of non-accidental injury.
- See Chapter 19 on Non-accidental Trauma for details.

Neurologic Examination

- Cannot be accurately performed in the patient with ongoing hypovolemia and hypoxia.
- Head-injured children extremely sensitive to hypoxia.
  - Prevent hypotension and hypoxia.
  - See Chapter 5 on Medical Management of Head Injuries for details.
- Check pupils.
- Persistent emesis with gastric drainage suggestive of raised ICP.
- GCS useful in school-age children or older.
- Toddlers and infants best motor score on GCS (Table 2-2) or pediatric verbal score (Table 2-3) more useful.
- Lower spinal injuries uncommon in infants and pre-school-age children.
- Assessment of neurologic deficits secondary to spinal injury in infants and young children based on tone/flaccidity and sensation—any deficits warrant neurosurgical consultation.
- See Chapter 13 on Thoracic and Lumbar Spine Injuries for details.

Interventions During the Secondary Survey

- In addition to ongoing resuscitation, the following common medications may be given during initial survey:
  - Antibiotics for open fractures, craniofacial injuries:
    - Cefazolin (25 mg/kg/dose IV) or
    - Clindamycin if penicillin-allergic (10 mg/kg/dose IV).
    - See Chapter 12 on Orthopedic Trauma for details.
  - Tetanus prophylaxis (0.5 mL tetanus toxoid IM).
  - Splinted long bone fractures should be assessed, traction splints placed, and analgesia given.
  - Antibiotics for abdominal trauma:
    - Cefoxitin (30 mg/kg/dose IV) or
    - Clindamycin (10 mg/kg/dose IV) and gentamicin (2.5 mg/kg/dose IV).
    - See Chapter 11 on Abdominal and Pelvic Trauma for details.
  - Analgesia:
    - Morphine (0.1 mg/kg/dose IV).
    - Fentanyl (1 μg/kg/dose IV)

TABLE 2-2

Glasgow Coma Scale (GCS)

	Score
Eye Opening	
Spontaneous	4
To voice	3
To pain	2
None	1
Verbal Response (Pediatric)	
Appropriate	5
Cries, consolable	4
Persistently irritable	3
Restless, agitated	2
None	1
Motor Response	
Obeys commands	6
Localizes pain	5
Withdraws (pain)	4
Flexion (pain)	3
Extension (pain)	2
None	1

TABLE 2-3

Pediatric Verbal Score

Verbal Response	V-Score
Appropriate words or social smile, fixes and follows	5
Cries, but consolable	4
Persistently irritable	3
Restless, agitated	2
None	1

(From American College of Surgeons' Committee on Trauma. *Advanced Trauma Life Support for Doctors (ATLS) Student Manual.* 7th ed. Chicago: American College of Surgeons; 2004, with Permission).

- Acetaminophen (15 mg/kg/dose PO/NG/PR).
- See Chapter 18 on Pain Management for details.
- Steroids are not currently recommended in spine injury. Consult your local referral center.
    - See Chapter 13 on Thoracic and Lumbar Spine Injuries for details.
- Keep patient warm—cover with warm blankets, Bear-Hugger, warm fluids.

Foley Catheter
- Contraindications for Foley catheter insertion:
    - Unstable pelvic fracture.
    - Blood at urethral meatus.
    - Perineal or scrotal ecchymoses.
    - High-riding or nonpalpable prostate.
- May require urethrogram and urology to insert Foley catheter.
- Insert only if concerned about adequacy of perfusion and duration of resuscitation or patient unable to mobilize for urination.
- Weighing diaper of incontinent infants/toddlers equally accurate for assessment of urine output.
- Adequacy of urine output based on age:
    - Infants age <1 year: 2 mL/kg/hr.
    - Toddlers to grade school age: 1.5 mL/kg/hr.
    - Older than 12 years: 1 mL/kg/hr.
- Evidence of gross hematuria → suspect renal or collecting system injuries, especially if pelvic fracture present.
    - Additional imaging (CT abdomen + pelvis with IV contrast, delayed views for CT cystogram).

Need for Further Interventions: Laparotomy/Thoracostomy
- A child who fails to stabilize with aggressive resuscitation and who has blood detected in the chest or peritoneal cavities requires operative intervention.
- Unless your center can manage pediatric trauma patients operatively, avoid additional imaging or interventions that delay patient transfer for definitive care (e.g., laparotomy, thoracotomy, sternotomy, craniotomy).
    - See Chapter 22 for Transport of the Critically Ill Child.
- Penetrating abdominal trauma with evisceration:
    - Reduce contents.
    - Cover site with moist dressing.
    - Decompress with gastric tube.
    - Start IV antibiotics.

- Chest tube drainage in excess of acceptable amounts (see page 14) requires ongoing fluid and blood replacement.
- Large air leaks with ongoing respiratory compromise may warrant 2nd chest tube placement.
- See Chapter 22 on Transport for details.

Need for Further Imaging

- Additional imaging **must not delay transfer** if patient's injuries already exceed the scope of care provided at the sending institution.
- Additional imaging should only be performed in stable patients who may warrant transfer to a pediatric trauma center pending the results of these investigations (e.g., intra-abdominal solid organ/hollow viscus injuries) and only if expertise available to interpret the results.
- Imaging studies performed outside the ER (such as CT scans) require an accompanying physician and should never be performed in the unstable patient.
- Extremity x-rays to investigate long bone fractures can be taken while awaiting transfer of a stable patient.
  - Obtaining these x-rays **should never delay transport.**
- CT is far superior to contrast x-rays and ultrasound for thoracic/abdominal/pelvic trauma.
  - Higher dose of radiation exposure.
  - Avoid these studies if poor-quality CT scan and plan is to transfer patient.
  - Head CT warranted for any suspected head injuries.
  - Orbital and maxillofacial windows on head CT useful for assessing injuries.
  - Abdominal/pelvic CT with IV and oral contrast exceedingly sensitive for abdominal and pelvic soft tissue and bony injuries.
  - C-spine CT accurate and sensitive for C-spine injuries.
  - See Chapter 4 on Diagnostic Imaging for more details on radiology.
- No role for endoscopy in the trauma room.
  - Bronchoscopy to rule out large airway injury if persistent large air leak via chest tube.
  - Esophageal perforations identified by contrast study—no role for UGI endoscopy.

Thoracic and Lumbar Spine X-Rays

- Presence of palpable thoracic or lumbar spinal misalignment (palpable step or tenderness) or neurologic deficits without extremity fractures, requires additional spinal x-rays if CT imaging of chest, abdomen, and pelvis not planned.
- AP and lateral views of spine easily obtained in trauma room.
- CT/MRI imaging eventually required.
- See Chapter 13 on Thoracic and Lumbar Spine Injuries for details.

CLINICAL PEARLS

DO
- Control ABCs early—intubate, IVs, fluids.
- Protect patient from hypothermia during primary and secondary surveys.
- Consider lung injuries in children with blunt trauma—pliable chest wall means rare rib fractures or chest wall signs but significant contusion and respiratory compromise in infants and children.[1]
- Contact and refer pediatric patients **EARLY** for definitive care at a pediatric trauma center, because most solid organ injuries in children can be managed through non-operative treatment in experienced pediatric trauma centers.[2]
- Contact and refer pediatric patients with head injuries, multisystem injuries, and burns as these injuries are associated with high risk of mortality.[3]
- Apply direct pressure over bleeding sites.

DON'T
- Leave pediatric patient exposed and predisposed to hypothermia.
- Keep a pediatric patient who clearly warrants care exceeding your institution's capabilities.
- Delay transfer to definitive treatment with investigations that will likely need to be repeated and will not aid your management plans.
- Apply tourniquets for bleeding sites in extremities.

REFERENCES

1. Sartorelli KH, Vane DW. The diagnosis and management of children with blunt injury of the chest. *Semin Pediatr Surg* 2004;13:98–105.
2. Upadhyaya P, Simpson J. Splenic trauma in children. *Surg Gynecol Obstet* 1968;126:781–790.
3. DeRoss AL, Vane DW. Early evaluation and rsuscitation of the pediatric trauma patient. *Semin Pediatr Surg* 2004;13:74–79.
4. Haller J. Pediatric trauma. The no. 1 killer of children. *JAMA* 1983;249:47.
5. Sharma O, Oswanski M, Stringfellow K, et al. Pediatric blunt trauma: a retrospective analysis in a level I trauma center. *Am Surg* 2006;72:538–543.
6. Hall J, Reyes H, Meller J, et al. Traumatic death in urban children, revisited. *Am J Dis Child* 1993;147:102–107.
7. Durkin M, Olsen S, Barlow B, et al. The epidemiology of urban pediatric neurological trauma: evaluation of, and implications for, injury prevention programs. *Neurosurgery* 1998;42:300–310.
8. Densmore JC, Lim HJ, Oldham KT, et al. Outcomes and delivery of care in pediatric injury. *J Pediatr Surg* 2006;41:92–98.
9. Tomashek T, Hsia J, Iyasu S. Trends in postneonatal mortality attributable to injury, United States, 1988–1998. *Pediatrics* 2003;111:1219–1225.
10. American College of Surgeons Committee on Trauma. *Advanced trauma life support for doctors*. 7th ed. Chicago: American College of Surgeons; 2005.
11. Bliss D, Silen M. Pediatric thoracic trauma. *Crit Care Med* 2002;30:S409–S415.
12. Keller MS. Blunt injury to solid abdominal organs. *Semin Pediatr Surg* 2004;13:106–111.
13. Gaines BA, Ford HR. Abdominal and pelvic trauma in children. *Crit Care Med* 2002;30:S416–S423.

CHAPTER 3

Airway Management

Cengiz Karsli, BSc, MD, FRCPC

INTRODUCTION

- Twenty percent of pediatric multiple trauma patients will require urgent invasive airway management.[1]
- Pediatric trauma airway management goals:
  - Maintain adequate oxygenation and ventilation.
  - Prevent pulmonary aspiration of blood, gastric contents, or other foreign bodies.
  - Maintain cervical spine immobilization.
  - Ensure airway safety prior to transport or undertaking diagnostic procedures such as CT.
- Hypoventilation leads to rapid oxygen desaturation in the child.
  - Supplemental oxygen should be administered to every traumatized child.
- Head-injured patients:
  - More than 50% of pediatric trauma victims present with head trauma.
  - Airway support measures must not decrease cerebral perfusion pressure (CPP) or increase intracranial pressure (ICP).
  - Direct laryngoscopy and tracheal intubation may be associated with increases in ICP of >40 mmHg in patients with decreased intracranial compliance.
  - ICP spikes are preventable with appropriate administration of anxiolytics, analgesics, and/or anesthetic agents prior to laryngoscopy.[2]

ANATOMIC CONSIDERATIONS[1,2]

- Pediatric airway matures from neonatal period until 8 years old.
- After 8 years of age it resembles the adult airway.
- Neonates and infants have a prominent occiput that raises the head into the "sniffing" position when supine.
  - Facilitates direct laryngoscopy and tracheal intubation.
- A pillow under a neonate's head will flex the neck and may cause airway obstruction.
- A roll under a small child's shoulders alleviates upper airway obstruction.
  - Line up upper-airway axes to make direct laryngoscopy easier (Fig. 3-1).
- Neonates and infants up to 4 months are obligate nasal breathers.
  - The relatively large tongue can partially obstruct the oral cavity.
  - If nares are obstructed (by blood, mucous, or a nasogastric tube), neonates may not readily convert to oral breathing.
  - Treat nasal obstruction by suctioning or bypassing with an oral airway, nasal airway, or endotracheal tube.
- The pediatric epiglottis is floppy and narrower than an adult, and angles over the vocal cords, as illustrated in Figure 3-2.
- Larynx is more cephalad and angled; it appears more anterior than an adult's.

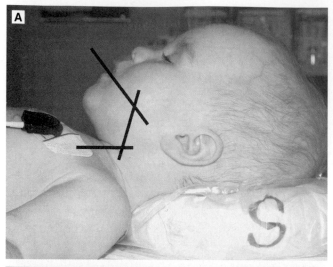

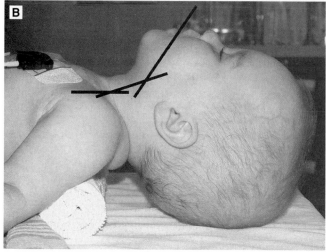

FIGURE 3-1 ●   **A:** Improper (flexed) Airway positioning in infant/small child. **B:** Proper (sniffing) Airway positioning in infants and small children.

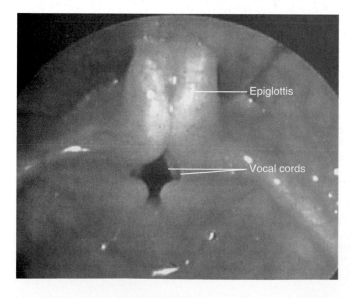

FIGURE 3-2 ●   The pediatric airway: floppy epiglottis is angled over the vocal cords.

- To improve the laryngoscopic view in children <8 years of age:
  - Use a straight laryngoscope blade.
  - Insert at the extreme right side of the mouth (Fig. 3-3).
  - Place tip under the epiglottis rather than in the vallecula.
- The cricoid ring:
  - Is the narrowest portion of the child's upper airway.
  - An endotracheal tube that passes through a child's vocal cords may not fit through the cricoid ring.
  - If ETT does not fit, a tube one-half size smaller should be inserted.
- Traditionally, uncuffed endotracheal tubes are used in children under the age of 8.
- The tube is sized so that a leak is detectable at 20 cm H_2O of pressure.
  - Decreases risk of causing mucosal ischemia at the cricoid ring.
  - *Uncuffed* tube size is calculated by the following formula: **(Age in years/4) + 4.**

- PALS 2005 Guidelines allow use of cuffed endotracheal tubes for ALL children.[3]
  - *Cuffed* tube size can be calculated by the following formula: **(Age in years/4) + 3.**

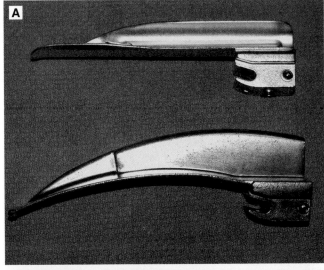

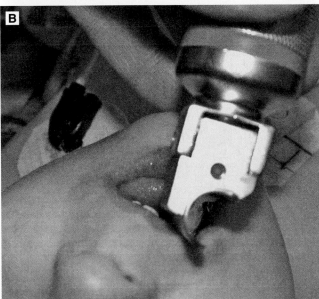

FIGURE 3-3 ● Straight versus curved laryngoscope blades. Note: Inserting straight blade in the extreme right side of the mouth in small children keeps the tongue to the left of the blade.

AIRWAY ESSENTIALS

- Airway assessment in uncooperative pediatric trauma patients is challenging and potentially unreliable.
- The Mallampati classification is not useful in small children[4] but may be used in older children as a predictor of difficult tracheal intubation (Fig. 3-4).
- Risk factors for difficult airway in pediatric trauma include:
  - Presence of C-spine collar.
  - Maxillofacial trauma.
  - Inhalation injury (burn).
  - Congenital syndromes (Pierre–Robin, Treacher–Collins, Goldenhar, mucopolysaccharidoses, etc.).
- Patients with trisomy 21 may have subglottic stenosis and are prone to upper airway obstruction due to macroglossia; however, tracheal intubation is rarely challenging.
- The ability to properly maintain a mask fit, provide continuous positive airway pressure (CPAP), and bag-mask ventilate is a more valuable skill than being able to intubate the trachea.
- Do not sedate a child without adequate skill, experience, and equipment to support and manage the airway.
  - Don't "burn any bridges" without a proper backup plan.
  - If active measures are required to maintain the airway, the first step is proper face-mask application.
- Ensure a tight fit and use high-flow oxygen.
  - In the event of partial or complete airway obstruction apply CPAP, as well as jaw thrust and chin lift.
  - An oral airway may also help by lifting the tongue off the posterior pharyngeal wall.
  - Overcome a difficult mask fit by using a two-hand technique (Fig. 3-5).

TRACHEAL INTUBATION

Indications

- Indications for immediate tracheal intubation in pediatric trauma management include:
  - Airway obstruction, unrelieved by simple maneuvers.
  - Apnea.
  - Cardiac arrest.
  - Major shock.
  - Decreasing LOC (airway protection and control of CO_2 tension).
  - Severe maxillofacial trauma.
  - Inhalation injury.

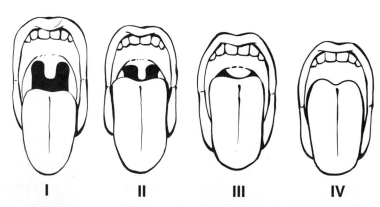

FIGURE 3-4 ●   Mallampati classification. Grade I: Soft palate, fauces, uvula and pillars visualized. Grade II: Soft palate, fauces and portion of uvula visualized. Grade III: Soft palate and base of uvula visualized. Grade IV: Hard palate only visualized.

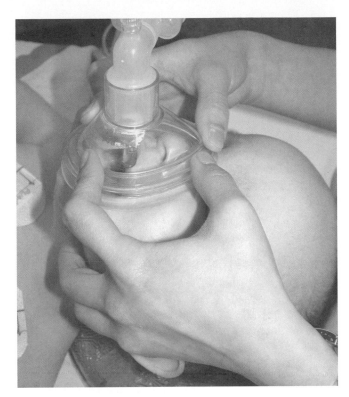

FIGURE 3-5 ● Demonstration of two-hand technique of mask ventilation. Note presence of oropharyngeal airway.

- In cases of maxillofacial trauma or inhalation injury, the pediatric airway may rapidly progress from fully patent to completely obstructed. Intubate the trachea immediately.
- Prophylactic tracheal intubation should also be considered in the child with chest trauma or head injury if that child is to be transported to another facility or to a more remote area of the hospital (such as the radiology suite for CT scan).
- Contraindications to tracheal intubation include lack of experience, equipment, or expertise in pediatric airway management.

Equipment and Technique
Table 3-1 outlines the equipment necessary to manage the pediatric airway. Suggested sizing guidelines for pediatric airway equipment are listed in Table 3-2 (Fig. 3-6).

Rapid-Sequence Induction (RSI)
- Assemble needed equipment and personnel to proceed with RSI.
- This process is outlined below:
    1. Preoxygenation with 100% FiO_2.
    2. Assistant applies in-line manual stabilization.
    3. Removal of anterior portion of C-spine collar.
    4. Premedication as necessary:
        - Atropine 0.02 mg/kg for children <6 years of age.
        - Lidocaine 1-2 mg/kg in head-injured patients.
    5. Administration of a predetermined dose of induction agent (see Table 3-3).
    6. Second assistant applies cricoid pressure.
    7. Administer fast-acting muscle relaxant (usually succinylcholine).
    8. Laryngoscopy and tracheal intubation 20 to 30 seconds after drug administration without bag-mask ventilation.

TABLE 3-1

Equipment and Supplies Needed at Bedside and Immediately Available to Secure the Pediatric Airway

Mandatory (at Bedside)	Immediately Available
Oxygen with high flow capacity	Laryngeal mask airways
Suction with appropriate tip	Surgical airway
Laryngoscope handle and blades	Sedatives/analgesics/anesthetic agents
Bag-mask device	
Face masks	
Oropharyngeal airways	
Nasopharyngeal airways	
Endotracheal tubes	
Stylets	
Resuscitation drugs:	
Atropine, epinephrine	

9. Confirm proper endotracheal tube placement:
   - Visualize tube pass through vocal cords.
   - Auscultation of the lungs with positive-pressure ventilation.
   - End-tidal CO_2 detector (Fig. 3-7).
10. Release of cricoid pressure.
11. Securing of tube with tape, replacing C-spine collar.
12. Continue ventilation (manual or ventilator).
13. Chest x-ray.

TABLE 3-2

Suggested Sizing Guidelines for Pediatric Airway Equipment

Type of Airway	Sizing Guideline	
Oropharyngeal	Distance between the lips and the angle of the mandible	
Nasopharyngeal	Tip of the nose to the tragus of the ear	
Face mask	Should form a seal around nasal bridge, cheeks, and mandible	
Laryngeal mask	1: <5 kg	2.5: 20–30 kg
	1.5: 5–10 kg	3: 30–50 kg
	2: 10–20 kg	4: >50 kg
Endotracheal tube	2.5: preemie <1.5 kg	3.5: Neonate–9 months
	3.0: preemie 1.5–2.5 kg	4.0: 9–15 months
	Thereafter. ETT size uncuffed = [Age (yrs)/4] + 4[a]	
	ETT size cuffed = [Age (yrs)/4] + 3[a]	
Laryngoscope blade	Preemie–full-term neonate: straight 0	
	Neonate–5 years: straight 1	
	5–8 years: straight 2	
	>8 years: straight or curved 2 or 3	

[a]ETT, endotracheal tube. Have one-half size larger and smaller prepared.

TABLE 3-3

Common Pharmacologic Agents Used in the Pediatric Trauma Setting for Acute Management and Ongoing Post-Intubation Care

Drug	Dose (IV)	Comments
Sedatives/Analgesics		
Midazolam	50–100 µg/kg prn 2–5 µg/kg/min	Effects additive when combined with narcotics.
Fentanyl	0.5–1.0 µg/kg prn 1.0–3.0 µg/kg/hr	Respiratory depression, apnea, chest wall rigidity, bradycardia.
Morphine	50–100 µg/kg prn 10–40 µg/kg/hr	Respiratory depression, bradycardia, apnea, histamine release.
Etomidate	0.3 mg/kg IV	Short-acting sedative-hypnotic, no analgesic properties, minimal cardiovascular changes.
Muscle Relaxants		
Succinylcholine	1.0–2.0 mg/kg	Fastest onset and shortest acting. Avoid repeated doses. Many side effects.[a]
Rocuronium	0.6–1.2 mg/kg 1.0 mg/kg/hr	Medium-acting. Rare anaphylaxis.
Pancuronium	0.1 mg/kg 0.05 mg/kg/hr	Tachycardia, long-acting.
Anesthetics		
Sodium Thiopental	2-4 mg/kg	Cardiovascular collapse if hypovolemic, potent cardiorespiratory depressant, histamine release.
Propofol	1–5 mg/kg 50–200 µg/kg/min	Potent cardiorespiratory depressant, propofol infusion syndrome. Limit infusion to less than 6 hours.
Ketamine	1–2 mg/kg 10–20 µg/kg/min	Increases intracranial pressure, maintains systemic blood pressure, bronchodilator.
Lidocaine	1.0–1.5 mg/kg	Blunts ICP and bronchoconstrictive response to laryngoscopy. Reduce dose in infants.

[a]Side effects of succinylcholine include hyperkalemia, dysrhythmias, malignant hyperthermia, masseter muscle rigidity, increased intracranial pressure (ICP), increased intraocular pressure, and myalgias.

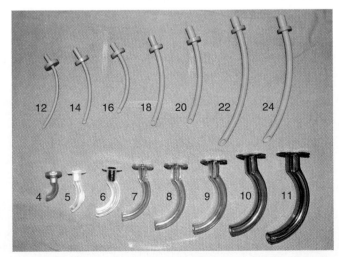

FIGURE 3-6 ● Nasopharyngeal and oropharyngeal airways commonly used in pediatric practice.

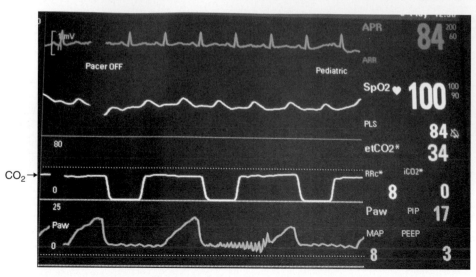

FIGURE 3-7 ● Normal CO_2 tracing (third from top) confirming tracheal intubation. End-tidal CO_2 would be zero with an esophageal intubation.

- Normal CO_2 tracing (third from top) confirms tracheal intubation. End-tidal CO_2 would be zero with an esophageal intubation.
- Administration of a sedative and/or analgesic along with a long-acting (and hence slow-onset) muscle relaxant does NOT constitute an RSI and is discouraged.
- Only personnel experienced in airway management should administer anesthetic agents or sedatives and muscle relaxants to secure the airway.
- Common pharmacologic agents used in the trauma setting are listed in Table 3-3.

Failed Intubation
- In the event of a failed tracheal intubation take immediate measures to:
  1. Ensure adequate oxygenation and ventilation.
  2. Prevent aspiration of gastric contents.
  3. Elicit experienced help.
  4. Consider alternatives to tracheal intubation.
- Apply simple maneuvers to ensure an adequate mask fit, patent airway, and adequate bag-mask ventilation.
- Maintain cricoid pressure unless it affects ventilation.
- Avoid repeated attempts at tracheal intubation.
- Consider an alternative airway management strategy if more than 3 attempts have been made to intubate the trachea.
- For failed intubation, options include continuation of bag-mask ventilation until spontaneous respirations return or insertion of a laryngeal mask airway (Fig. 3-8).
- Other airway tools such as the fiber-optic bronchoscope, Bullard laryngoscope, lighted stylet, esophageal combitube, or retrograde intubation require user experience.
- May require needle or surgical cricothyroidotomy in the "can't intubate, can't ventilate" situation.
- Commercially prepared cricothyroidotomy kits are available; however, one may also be easily assembled using existing equipment (see Chapter 21 on Procedures for details).
  - An intravenous catheter of any size is inserted through the cricothyroid membrane and the needle removed.
  - Verify proper placement by aspirating air bubbles into a syringe partially filled with saline or water.
  - The 15-mm adapter from a size 3.0 endotracheal tube will fit snugly into the hub of the IV catheter and may be attached to any standard bag-mask ventilation system.

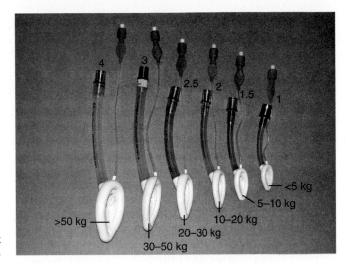

FIGURE 3-8 ● Laryngeal mask airway sizing recommendations.

Post-Intubation Care

- Once airway is secured, constant vigilance is essential to ensure oxygenation and ventilation are adequate and that appropriate sedation and/or analgesia is provided.
- Ongoing sedation may be achieved with intermittent boluses or continuous infusion (Table 3-3).
- Continuously monitor vital signs.
- Any equipment necessary to reintubate the trachea should be available, including during patient transport.
- The preferred mode of ventilation depends on nature and extent of injuries sustained.
- Due to the high incidence of head injuries in pediatric trauma, positive-pressure ventilation (with volume or pressure control) should be instituted to achieve normocapnia (see Chapter 5 on the Medical Management of Head Injury for details).
- Positive end-expiratory pressure (PEEP, starting at 5 cm H_2O) is required to prevent atelectasis and maintain adequate minute ventilation, although excessive PEEP (>10 cm H_2O) may impair venous return to the heart in the hypovolemic patient.
- An example of an initial ventilatory setting: volume control 7 mL/kg, rate 15/min, PEEP 5 cm H_2O. Adjust rate to achieve end-tidal CO_2 (or pCO_2) of 35 mmHg.
- A high FiO_2 should be provided initially to ensure adequate cerebral and systemic oxygenation.
- In the absence of head injury, limiting ventilatory pressures and allowing for permissive hypercapnia reduces ventilator-induced lung injury.[5]

CLINICAL PEARLS

DO
- Maintain oxygenation, ventilation.
- Elicit experienced help.
- Prevent pulmonary aspiration.
- Maintain cervical spine immobilization.
- Prevent increases in intracranial pressure.

DON'T
- Paralyze without backup plan.
- Persist with repeated intubation attempts.

REFERENCES
1. McBrien MF, Pollok AJ, Steedman DJ. Advanced airway control in trauma resuscitation. *Arch Emerg Med* 1992;9:177–180.
2. Marraro G. Airway management. In: Bissonnette B, Dalens B, eds. *Pediatric anesthesia: principles and practice*. New York: McGraw-Hill; 2002:778.
3. Pediatric basic and advanced life support. *Circulation* 2005;112:73–90.
4. Koop VJ, Baily A, Vally RD, et al. Utility of Mallampati classification for predicting difficult intubation in pediatric patients. *Anesthesiology* 1995;83A:1146.
5. Kavanagh BP, Roy L. Pediatric ventilation—towards simpler approaches for complex diseases. *Paediatr Anaesth* 2005;15:699–702.

CHAPTER 4

Diagnostic Imaging of the Pediatric Trauma Patient

Stephen F. Miller, MD, FRCPC

DIAGNOSTIC IMAGING IN THE PEDIATRIC TRAUMA ROOM
- The primary radiographic series for the pediatric trauma patient consists of:
  1. Lateral cervical spine.
  2. AP supine chest.
  3. AP supine pelvis.
- Extremity fractures can be imaged after the primary series.
- Abdominal radiographs have no role in this setting.
- Patients with clinically suspected cranial, thoracic, or abdominal trauma should undergo CT.
- The role of ultrasound (FAST) in pediatric trauma is not well established, and is not routine at SickKids.
  - FAST does not serve as a substitute for CT and is of questionable prognostic value.

CT Imaging
Head CT
- Noncontrast head CT is used to search for fractures, intracranial hemorrhage, or mass effect.
- IV contrast may be administered to evaluate for vascular injuries and thromboses.

Abdominal CT
- Abdominal CT is always performed with IV contrast.
  - Ensure that there is no preexisting allergy or profound renal impairment.
  - Use of oral contrast is controversial.
- See Chapter 11 on Abdominal and Pelvic Trauma for discussion.
- Should not administer oral contrast if patient is hemodynamically unstable or has conditions warranting emergency surgery, in order to prevent undue delay.

Thoracic CT
- Thoracic CT is always performed with IV contrast.
  - Ensure that there is no preexisting allergy or profound renal impairment.
- Used to search for vascular injuries such as aortic dissection, aortic rupture, pulmonary arterial or venous injuries.

Other Imaging
- Standard contrast studies, such as upper GI series and contrast enema, are rarely used in the trauma setting.
- Upper GI studies, using iso- or hypo-osmolar, water-soluble contrast, may help confirm or refute suspected duodenal hematoma or rupture.
- Retrograde urethrography is the study of choice in suspected urethral injury in males.

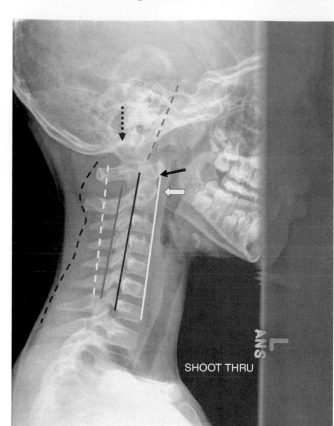

FIGURE 4-1 ● Normal lateral cervical spine radiograph. Prevertebral soft tissue (*white arrow*); clivodental line (*gray dashed line*); predental interspace (*black arrow*); craniocervical junction (*black dashed arrow*); anterior spinal line (*white line*); posterior spinal line (*black line*); facet joints (*gray line*); posterior arches (*white dashed line*); spinous processes (*black dashed curve*). (© Hospital for Sick Children, Toronto.)

- Obtain spinal MRI for all patients with clinically suspicious injuries, especially those with neurologic deficits attributable to the spinal cord.
  - Rapid sequences can delineate with exquisite detail cord edema/contusion, cord discontinuity, and epidural hematomas.
  - MRI is indispensable for evaluating patients with craniocervical junction trauma.

LATERAL CERVICAL SPINE RADIOGRAPHS
- 5-line, 3-column approach to the vertebrae (Fig. 4-1).
- Prevertebral soft-tissue thickness anterior to C2-C3 is age-dependent and can vary with inspiration/expiration:
  - Age 0 to 2 years, allow 1 AP vertebral body thickness.
  - Age >2 years, prevertebral thickness anterior to C2-C3 should be less than 4 mm.
- The clivodental line, drawn along the posterior aspect of the clivus, should intersect the posterior aspect of the dens.
- Predental interspace should be less than 5 mm.
- Using the 5-line approach, all lines should be regular, without stepoff or interruption, except for the most posterior, which undulates with the spinous processes (See Fig. 4-1).
- In young patients, often see <3 mm gap at the craniocervical junction; if 5 mm or more, especially in high-speed MVA, obtain MRI.
- Once the lateral view is judged to be normal, obtain frontal and open-mouth odontoid views.
- The value of the open-mouth odontoid view in young children is questionable. This view is often quite difficult to obtain in children younger than 5 years.[1]

- In young children, most C2 fractures occur through the dens-body synchondrosis (synchondrotic slip)—this is usually readily apparent on the lateral view.[1]
- In older children, once the lateral has been cleared, AP radiograph of the cervical vertebral column and an open-mouth odontoid view should be obtained. Oblique views are also recommended.[1]
- If adequate plain radiographs cannot be produced, proceed to CT with sagittal and coronal reformatting.[1]
- At SickKids, all cranial CT examinations begin at C2—pay close attention to the upper cervical spine on the lateral tomogram and on the axial images.
- If there are multiple fractures, most occur at contiguous levels.[2]
- AP and lateral views of clinically suspicious areas should be obtained—lateral views at minimum.
- Assess vertebrae and disk interspaces for height and regularity—discrepant sizes of contiguous vertebrae or disks are suggestive of acute fracture and should be investigated with CT initially; MRI can follow to assess potential cord injury.
- Significant spinal cord injury can occur in the absence of readily apparent vertebral trauma, due to ligamentous hypermobility.
- Patients with neurologic deficits attributable to the spinal cord require MRI and CT to determine potential operative management.
- Most pediatric vertebral fractures are in the thoracic region[2]:

T2-T10:	28.7%
L2-L5:	23.2%
Midcervical:	18.9%
Thoracolumbar junction:	14.6%
Cervicothoracic junction:	7.9%
Craniocervical junction:	6.7%

- See Figs. 4-2 to 4-11 for interesting images of injuries of the C-spine.

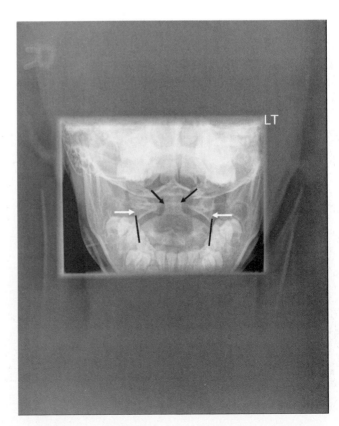

FIGURE 4-2 ● Normal open-mouth odontoid view. The odontoid process (*black arrows*) is intact. The lateral masses of C1 (*white arrows*) align vertically with those of C2 (*black lines*). (© Hospital for Sick Children, Toronto.)

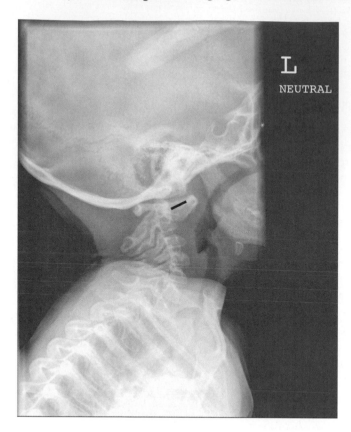

FIGURE 4-3 ● Increased predental interspace. Lateral radiograph demonstrates increased predental interspace (*black line*), indicating a torn transverse ligament. This is an unstable injury. (© Hospital for Sick Children, Toronto.)

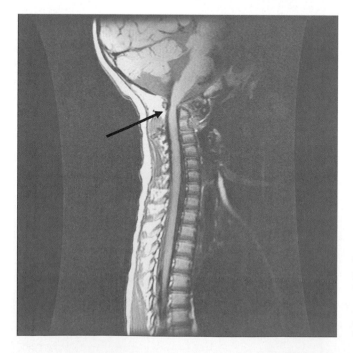

FIGURE 4-4 ● Increased predental interspace. Sagittal T1-weighted MRI image from same patient as Fig. 4-3 demonstrates marked narrowing of the cervical spinal canal at the C1-C2 level (*black arrow*). (© Hospital for Sick Children, Toronto.)

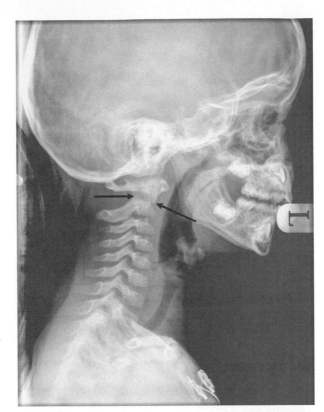

FIGURE 4-5 ● C2 synchondrotic fracture. There is abnormal anterior angulation of the odontoid process, due to synchondrotic fracture at base of the dens (*black arrows*). (© Hospital for Sick Children, Toronto.)

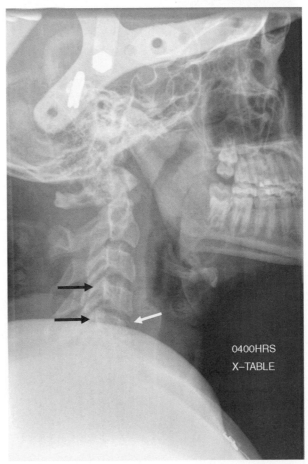

FIGURE 4-6 ● C5 fracture. Lateral view demonstrates anterior wedging of C5 (*white arrow*) and anterior translation of C4 onto C5 (*black arrows*). This is a hyperflexion injury. (© Hospital for Sick Children, Toronto.)

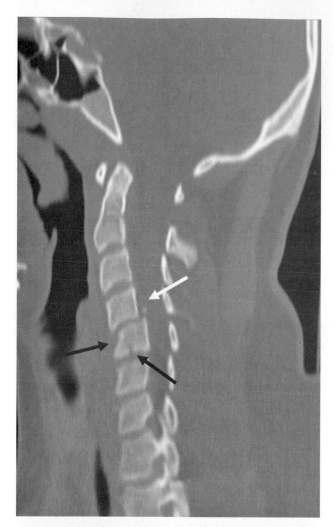

FIGURE 4-7 ● C5 fracture. Sagittal reformatted images from CT of same patient as Fig. 4-6 demonstrate anterior compression fracture of the body of C5 (*black arrows*) and small retropulsed fragment posterior to the C4-C5 disk (*white arrow*). (© Hospital for Sick Children, Toronto.)

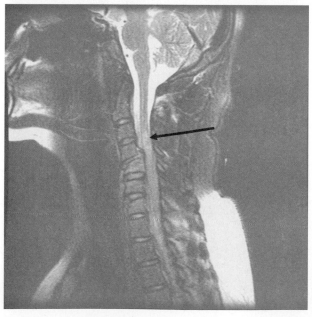

FIGURE 4-8 ● C5 fracture. Sagittal T2 MRI from same patient as Fig. 4-6 and 4-7 shows increased intramedullary signal within the spinal cord at C4-C5 (*black arrow*). Note the increased signal in the C5 vertebral body, consistent with edema/hemorrhage. The anterior compression fracture deformity at C5 is well demonstrated. (© Hospital for Sick Children, Toronto.)

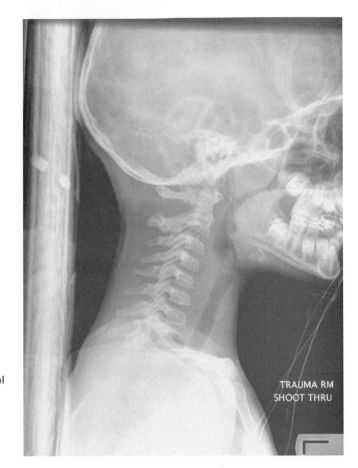

FIGURE 4-9 ● Craniocervical junction injury. Lateral radiograph shows no definite abnormality. Patient was passenger in a high-speed MVA. (© Hospital for Sick Children, Toronto.)

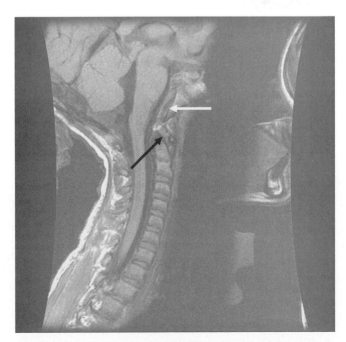

FIGURE 4-10 ● Craniocervical junction injury. Sagittal T1 MRI image demonstrates hematoma subtending tectorial membrane (*white arrow*) and abnormal tissue interposed between dens and anterior arch of C1 (*black arrow*). (© Hospital for Sick Children, Toronto.)

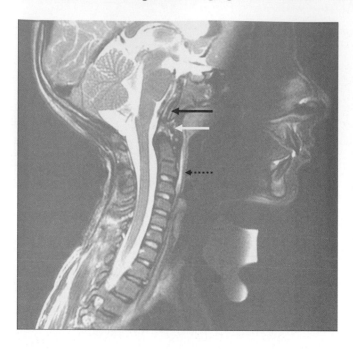

FIGURE 4-11 ● Craniocervical junction trauma. Sagittal T2 MRI image from same patient as Fig. 4-10 shows abnormally hyperintense tissue (*black arrow*) between clivus and tectorial membrane, consistent with hemorrhage. Abnormal signal at tip of dens (*white arrow*) is also consistent with hemorrhage. Minimal prevertebral edema is seen (*black dashed arrow*). (© Hospital for Sick Children, Toronto.)

PEDIATRIC THORACIC TRAUMA IMAGING

- Anteroposterior (AP) chest radiograph is integral to the radiographic trauma series.
  - Indispensable for evaluating pneumothorax, presence and position of support catheters, detecting significant pleural effusions, and fractures.
- AP chest radiograph is often inadequate in patients with significant blunt chest trauma, and may need to be followed with a contrast-enhanced chest CT if clinically indicated.

Chest Radiographs in the Pediatric Trauma Setting

- AP (supine) chest radiograph is a component of the primary trauma series.
- Assess for:
  1. Pneumothorax/pneumomediastinum.
  2. Hemothorax.
  3. Fractures of vertebrae, shoulder girdles, ribs.
  4. Position of support catheters.
  5. Foreign bodies.
  6. Pneumoperitoneum.
  7. Cardiomegaly.
  8. Atelectasis.
  9. Pulmonary contusion.
  10. Mediastinal widening.
  11. Diaphragmatic integrity and position.
  12. Upper abdominal viscera.
- Pneumothorax is delineated from aerated lung by the presence of a thin dense line confined to the expected pleural space.
- May be difficult to appreciate small pneumothoraces on supine films.
- Pneumomediastinum will outline the thymus, cardiac borders, trachea, esophagus, and can extend into the neck, axilla, subcutaneous tissues, and abdomen.
- Hemothorax is seen as a meniscus between aerated lung and the chest wall laterally or the diaphragm inferiorly. The supine film will show opacification/haziness of the hemithorax.
- Carefully assess the position of endotracheal tube, naso/orogastric catheter, and vascular support catheters. If position is in question, obtain lateral radiographs.
- AP technique causes artifactual enlargement of the cardiac and mediastinal silhouettes.

- If cardiomegaly or pericardial effusion is suspected, obtain prompt echocardiography.
- Evaluate suspected mediastinal widening with contrast-enhanced CT.

CT of Chest Trauma in Children[3,4]

- Children with clinically significant blunt or penetrating chest trauma should also undergo chest CT if hemodynamically stable.
- Multislice CT scanners, with proper timing of IV contrast administration, allow for excellent depiction of thoracic vascular structures.
- The most common CT finding in blunt thoracic trauma is pulmonary contusion.
    - Presents as nonsegmental, hyperdense, often crescentic foci that parallel the anterior, lateral, or posterior chest wall.
    - Majority (75%) of patients with significant contusions to the RML or RLL have concomitant right hepatic lobar or right renal trauma.
    - Minority (33%) of patients with significant contusions to the lingula or LLL have concomitant injury to the spleen or left kidney.
- Pulmonary lacerations are often not appreciated on AP CXR, but can be detected on CT.
- CT can help confirm adequacy of chest tube placement.
- Rib fractures are uncommon, due to the extraordinary compliance of the pediatric chest wall.
- Traumatic rupture of the diaphragm is present in 4% to 6% of children with significant thoracoabdominal trauma, usually in high-speed MVA.
- Diaphragmatic injuries are accurately depicted on CT, although usually suspected on CXR.
- Most patients with diaphragmatic rupture have severe concomitant injuries (closed head trauma, visceral/mesenteric trauma, major extremity trauma, vascular interruption).
- On CXR and CT, suspect diaphragmatic trauma if:
    - Hemidiaphragm is indistinct.
    - Elevated hemidiaphragm.
    - Large pleural effusion.
    - Bowel or nasogastric tube projects over chest.
- See Figs. 4-12 to 4-18 for imaging of thoracic trauma.

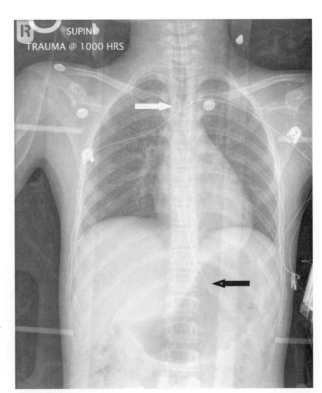

FIGURE 4-12 ● Normal AP chest radiograph. AP chest radiograph demonstrating well-positioned endotracheal tube (*white arrow*) and nasogastric catheter (*black arrow*). No acute abnormalities are seen. (© Hospital for Sick Children, Toronto.)

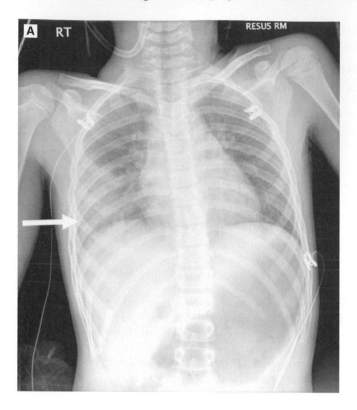

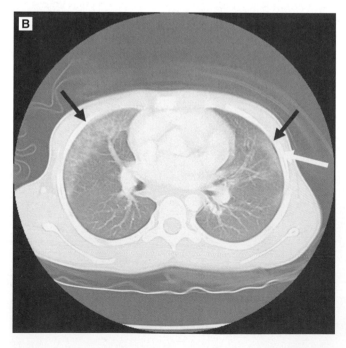

FIGURE 4-13 ● **A.** Pulmonary contusion. AP radiograph demonstrating a right-sided pulmonary contusion (white arrow). **B.** Pulmonary contusion. CT with lung window demonstrates pulmonary contusions (*black arrows*) and small left pneumothorax (*white arrow*). (© Hospital for Sick Children, Toronto.)

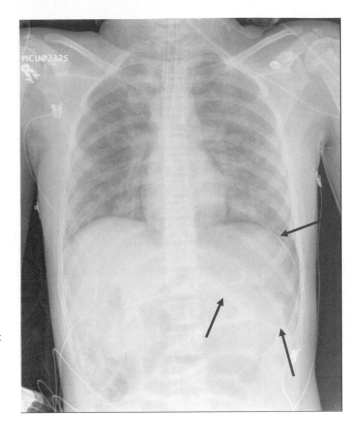

FIGURE 4-14 ● Pulmonary contusions and pneumothorax. AP CXR demonstrates multifocal opacities in child with blunt trauma, consistent with contusions. Radiographically subtle yet large left pneumothorax is subpulmonic in location (*black arrows*). (© Hospital for Sick Children, Toronto.)

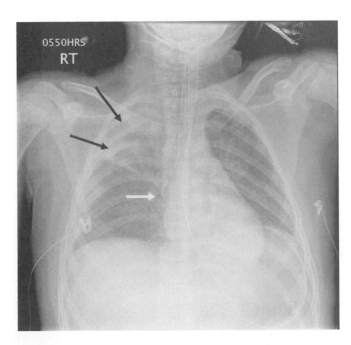

FIGURE 4-15 ● Malpositioned catheter. Portable radiograph demonstrates right apical pleural effusion (*black arrows*) and malpositioned esophageal lead within the right lower lobar bronchus (*white arrow*). Effusion due to T4 fracture not well depicted on this study. (© Hospital for Sick Children, Toronto.)

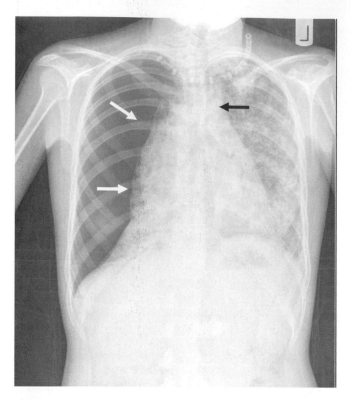

FIGURE 4-16 ● Tension pneumothorax. Upright radiograph demonstrates a large right tension pneumothorax (*white arrows*) in a child with underlying cystic fibrosis and respiratory difficulty after minor trauma. Note that the right lung is completely collapsed and the right diaphragmatic leaflet is depressed. The trachea (*black arrow*) is displaced to the left of midline. (© Hospital for Sick Children, Toronto.)

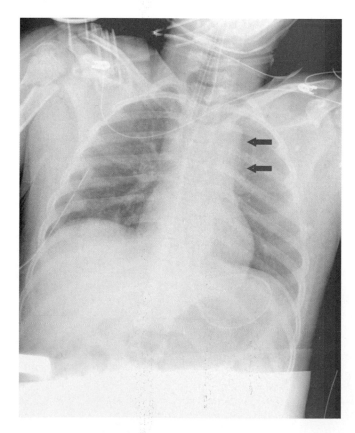

FIGURE 4-17 ● Mediastinal widening. AP CXR demonstrating mild widening of superior mediastinum, suggestive of mediastinal hematoma (*black arrows*). Note displaced fracture of right humerus. (© Hospital for Sick Children, Toronto.)

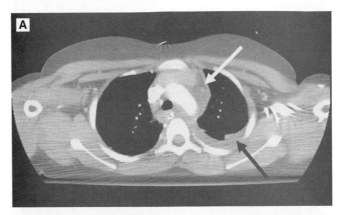

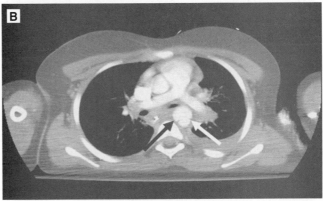

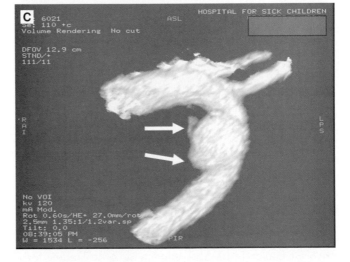

FIGURE 4-18 ● Traumatic aortic pseudoaneurysm. **A.** Left pleural effusion (*black arrow*) and mediastinal hemorrhage (*white arrow*). **B.** Aortic pseudoaneurysm (*black and white arrows*). **C** 3D reformatted image showing aortic pseudoaneurysm (*white arrows*). (© Hospital for Sick Children, Toronto.)

IMAGING OF PEDIATRIC ABDOMINAL AND PELVIC TRAUMA

- Patients with physical or laboratory indicators of abdominal or pelvic injury should undergo CT.
  - Plain radiographs are of little to no value in these patients.
- Ultrasound (FAST) has not been validated in the pediatric trauma setting.
  - Can be performed to search for free fluid, but is of questionable value, as most solid visceral organ injuries resulting in hemoperitoneum are managed nonoperatively.
  - Ultrasound is of little value in the search for injury to the hollow viscera, retroperitoneum, and is of no value in assessing possible skeletal trauma.

- Few individuals outside major pediatric imaging departments possess requisite skill set for this modality.
- Pelvic radiographs are useful in detecting pelvic fractures.
  - They remain part of the primary radiologic series; however, a review suggests that routine pelvic radiographs, in the absence of hematuria or clinically obvious findings, are of limited value.[5]
- CT of the abdomen and pelvis should always be performed with intravenous contrast in the absence of a documented allergy to contrast or severe renal failure.
  - Oral contrast is often administered, but should be omitted in the clinically unstable child likely to require emergency surgery.
- Modern multislice CT scanners, along with proper timing of IV contrast administration, provide excellent evaluation of the abdominal and pelvic vasculature.
  - Data from these studies may be reprocessed to produce CT angiographic images.
- Coronal and sagittal reformatting is valuable for evaluating diaphragmatic integrity, pelvic and vertebral fractures, and bladder and vascular injuries.
- Suspected duodenal hematoma can be evaluated after CT with a limited upper GI series (UGI) using water-soluble contrast.
  - Sonography can also be valuable in this setting.
- CT of the abdomen and pelvis can be performed in conjunction with CT of the brain, cervical spine, and/or chest in the victim of polytrauma.
- Males with straddle injuries or with ischial fractures and hematuria require retrograde urethrography.
  - Perform in the trauma room using water-soluble contrast (same IV contrast used for CT).
- Liver, spleen, and kidney injuries are graded according to severity as seen on CT.
- See Chapter 11 on Abdominal and Pelvic Trauma for details.
- Hemodynamically stable children are usually managed nonoperatively, despite CT findings, in the absence of hollow visceral injuries.
- Children with CT findings of devascularization of spleen or kidney are managed operatively.
- Ultrasound is often used for follow-up imaging of patients with documented solid visceral trauma.

Liver[6,7]

- Hepatic injuries are seen in 10% to 27% of pediatric abdominal trauma.
- Most common injuries are parenchymal hematomas and lacerations.
- Most common site is the right hepatic lobe.
- The normal contrast-enhanced liver is homogeneous, with the appearance of the hepatic veins, portal venous branches, and hepatic arteries varying with the timing of IV contrast injection and image acquisition.
- CT findings of acute hepatic injury include:
  - Intraparenchymal hematoma/laceration.
  - Subsegmental/segmental devascularization.
  - Perihepatic/subcapsular fluid.
  - Intraparenchymal "blush" = site of active bleeding.
- See Chapter 11 on Abdominal and Pelvic Trauma for AAST Liver Injury Grading Scale.
- See Fig. 4-19 for liver lacerations.

Spleen[8–10]

- Timing of contrast administration and image acquisition often results in unusual appearance of the spleen—it is important to recognize these artifacts and not interpret them as evidence of splenic trauma:
  - Tigroid or zebra appearance.
  - Focal round areas of differing densities.
- Signs of splenic injury are similar to those for the liver:
  - Intraparenchymal hematoma/laceration.
  - Focal devascularization.

- Perisplenic/subcapsular fluid.
- Intraparenchymal "blush."
- In the literature, focal "blush" is seen in up to 30%.
- Blush is indicative of active bleeding, which may indicate need for operative management in some patients.
  - The majority of pediatric patients with this sign have been managed successfully without requiring surgery.
- See Chapter 11 on Abdominal and Pelvic Trauma for AAST Splenic Injury Grading Scale.
- See Fig. 4-20 for splenic laceration.

Kidney[11]

- Renal trauma is usually managed conservatively if child remains hemodynamically stable.
- Urinomas are frequent, usually surround the kidney or are located along medial/lateral aspect of kidney.
- Kidneys should enhance symmetrically.
  - Timing of contrast injection and image acquisition will determine pattern of renal enhancement.

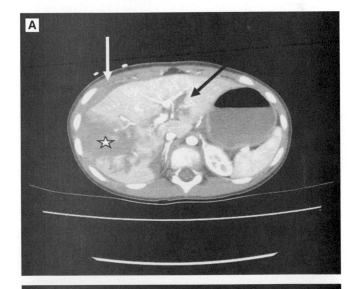

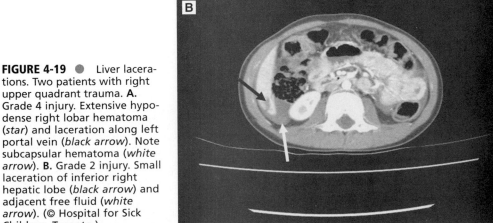

FIGURE 4-19 ● Liver lacerations. Two patients with right upper quadrant trauma. **A.** Grade 4 injury. Extensive hypodense right lobar hematoma (*star*) and laceration along left portal vein (*black arrow*). Note subcapsular hematoma (*white arrow*). **B.** Grade 2 injury. Small laceration of inferior right hepatic lobe (*black arrow*) and adjacent free fluid (*white arrow*). (© Hospital for Sick Children, Toronto.)

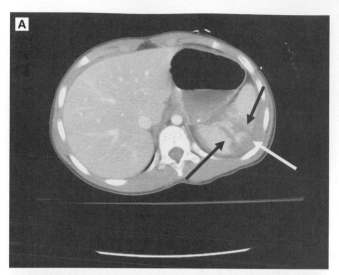

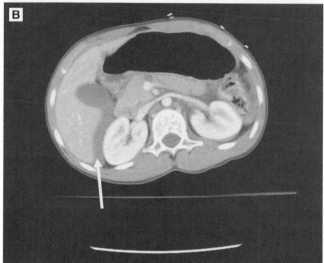

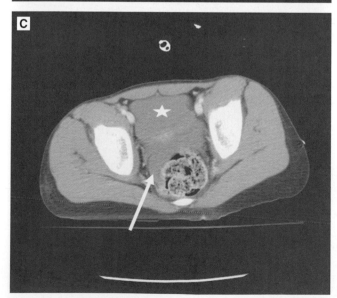

FIGURE 4-20 ● Splenic laceration. **A.** Linear lacerations of splenic parenchyma (*black arrows*), with free fluid (*white arrow*). **B.** Free fluid in right upper quadrant (*white arrow*). **C.** Free fluid in pelvis (*white arrow*). Note that free fluid and bladder (*star*) have similar density. (© Hospital for Sick Children, Toronto.)

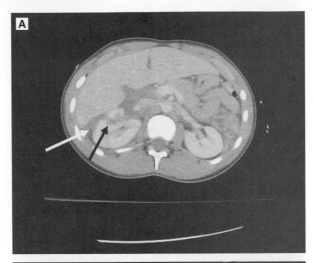

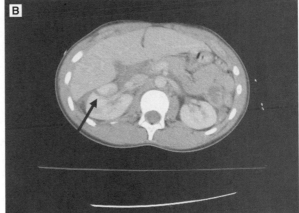

FIGURE 4-21 ● Renal laceration. Sequential CT images demonstrate a linear fracture of the right kidney (**A** and **B**, *black arrows*), with associated free fluid within the Morison pouch (**A**, *white arrow*). (© Hospital for Sick Children, Toronto.)

- Signs of renal trauma on CT include:
  - Asymmetrical enhancement may indicate renal arterial occlusion or an obstructed collecting system.
  - Focal areas of poor enhancement.
  - Linear clefts within renal parenchyma.
  - Perinephric fluid collections. Delayed images may demonstrate increased enhancement if due to urinary leak.
  - Hypodense mass in the bladder in this setting is usually hematoma.
- See Figs. 4-21 for renal laceration and 4-22 for renal artery dissection.

Pancreas[12]
- Trauma is the most common cause of pancreatitis in children.
- Pancreas is not usually damaged even in polytrauma; usually results from direct blow, as in:
  - Handlebar injury.
  - Seatbelt injury.
  - Blunt object (e.g., hockey stick, fist).
- Pancreatic trauma often results in pseudocyst formation later in course.
- On CT, pancreas usually enhances homogeneously, demonstrating either a smooth or mildly lobulated outer contour.
- Ultrasound is of no value in the acute setting.

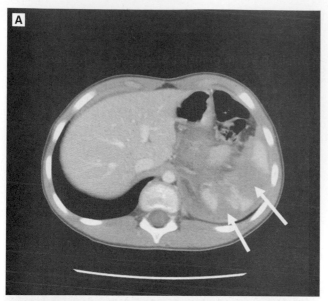

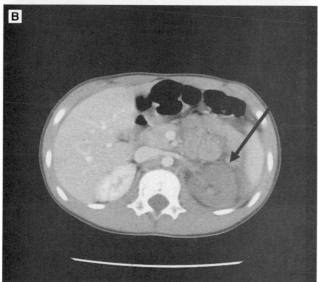

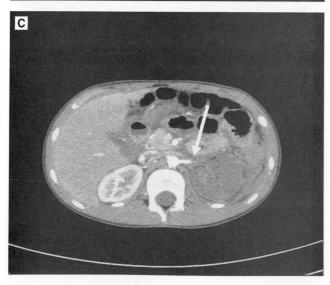

FIGURE 4-22 ● Renal arterial dissection. Patient with extensive splenic lacerations (**A,** *white arrows*) demonstrates absence of perfusion of left kidney (**B,** *black arrow*). CT angiogram shows abrupt cutoff of left renal artery (**C,** *white arrow*), consistent with renal arterial dissection. (© Hospital for Sick Children, Toronto.)

- CT signs of pancreatic injury include:
  - Peripancreatic fluid.
  - Fluid in lesser sac.
  - Mesenteric stranding.
  - Linear parenchymal clefts, often at junction of body and head.
  - Focal decreased parenchymal enhancement.
  - Associated duodenal hematoma is common.
- CT may be falsely negative early in course; if suspicion persists, obtain repeat imaging.
  - Thin-section reformatting, including coronal images, is helpful.
- See Fig. 4-23 for pancreatic laceration.

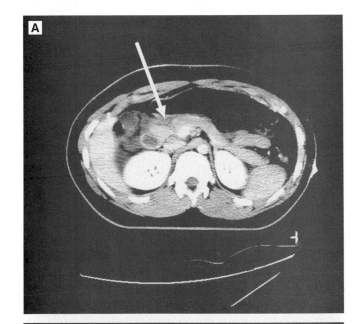

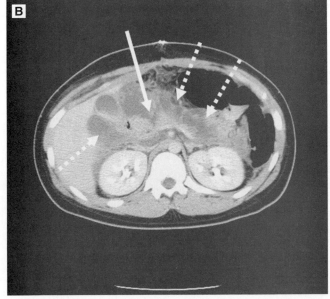

FIGURE 4-23 ● Pancreatic laceration. **A.** Initial study shows subtle cleft at lateral head of pancreas (*white arrow*), not appreciated initially. **B.** Study performed one week later, after repair of duodenal perforation, demonstrates widening of cleft (*white solid arrow*) and multiple low-density peripancreatic fluid collections (*white dashed arrows*), representing florid pancreatitis. (© Hospital for Sick Children, Toronto.)

Bowel/Mesentery[13,14]

- Duodenal hematoma is most often seen in lapbelt or handlebar injuries, blunt object trauma, and in Nonaccidental Trauma.
- Duodenal hematoma is best imaged utilizing fluoroscopy and water-soluble contrast.
- Up to 60% of bowel perforations occur in the proximal jejunum, just distal to the ligament of Treitz.
- Jameson and associates reported findings of 43 patients with GI tract perforation over a 10-year period:
  - CT was obtained in 22 patients.
  - Signs suggestive of significant bowel trauma include:
    - Extraluminal (free) air.
    - Intraperitoneal free fluid.
    - Bowel wall thickening.
    - Bowel wall enhancement.
    - Bowel dilatation.

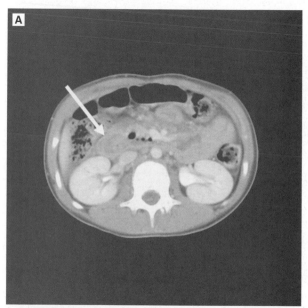

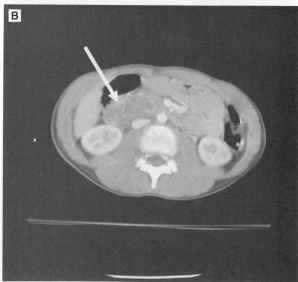

FIGURE 4-24 ● Duodenal hematoma. Two different patients with lapbelt injuries. The distal second and proximal third portions of duodenum are dilated, with hypodense wall thickening, consistent with intramural hemorrhage (*white arrows*). This finding may be confirmed with a limited upper GI series, utilizing water-soluble contrast. (© Hospital for Sick Children, Toronto.)

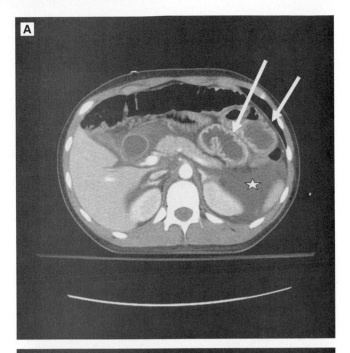

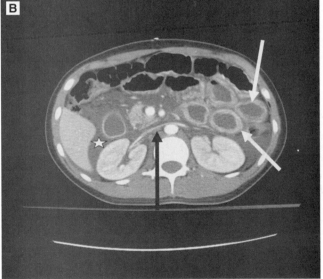

FIGURE 4-25 ● Shock bowel with hypotension. Two images from abdominal CT demonstrate intraperitoneal free fluid (*stars*), thickened, enhancing small bowel loops (*white arrows*), and narrow, collapsed IVC (**B,** *black arrow*). (© Hospital for Sick Children, Toronto.)

- CT documented free air in 47%.
- 18% had all five of the above signs and perforation.
- Intraperitoneal free air may not be seen in all patients with bowel perforation.
- Duodenal perforations may be retroperitoneal.
- See Figs. 4-24 for duodenal hematoma and 4-25 for shock bowel.

Bladder/Pelvis[15]
- Pelvic injuries most common in high-speed MVAs, snowboarding/skiing accidents, straddling injuries.
- Pelvic fractures often underevaluated with standard AP pelvic radiographs, especially complex acetabular fractures, sacral fractures, and sacroiliac joint diastatic injuries.

- CT, with sagittal and coronal reformatted images, is the study of choice to evaluate for pelvic and acetabular fractures, as well as sacral/sacroiliac joint trauma.
- Pelvic fractures are associated with potentially large pelvic hematomas; these may be suspected if the bladder catheter is displaced from the midline, or if vascular access catheters assume an unusual course.
- CT with IV contrast may demonstrate a contrast blush in actively bleeding pelvic hematomas; if seen, consider angiographic embolization for achieving hemostasis.
- The full urinary bladder may rupture, usually at the posterior aspect of the dome, which is its weakest point.
- Intraperitoneal bladder rupture is more common than retroperitoneal rupture in children (opposite to adult bladder rupture).
- Bladder rupture may be seen with or without pelvic fractures.
- CT cystography, performed with instillation of water-soluble or nonionic contrast into the bladder via a Foley catheter, is the study of choice to confirm or refute bladder rupture.
- Male urethra may be transected in straddle injuries, usually with diastasis or fractures at pubic symphysis.
- Male urethra usually transected at membranous level, immediately distal to the fixed prostate gland.
- Retrograde urethrography, usually performed in the trauma room, utilizing nonionic contrast, is the study of choice to evaluate the potentially transected urethra.
- See Figs. 4-26 for intraperitoneal bladder rupture and 4-27 for urethral transection.

IMAGING OF PEDIATRIC EXTREMITY TRAUMA
- Many victims of polytrauma exhibit clinically obvious extremity fractures.
- Attempt to obtain AP and lateral views of suspicious areas.
- Intra-articular fractures, especially at the hip, knee, and ankle level, are best evaluated with CT, with sagittal and coronal reformatted images useful for full depiction of fracture displacement, angulation, and comminution.
- Marked displacement at fracture site may predispose to neurovascular compromise, particularly at the shoulder, elbow, hip, and knee.
- CT angiography, using multislice CT with IV contrast administration, can accurately depict posttraumatic arteriovenous fistulae, pseudoaneurysms, thromboses, and transections.
- This technique is valuable in patients with markedly displaced fractures, crush injuries, and degloving injuries.
- Prior to physeal closure, articular or periarticular fractures are classified according to the Salter–Harris nomenclature (Fig. 4-28):
  Salter–Harris 1:   Transverse fracture of the physis.
  Salter–Harris 2:   Transverse fracture of the physis, extending into the metaphysis.
  Salter–Harris 3:   Transverse fracture of the physis, extending into the epiphysis.
  Salter–Harris 4:   Transverse fracture of the physis, extending into the metaphysis and epiphysis.
  Salter–Harris 5:   Crush injury of metaphysis, physis, and epiphysis.
- See Chapter 12 on Orthopedic Trauma for further details.
- Complex intraarticular fractures are best assessed with CT.
- CT angiography is indicated in patients with suspected vascular injury or thrombosis.

CRANIAL IMAGING IN THE TRAUMA SETTING
- Plain radiographs are of little utility in the initial evaluation.
- CT of the upper cervical spine and brain is indicated in patients with history of significant impact, deceleration, penetrating trauma, or history of loss of consciousness.
- CT can be performed even in unstable patients and is the initial study of choice.
- Initially, CT is always performed without IV contrast; contrast may then be given to evaluate for vascular injury/thrombosis.

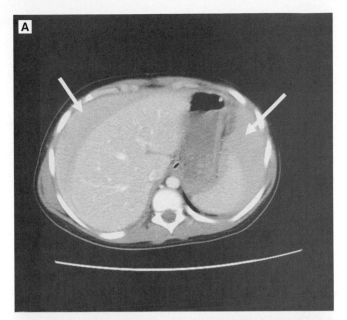

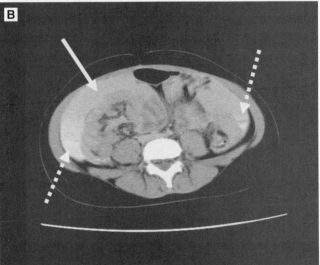

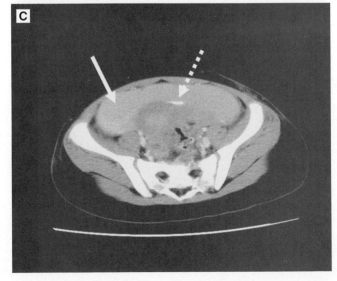

FIGURE 4-26 ● Intraperitoneal bladder rupture. Hyperintense intraperitoneal fluid (*white solid arrows*), with markedly hyperintense fluid (**B** and **C,** *white dashed arrows*) layering in paracolic gutters and anterior to bladder dome. Note the progressively hyperintense nature of the fluid in the right paracolic gutter. (© Hospital for Sick Children, Toronto.)

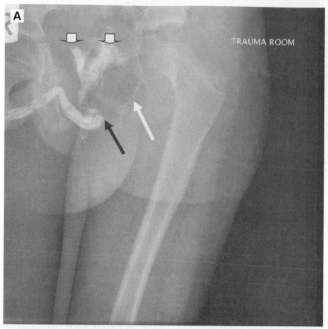

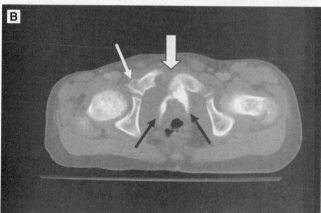

FIGURE 4-27 ● Urethral transection. **A.** Retrograde ure-throgram demonstrates ure-thral transection (*black arrow*) with retroperitoneal (*arrow-heads*) and vascular extravasa-tion (*white arrow*). **B.** CT with bone windows shows right ischial fracture (*narrow white arrow*), diastasis of pubic sym-physis (*wide white arrow*), and retroperitoneal contrast (*black arrows*). (© Hospital for Sick Children, Toronto.)

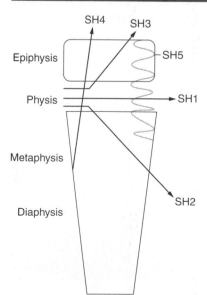

FIGURE 4-28 ● Salter–Harris fracture classification. SH1; SH2; SH3; SH4; and SH5. (© Hospital for Sick Children, Toronto.)

- Urgent MRI is indicated in patients with suspected injury to the spinal cord; a tailored study can be performed in patients too unstable to withstand a full examination.
- CT is indispensable for the evaluation of:
  - Fractures of the facial structures, craniocervical junction, petrous bones, and calvarium.
  - Subgaleal and subcutaneous hematoma.
  - Subarachnoid, subdural, and epidural hemorrhage.
  - Intraparenchymal hemorrhage and contusion.
  - Cerebral edema.
  - Hydrocephalus.
  - Herniation, including uncal, transtentorial, and transfalcine varieties.
  - Foreign bodies.
- See Figs. 4-29 to Fig. 4-33 for images of intracranial injuries.

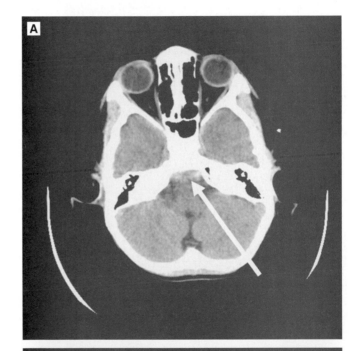

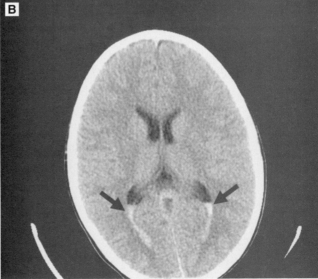

FIGURE 4-29 ● Tectorial hematoma with intraventricular hemorrhage. **A.** *White arrow* demonstrates hyperdense blood posterior to the clivus, subtending the tectorial membrane. This indicates trauma at the craniocervical junction. **B.** *Black arrows* indicate dependent hyperdense blood within the occipital horns of the lateral ventricles. (© Hospital for Sick Children, Toronto.)

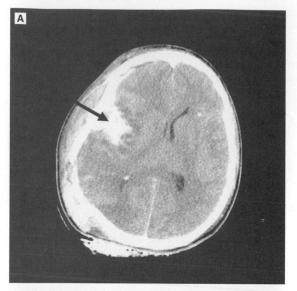

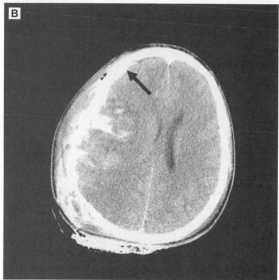

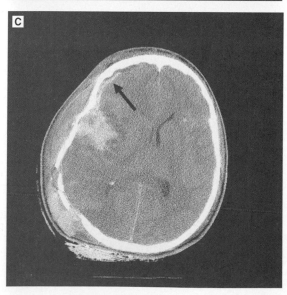

FIGURE 4-30 ● Parenchymal and subdural hemorrhage. Acute right posterior
frontal lobar hemorrhage (**A,** *black
arrow*) and right anterior frontal subdural
hematoma (**B,C,** *black arrows*). There
is compression of right lateral ventricle.
(© Hospital for Sick Children, Toronto.)

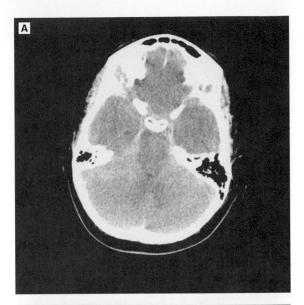

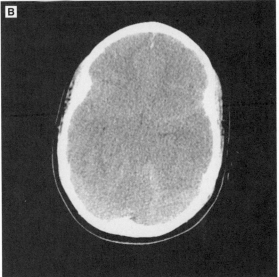

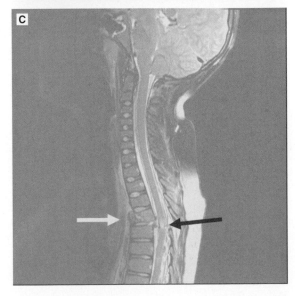

FIGURE 4-31 ● Reversal sign. **A, B.** Axial CT images demonstrate abnormally low density (edema) of the temporal and frontal lobes, with normal density of cerebellar hemispheres. There is uncal herniation with effacement of basilar cisterns. **C.** Note associated fracture of T4 on MRI (*white arrow*) and cord edema (*black arrow*). (© Hospital for Sick Children, Toronto.)

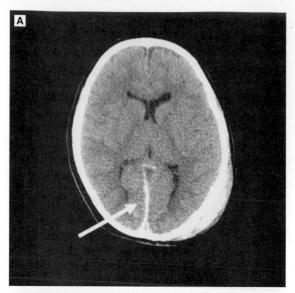

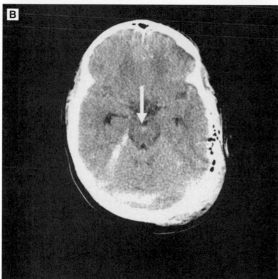

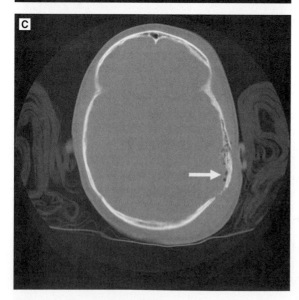

FIGURE 4-32 ● Subdural and sub-arachnoid hemorrhage. Acute hyper-dense posterior falcine subdural hemorrhage (**A**, *white arrow*) and acute subarachnoid blood within the prepontine cistern (**B**, *white arrow*). Bone window image demonstrates pneumocephalus (**C**, *white arrow*) due to left temporal fracture. (© Hospital for Sick Children, Toronto.)

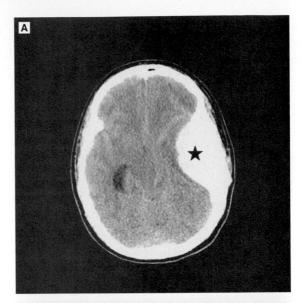

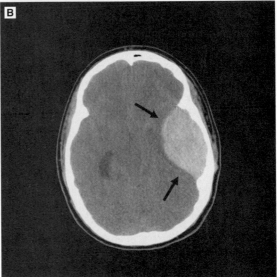

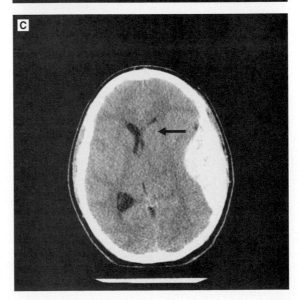

FIGURE 4-33 ● Epidural hematoma. Large hyperdense, acute left temporal epidural hematoma (**A,** *star*). Changing the window settings allows the hematoma to be distinguished from the calvarium (**B,** *black arrows*). Note mass effect on the compressed left frontal horn (**C,** *black arrow*). There is left uncal and subfalcine herniation. (© Hospital for Sick Children, Toronto.)

CLINICAL PEARLS

DO
- Look "through" the heart for posteromedial pulmonary atelectasis/contusion, vertebral fractures, and rib fractures.
- Note that extensive or persistent subcutaneous/mediastinal air, and/or persistent pneumothorax, is suggestive of tracheobronchial injury.
- Remember to search for Chance fractures of the upper lumbar vertebrae in patients with lapbelt injuries. Sagittal and coronal reformatted CT images are of paramount importance to detect these injuries.
- Suspect bladder rupture if bladder is small or empty, or if high-density fluid is seen in low pelvis or in paracolic gutters.

DON'T
- Confuse a skinfold for a pneumothorax.
- Interpret air surrounding the heart on AP supine radiograph as being pneumopericardium. It is almost always pneumomediastinum.
- Forget to consider nonaccidental injury when managing pediatric trauma, especially with pancreatic, bowel, and mesenteric injuries.

REFERENCES
1. Swischuk LE, John SD, Hendrick EP. Is the open-mouth odontoid view necessary in children under 5 years? *Pediatr Radiol* 2000;30:186–189.
2. Reddy SP, Junewick JJ, Backstrom JW. Distribution of spinal fractures in children: does age, mechanism of injury, or gender play a significant role? *Pediatr Radiol* 2003;33:776–781.
3. Manson DE, Babyn PS, Palder S, et al. CT of blunt chest trauma in children. *Pediatr Radiol* 1993;23:1–5.
4. Koplewitz BZ, Ramos C, Manson DE, et al. Traumatic diaphragmatic injuries in infants and children: imaging findings. *Pediatr Radiol* 2000;30:471–479.
5. Rees MJ, Aicken R, Kolbe A, et al. The screening pelvic radiograph in pediatric trauma. *Pediatr Radiol* 2001;31:497–500.
6. Navarro O, Babyn PS, Pearl RH. The value of routine follow-up imaging in pediatric blunt liver trauma. *Pediatr Radiol* 2000;30:546–550.
7. Basile KE, Sivit CJ, O'Riordan MA, et al. Acute hemoperitoneum in children: prevalence of low attenuation fluid. *Pediatr Radiol* 2000;30:168–170.
8. Lutz N, Mahboubi S, Nance ML, et al. The significance of contrast blush on computed tomography in children with splenic injuries. *J Pediatr Surg* 2004;39:491–494.
9. Nwomeh BC, Nadler EP, Meza MP, et al. Contrast extravasation predicts the need for operative intervention in children with blunt splenic trauma. *J Trauma* 2004;56:537–541.
10. Mooney DP, Downard C, Johnson S, et al. Physiology after pediatric splenic injury. *J Trauma* 2005;58:108–111.
11. Wilkinson AG, Haddock G, Carachi R. Separation of renal fragments by a urinoma after renal trauma: percutaneous drainage accelerates healing. *Pediatr Radiol* 1999;25:503–505.
12. Nijs E, Callahan MJ, Taylor GA. Disorders of the pediatric pancreas: imaging features. *Pediatr Radiol* 2004;35:358–373.
13. Jamieson DH, Babyn PS, Pearl R. Imaging gastrointestinal perforation in pediatric blunt abdominal trauma. *Pediatr Radiol* 1996;26:188–194.
14. Shah P, Applegate KE, Buonomo C. Stricture of the duodenum and jejunum in an abused child. *Pediatr Radiol* 1997;27:282–283.
15. Brown D, Magill HL, Black TL. Delayed presentation of traumatic intraperitoneal bladder rupture. *Pediatr Radiol* 1986;16:252–253.

CHAPTER 5

Head Trauma: Medical Management

James Hutchison, MD, FRCPC, FAAP
Anne-Marie Guerguerian, MD, FAAP, FRCPC

EPIDEMIOLOGY AND ETIOLOGY

- Severe head trauma in children has a mortality of 20% to 30%.[1,2]
- Most children with multiple trauma are at risk of secondary hypoxic-ischemic brain injury due to shock, hypotension, hypoxia, and intracranial hypertension.[3–9]
- Injuries are most commonly due to motor vehicle collisions, falls, and bicycle and sports related injuries.[1]
- Most head injuries are caused by blunt trauma.
- Head trauma secondary to child abuse is most common in infants and is associated with a higher mortality.[10]
- Males are more commonly injured than females.
- The peak incidences occur in toddlers and adolescents.
- Diffuse axonal injury (shear injury of the white matter) is more common and intracranial hematomas requiring surgical evacuation are less common in children than in adults.
  - Current CT imaging techniques underestimate diffuse axonal injury; therefore children can have severe diffuse axonal injury with only subtle or no focal white matter lesions visible on CT imaging.
- Epidural hematomas are a neurosurgical emergency and most often follow trauma to the temporal region.
  - There may be a period of consciousness followed by rapid deterioration and coma.
  - See Chapter 6 on Surgical Management of Head Trauma for details.
- Survivors of head trauma have a high incidence of functional and neuropsychological dysfunction.[1,11–13]
- Children who have coma need early comprehensive assessment and care by a multidisciplinary rehabilitation team.

PATHOPHYSIOLOGY

Intracranial Compliance Curve

- The intracranial vault contains brain matter, blood, and cerebrospinal fluid (CSF) in a closed space.
- An expanding mass, such as a hematoma or cerebral contusion, will first displace venous blood and CSF, and intracranial pressure will initially remain stable.
- As a mass expands, eventually no space remains and the intracranial pressure (ICP) rises exponentially (Munroe–Kellie doctrine; see Fig. 5-1).
  - The brain is said to be "tight" when relatively small increases in intracranial volume lead to relatively large increases in intracranial pressure.
  - Open fontanelles in an infant do not protect the brain from increased ICP.[3]

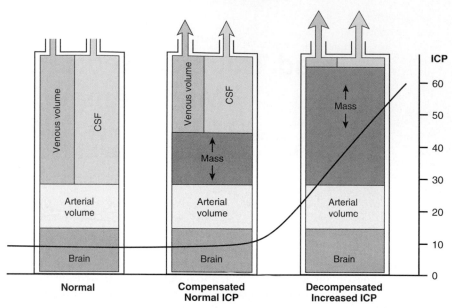

FIGURE 5-1 ● Munroe–Kellie doctrine. As a mass expands within the cranium, CSF and venous blood are displaced. Eventually the compensatory mechanisms are overcome and the intracranial pressure (ICP) begins to rise. (Adapted from Poss WB, Brockmeyer DL, Clay B, et al. Pathophysiology and management of the intracranial vault. In: Rogers MC, Nichols DG, eds. *Textbook of pediatric intensive care.* 3rd ed. Baltimore: Williams & Wilkins; 1996:646.)

Cerebral Blood Flow and Edema

- Arterial oxygen tension (PaO_2), arterial carbon dioxide tension ($PaCO_2$), and blood pressure have important effects on cerebral blood flow (Fig. 5-2).
- High cerebral blood flow may result in intracranial hypertension.
- Low cerebral blood flow results in cerebral ischemia.

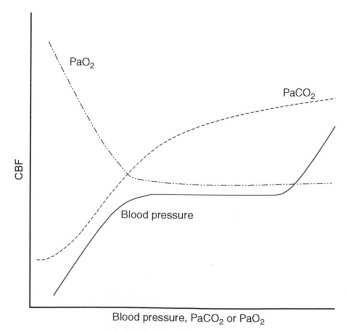

FIGURE 5-2 ● The relationship between PaO_2, $PaCO_2$, and blood pressure and cerebral blood flow (CBF).

- Cerebral blood flow is relatively constant (autoregulation) over a broad range of blood pressures in healthy viable brain.
- Autoregulation is lost in injured brain areas.
  - These areas are susceptible to further ischemic injury during hypotension.
  - Infants and young children have a relatively high baseline cerebral blood flow compared to older children and adolescents, which may increase risk of rapid cerebral edema and intracranial hypertension.
- Brain edema occurs due to vasogenic (disruption of the blood–brain barrier) and cytotoxic edema.
- As PaO_2 drops below 60 mmHg, cerebral blood flow rises exponentially.
  - **Therefore keep PaO_2 > 80 mmHg or SaO_2 > 95%.**
- Hypercarbia results in cerebral hyperemia but aggressive hyperventilation results in cerebral ischemia.
  - **Maintain $PaCO_2$ 35 to 40 mmHg and monitor end-tidal CO_2 continuously.**
- Areas that are injured may lose autoregulation.
  - **Measure blood pressure and maintain blood pressure in the high normal range for age.**

Cerebral Metabolic Rate

- Cerebral metabolic rate will be increased by fever, seizures, pain, and agitation, which may lead to increased cell death, hyperemia, and intracranial hypertension.
- There is a massive inflammatory response following head trauma. Fever develops in the majority of children and adolescents within hours of the injury.[14,15]
  - **Maintain normothermia, give prophylactic anticonvulsants, and maintain deep sedation and analgesia after ensuring a secure airway.**

Brain Cell Death

- Brain cell death occurs in contusions and in areas of shear injury.
- Contusions are often seen in a "coup and contre-coup" distribution.
- Many viable cells are selectively vulnerable to subtle insults such as hypoxia and hypotension.
  - **Great care must be taken to rapidly recognize and treat hypoxia, shock, and hypotension.**

DEFINITION/RISK FACTORS

- Severe traumatic brain injury is defined as those children with a Glasgow Coma Score (GCS) of ≤8 following head trauma.
- Patients with a GCS of 3 to 4, cardiac arrest, or severe hypotension, shock, or hypoxia have a worse prognosis.

INITIAL MANAGEMENT

Indications to perform early intubations:
1. Upper airway obstruction from:
   - Actual or potential loss of pharyngeal muscle tone.
   - Inability to clear oral secretions or vomit.
   - Seizures.
   - Foreign body.
2. Coma or decreasing level of consciousness with a GCS ≤ 8 or deteriorating GCS.
3. Loss of protective airway reflexes such as cough and gag.
4. Respiratory arrest, failure, or depression; hypoxia: inability to maintain PaO_2 > 60 mmHg or SaO_2 > 93% despite supplemental oxygen; respiratory acidosis.
5. To facilitate hyperventilation if severe increased ICP is suspected (rapidly deteriorating GCS or herniation syndrome).
6. Seizures or status epilepticus.
7. Decompensated shock.

ABC MANAGEMENT
- 100% oxygen by non-rebreathing face mask.
- C-spine precautions with rigid C-spine collar properly fitted for age and size.
- Early intubation using rapid-sequence induction (RSI) of anesthesia by skilled personnel to prevent complications.[16-20]
- Bag-mask ventilation with cricoid pressure may need to be initiated until tracheal intubation is performed in the presence of deep coma, respiratory depression, and/or hypoxia.
  - Otherwise, cricoid pressure is performed after medications are delivered.

RSI of the Head Injured Patient
Premedication
- Atropine (10–20 μg/kg IV) in children <6 years of age or in patients who will receive succinylcholine as a neuromuscular blocking agent.
- Lidocaine (1–2 mg/kg IV) as intravenous dose 2 to 5 minutes before laryngoscopy blunts the hemodynamic responses to intubation.
  - Primarily used in hemodynamically unstable patients.
  - Often administered as an adjunct medication with low-dose thiopental, fentanyl, and/or midazolam.

Administer IV Anesthetic
- Choices are thiopental, fentanyl, and etomidate.
- Propofol is used in adults but is not recommended in children.
- Thiopental (4 to 2–4 mg/kg IV).
  - Short-acting barbiturate and a general anesthetic without analgesic properties that blunts ICP elevation in response to intubation.
  - Decreases brain metabolism and used to lower increased ICP acutely.
  - Potent negative inotrope.
  - Dramatic falls in blood pressure can occur in hypovolemic patients.
  - Lower-dose thiopental should be used if risk of hypotension.
  - Thiopental is contraindicated in shock.
- Fentanyl (1–3 μg/kg IV).
  - Short-acting opiate analgesic.
  - Has the fewest hemodynamic side effects.
  - Rapid IV administration can produce chest wall rigidity, making ventilation impossible (treat with succinylcholine or naloxone).
  - Fentanyl may lower ICP by blunting the response to intubation and by decreasing pain associated with other injuries found in trauma patients.
  - Lower-dose fentanyl should be used if risk of hypotension.
- Etomidate (0.3 mg/kg IV).
  - Short-acting sedative-hypnotic, without analgesic properties.
  - Causes minimal cardiovascular changes.
  - It decreases ICP, cerebral blood flow, and cerebral metabolic rate.
  - A single dose can suppress cortisol production; contraindicated in adrenal insufficiency.

Neuromuscular Blockade to Facilitate Intubation with RSI
- Rapid paralysis of patients prevents cough-induced ICP rises, facilitates intubation, and reduces risk of vomiting and aspiration pneumonia.
- Two choices are:
  - Succinylcholine (1–2 mg/kg IV).
    - Depolarizing agent.
    - Rapid acting and short-lived.
    - Contraindicated in open globe injury, crush injuries, and burns.
    - Should never be used to maintain paralysis after intubation.
  - Rocuronium (0.6–1.2 mg/kg IV).
    - Nondepolarizing agent, with onset of action within 60 seconds.

- Caution should be taken to flush intravenous line well with 10 mL of NaCl 0.9% after thiopental if it is given before rocuronium.
    - This avoids crystallization of the drugs.
- When paralyzed, orally intubate with C-spine precautions.
- Maintain SaO_2 > 95% and $PaCO_2$ 35–40 mmHg.
- End-tidal CO_2 monitor continuously.

Circulation

- Two large-bore peripheral IVs or intra-osseous needles.
- Treat shock or hypotension with an IV bolus of 20 mL/kg normal saline.
    - Reassess hemodynamic status and repeat IV normal saline bolus if necessary.
    - Blood transfusion if suspected hemorrhagic shock and hypotension.
    - Measure temperature and rewarm shocked hypothermic (<32°C), hypotensive patient with severe hemorrhage and coagulopathy.

Disability

- Assess GCS and pupils.
- If pupil(s) is/are nonreactive to light or dilated and you suspect **trans-tentorial herniation:**
    - Administer therapies **RAPIDLY** to reverse intracranial hypertension while organizing STAT CT scan and potential operation with neurosurgeon and anesthetist.
    - Hyperventilate and administer sedation, analgesia, mannitol, hypertonic saline, thiopental (see doses below under Definitive Management), until the pupil(s) begins to respond.
    - Be prepared to administer another bolus of IV normal saline and administer vasoactive medications if patient becomes hemodynamically unstable.
- Place an oral gastric tube and Foley catheter.

EVALUATION

History

- AMPLE history.
- When time permits, obtain details of the mechanism of injury (e.g., motor vehicle collision, mechanism, location in vehicle, belted/nonbelted. Any deaths in the crash? Time at scene? Alcohol or drug consumption?)
- Review transport/paramedic records/records from other hospital if referred.
- Review mental status, hemodynamics, oxygenation, and any images (x-rays/CTs) or blood work.

Physical Exam

- Complete secondary survey.
- Lab testing—CBC, type and cross-match, electrolytes, glucose, ABG, BUN, creatinine, LFTs, INR (or PT), PTT, fibrinogen, amylase, β-HCG in female adolescents, toxicology screen as needed.

Imaging

- Obtain chest x-ray after intubation, a lateral and A-P C-spine x-ray, and CT scan of brain.
- CT is the test of choice in the acute phase.
- MRI is not used in the acute phase unless spinal cord injury is suspected.

SPECIFIC INJURIES

- Should be described on the initial head CT by a radiologist.
- Hematomas, contusions, skull fractures—vault, depressed or basal, diffuse axonal injury.
- Describe state of gray-white differentiation, any midline shift—measure, and state of basal cisterns—normal, attenuated, obliterated.
- See Chapter 4 on Diagnostic Imaging for specific examples.

DEFINITIVE MANAGEMENT

- Patient should be cared for in an institution with a pediatric critical care unit, a trauma surgeon, and a neurosurgeon.
- Intracranial pressure (ICP) monitor—indications:

- GCS ≤8 and abnormal CT scan; patient at risk of intracranial hypertension.
- Patient will be anesthetized or deeply sedated for an extended period of time, making clinical assessment of neurologic status impossible.
- Various types of ICP monitors are available.[21]
- An external ventricular drain or intra-parenchymal pressure monitor are inserted to measure continuous intracranial pressure.
- Arterial and central venous catheters should be placed to measure continuous arterial and central venous pressure.

Objectives

- Attempt to maintain:
  - ICP < 20 to 25 mmHg.
  - SaO_2 > 95%.
  - Systolic BP ≥ 100 mmHg for age ≥10 years.
  - 80 + 2 (age in years) for age <10 years.

Factors That Can Provoke Raised ICP

- Hypercarbia, hypoxia, fever (lower esophageal temperature >37.5 °C), shivering, pain and inadequate sedation/analgesia, suctioning, seizures, or technical problem with ICP monitor.
- These should be excluded/corrected before proceeding with further treatment.
- Morphine infusion (start with 20 µg/kg/hr IV)[22] and lorazepam (0.1 mg/kg q4 hours as needed) for analgesia and sedation.
- Phenytoin 20 mg/kg IV over 20 minutes followed by 5 mg/kg/day IV divided q12 hours for seizure prophylaxis (phenytoin interval to be adjusted for age).
- Consider expanding mass or hematoma.

ICP >20–25 mmHg for >5 Minutes or Rapidly Rising ICP

- Always start with treatment 1 (below).
- Proceed to next therapy *only* if prior therapy ineffective.
  1. Drain CSF for 5 minutes—or if frequent drainage open drain and set threshold for drainage at 10 or 20 cm H_2O in consultation with neurosurgery. If CSF is drained continuously, 3-way stopcock should be closed to drainage intermittently for accurate ICP measurement.
  2. Mannitol 0.5 g/kg IV over 20 minutes q6 hours as needed.[23–27] Hold mannitol if osmolarity >320 mOsm/L.
  3. Hypertonic 3% saline[28] given in boluses of 3 mL/kg over 5 minutes. Repeat q 6 hours as needed (may develop hypernatremia and hyperchloremic metabolic acidosis). Hold 3% saline if severe hyperosmolar state develops (serum sodium >170 mEq/L). If hypernatremia develops, lower serum sodium slowly (<8 mEq/L/24 hr) when cerebral edema is resolving.
  4. Hypothermia[29,30]; staged approach—lower esophageal temperature to 35 ± 1°C, then 33 ± 1°C if necessary.
  5. Hyperventilation on the mechanical ventilator to a $PaCO_2$ range of <35 mmHg; staged approach—$PaCO_2$ 30 to 34 mmHg, then $PaCO_2$ < 30 mmHg if necessary.[31,32]
  6. Barbiturate therapy titrated to ICP, BP and continuous EEG if available (thiopental IV 4 mg/kg bolus and 2–4 mg/kg/hr infusion).[33]
- Use hyperventilation and/or barbiturate therapy only in cases where ICP remains >25 mmHg with evidence of increasing cerebral edema on CT scan.
- Acute hyperventilation with bag and 100% O_2 should be used transiently only if refractory severe intracranial hypertension and/or signs of transtentorial herniation develop.
- STAT head CT and neurosurgical consult if uncontrolled intracranial hypertension or herniation develop.
- Intermittent neuromuscular blockers may be necessary to facilitate oxygenation/ventilation, during painful or stressful procedures (e.g., suctioning) or during active cooling to prevent shivering.[34]
- Monitoring of jugular venous bulb saturations may be used during hyperventilation.[35,36]
- Treatment with steroids is not currently recommended.

Maintenance of Normal Blood Pressure (BP)

To maintain adequate cerebral blood flow, shock and hypotension must be corrected rapidly:

- If low systolic BP or suspected hypovolemia give 10–20 mL/kg normal saline intravenously over 5 to 10 minutes. Repeat as necessary until normal, age-dependent BP is restored.
- For ongoing hypovolemia despite aggressive volume resuscitation, suspect and search for unrecognized bleeding other than from head injury (e.g., abdominal CT).
- For ongoing hypotension after correction of hypovolemia (guided by CVP measurements), commence vasopressors (α-agonists).
- Phenylephrine and norepinephrine are the preferred vasopressors; they do not increase cerebral O_2 consumption ($CMRO_2$) or lead to cerebral vasoconstriction.
- Dopamine or epinephrine should only be considered if cardiac dysfunction is also suspected from trauma, sepsis, severe hypoxemia (e.g., diving accidents), or associated with intoxications.[37–39]

General Care

- Head in midline in neutral position.
- Avoid obstruction of jugular veins.
- Head of bed at 30-degree angle unless the patient is hypotensive.
- Nutrition—early enteral feeding if possible, parenteral if enteral feeds contraindicated or not tolerated.
- Prophylactic gastric protectants can be considered while patient is not receiving enteral feeds.
- Avoid pressure-induced injuries to skin.
- Prophylactic antibiotics not needed for intracranial pressure monitors.
- The indication to pursue or discontinue prophylactic anticonvulsants should be reviewed at 7 days after injury.

CLINICAL PEARLS

DO
- Maintain high oxygen saturations and normal blood pressure.
- Prevent hypoxia/hypotension.
- Use an end-tidal CO_2 monitor during initial stabilization and transport, and maintain normal CO_2.

DON'T
- Allow patient to remain hypoxic or hypotensive.
- Hyperventilate unless there is evidence of severe intracranial hypertension with herniation—e.g., a life-threatening emergency.

REFERENCES
1. Keenan HT, Bratton SL. Epidemiology and outcomes of pediatric traumatic brain injury. *Dev Neurosci* 2006;28:256–263.
2. Sharples PM. Head injury in children. In: Little RA, Platt W, eds. *Injury in the young.* Cambridge: Cambridge University Press; 1998:151–175.
3. Adelson PD, Bratton SL, Carney NA, et al. Guidelines for the acute medical management of severe traumatic brain injury in infants, children, and adolescents. *Pediatr Crit Care Med* 2003;4(suppl):S1–S75.
4. Stocchetti N, Furlan A, Volta F. Hypoxemia and arterial hypotension at the accident scene in head injury. *J Trauma* 1996;40:764–767.
5. Coates BM, Vavilala MS, Mack CD, et al. Influence of definition and location of hypotension on outcome following severe pediatric traumatic brain injury. *Crit Care Med* 2005;33:2645–2650.
6. Pigula FA, Wald SL, Shackford SR, et al. The effect of hypotension and hypoxia on children with severe head injuries. *J Pediatr Surg* 1993;28:310–314.
7. Kokoska ER, Smith GS, Pittman T, et al. Early hypotension worsens neurological outcome in pediatric patients with moderately severe head trauma. *J Pediatr Surg* 1998;33:333–338.
8. Chesnut RM, Marshall SB, Piek J, et al. Early and late systemic hypotension as a frequent and fundamental source of cerebral ischemia following severe brain injury in the Traumatic Coma Data Bank. *Acta Neurochir Suppl (Wien)* 1993;59:121–125.

9. Robertson CS, Valadka AB, Hannay HJ, et al. Prevention of secondary ischemic insults after severe head injury. *Crit Care Med* 1999;27:2086–2095.

10. Natale JE, Guerguerian AM, Joseph JG, et al. Pilot study to determine the hemodynamic safety and feasibility of magnesium sulfate infusion in children with severe traumatic brain injury. *Pediatr Crit Care Med* 2007;8:1–9.

11. Bowers SA, Marshall LF. Outcome in 200 consecutive cases of severe head injury treated in San Diego County: a prospective analysis. *Neurosurgery* 1980;6:237–242.

12. Alberico AM, Ward JD, Choi SC, et al. Outcome after severe head injury. Relationship to mass lesions, diffuse injury, and ICP course in pediatric and adult patients. *J Neurosurg* 1987;67:648–656.

13. Campbell CG, Kuehn SM, Richards PM, et al. Medical and cognitive outcome in children with traumatic brain injury. *Can J Neurol Sci* 2004;31:213–219.

14. Haqqani AS, Hutchison JS, Ward R, et al. Biomarkers and diagnosis: protein biomarkers in serum of pediatric patients with severe traumatic brain injury identified by ICAT-LC-MS/MS. *J Neurotrauma* 2007;24:54–74.

15. Natale JE, Joseph JG, Helfaer MA, et al. Early hyperthermia after traumatic brain injury in children: risk factors, influence on length of stay, and effect on short-term neurologic status. *Crit Care Med* 2000;28:2608–2615.

16. Gausche M, Lewis RJ, Stratton SJ, et al. Effect of out-of-hospital pediatric endotracheal intubation on survival and neurological outcome: a controlled clinical trial. *JAMA* 2000;283:783–790.

17. Cooper A, DiScala C, Foltin G, et al. Prehospital endotracheal intubation for severe head injury in children: a reappraisal. *Semin Pediatr Surg* 2001;10:3–6.

18. Meyer G, Orliaguet G, Blanot S, et al. Complications of emergency tracheal intubation in severely head-injured children. *Paediatr Anaesth* 2000;10:253–260.

19. Sing RF, Reilly PM, Rotondo MF, et al. Out-of-hospital rapid-sequence induction for intubation of the pediatric patient. *Acad Emerg Med* 1996;3:41–45.

20. Davis DP, Hoyt DB, Ochs M, et al. The effect of paramedic rapid sequence intubation on outcome in patients with severe traumatic brain injury. *J Trauma* 2003;54:444–453.

21. Mollman HD, Rockswold GL, Ford SE. A clinical comparison of subarachnoid catheters to ventriculostomy and subarachnoid bolts: a prospective study. *J Neurosurg* 1988;68:737–741.

22. Lauer KK, Connolly LA, Schmeling WT. Opioid sedation does not alter intracranial pressure in head injured patients. *Can J Anaesth* 1997;44:929–933.

23. Sayre MR, Daily SW, Stern SA, et al. Out-of-hospital administration of mannitol to head-injured patients does not change systolic blood pressure. *Acad Emerg Med* 1996;3:840–848.

24. Schwartz ML, Tator CH, Rowed DW, et al. The University of Toronto head injury treatment study: a prospective, randomized comparison of pentobarbital and mannitol. *Can J Neurol Sci* 1984;11:434–440.

25. Biestro A, Alberti R, Galli R, et al. Osmotherapy for increased intracranial pressure: comparison between mannitol and glycerol. *Acta Neurochir (Wien)* 1997;139:725–732.

26. Smith HP, Kelly DL Jr., McWhorter JM, et al. Comparison of mannitol regimens in patients with severe head injury undergoing intracranial monitoring. *J Neurosurg* 1986;65:820–824.

27. Kirkpatrick PJ, Smielewski P, Piechnik S, et al. Early effects of mannitol in patients with head injuries assessed using bedside multimodality monitoring. *Neurosurgery* 1996;39:714–720.

28. Simma B, Burger R, Falk M, et al. A prospective, randomized, and controlled study of fluid management in children with severe head injury: lactated Ringer's solution versus hypertonic saline. *Crit Care Med* 1998;26:1265–1270.

29. Biswas AK, Bruce DA, et al. Treatment of acute traumatic brain injury in children with moderate hypothermia improves intracranial hypertension. *Crit Care Med* 2002;30:2742–2751.

30. Hutchison J, Ward R, Lacroix J, et al. Hypothermia pediatric head injury trial: the value of a pretrial clinical evaluation phase. *Dev Neurosci* 2006;28:291–301.

31. Muizelaar JP, Marmarou A, Ward JD, et al. Adverse effects of prolonged hyperventilation in patients with severe head injury: a randomized clinical trial. *J Neurosurg* 1991;75:731–739.

32. Skippen P, Seear M, Poskitt K, et al. Effect of hyperventilation on regional cerebral blood flow in head-injured children. *Crit Care Med* 1997;25:1402–1409.

33. Pittman T, Bucholz R, Williams D. Efficacy of barbiturates in the treatment of resistant intracranial hypertension in severely head-injured children. *Pediatr Neurosci* 1989;15:13–17.

34. Hsiang JK, Chesnut RM, Crisp CB, et al. Early, routine paralysis for intracranial pressure control in severe head injury: is it necessary? *Crit Care Med* 1994;22:1471–1476.

35. Cruz J. The first decade of continuous monitoring of jugular bulb oxyhemoglobinsaturation: management strategies and clinical outcome. *Crit Care Med* 1998;26:344–351.

36. Goetting MG, Preston G. Jugular bulb catheterization: experience with 123 patients. *Crit Care Med* 1990;18:1220–1223.

37. Tuor UI, Edvinsson L, McCulloch J. Catecholamines and the relationship between cerebral blood flow and glucose use. *Am J Physiol* 1986;251:H824–H833.

38. Myburgh JA, Upton RN, Grant C, et al. A comparison of the effects of norepinephrine, epinephrine, and dopamine on cerebral blood flow and oxygen utilisation. *Acta Neurochir Suppl* 1998;71:19–21.

39. Darby JM, Yonas H, Marks EC, et al. Acute cerebral blood flow response to dopamine-induced hypertension after subarachnoid hemorrhage. *J Neurosurg* 1994;80:857–864.

CHAPTER 6

Head Trauma: Surgical Management

Sandrine de Ribaupierre, MD, FRCSC
Peter Dirks, MD, PhD, FRCSC

INTRODUCTION

- Pediatric head injury incidence is 2 per 1,000 under 15 years of age, and 3.4 per 1,000 for ages 15 and over.
- Neurologic injuries account for 18% of all pediatric injuries and 23% of traumatic deaths.[1]
- Closed head trauma has a fatality risk of 0.5 per 1,000.[2]
- Eight percent to nine percent of patients with a mild head injury (Glasgow Coma Scale 13–15) lacking neurologic symptoms will have an abnormal CT scan, and 1% to 4% will require a neurosurgical intervention.[3,4]
- Children have fewer mass lesions than adults, but more skull fractures.
- Severity of head injury is typically assessed with the Glasgow Coma Scale (GCS),
  - Mild head injury: GCS 13–15.
    - No or brief loss of consciousness (LOC).
  - Moderate head injury: GCS 9–12.
    - LOC from a few minutes to hours, confusion can last a few days.
  - Severe head injury: GCS ≤8.
    - Coma is defined by a profound state of unconsciousness.
    - Comatose patient fails to respond normally to voice, pain or light, does not have sleep–wake cycles, and does not take voluntary actions.

INITIAL MANAGEMENT

- Use ATLS protocol for initial evaluation of pediatric head injuries.
  - **DO NOT** rush to CT with a unilateral or bilateral mydriasis without completing the ABCs.
  - Hypoxia, hypoglycemia, and hypotension are associated with much worse outcome following severe head injury.
- Establish a secure airway.
  - Prevent secondary brain injuries by ensuring there are no breathing or circulatory problems in a head-injured child.
- If there is evidence of intracranial hypertension/herniation, give mannitol (0.5–1 g/kg) or hypertonic saline (3% NaCl at 3 mL/kg).
- Hyperventilation is not routinely recommended, unless clinical signs of acute herniation.
- Cervical spine trauma can be associated with significant head injuries.

EVALUATION

History

- Determine **mechanism of injury** as per patient, witness, parents, paramedics:
  - Acceleration/deceleration mechanism (MVA, falls).
  - Blunt trauma (falls, blows).
  - Crush injury.

- Penetrating injury (falls, blows, toys, missile).
  - Children can have bizarre mechanisms of accidental injury.
- Determine if **loss of consciousness** occurred and its duration.
  - Did patient talk at any time?
  - Does patient recall the accident?
- Determine if there has been a fluctuating level of consciousness or progressive deterioration/amelioration.
- Determine **amount of time** elapsed from time of injury.
- Did a **seizure** occur following the trauma?
- Did **hypoxia or hypotension** occur at any time?
- How much bleeding resulted from the head injury (scalp, sinus, carotid, ear, nose)?
- Any other injuries?

Physical Exam

- Assess **pupil size and reactivity** to light.
  - Should occur during primary survey with the GCS.
- Check for **local signs of trauma,** such as contusion/laceration/skin mark above the clavicles.
- Use the **GCS** to record level of consciousness and fluctuations in time (Table 6-1).
  - **Motor assessment** is most reliable indicator in infant and younger children (unless associated spinal cord injury).
  - GCS may be unreliable in young children because different scales can make assessment difficult.
  - Document each of 3 scores (eyes, motor, verbal) leading to final GCS.
  - GCS score has not been fully validated in pediatric patients but it is important to document initial GCS and follow trends over time.[5]
- Assess for:
  - Motor deficits.
  - Sensory deficits.
  - Change in reflexes.
- Evaluate for signs of basal skull fracture:
  - Battle sign.
  - Raccoon eyes
  - Hemotympanum.
  - CSF leak (otorrhea, otorrhagia, rhinorrhea).
- Monitor heart rate.
  - Bradycardia may precede decreased level of consciousness in the presence of an expanding mass lesion.
- Evaluate for signs of herniation:
  - Progressive obtundation.
  - Mydriasis (unilateral, bilateral pupil dilatation). Pupil dilation is a critical lateralizing sign.

TABLE 6-1

GCS Scores As Determined by Best Responses by Age

Age	Best Motor	Best Verbal	Best Score
<6 mo	Flexion (4)	Smiles/cries (2)	10
6–12 mo	Localizes (5)	Smiles/cries (2)	11
1–2 yr	Localizes (5)	Sounds/words (4)	13
2–5 yr	Obeys (6)	Words/phrases (4–5)	15

- ▪ Medication (atropine) can be a confounding factor (pupils, HR).
- ▪ Pupil dilatation can also be from direct trauma or contusions to the optic nerve.
- ▪ **In general, pupil dilatation is more lateralizing than limb weakness.**
- Contralateral hemiparesis (unilateral hemiparesis = Kernohan notch phenomenon).
- Cushing's triad (bradycardia, hypertension, irregular respirations): Most often late signs.
- In infants: Check fontanel when assessing intracranial pressure (sunken, flat, full, bulging, tense).

Laboratory Investigations

- Hemoglobin:
  - Initial hemoglobin level may not reflect intravascular volume status.
  - In older patients, hypovolemia must be excluded from other sources (abdominal, thoracic, and pelvic).
  - In older children and teenagers, intracranial bleeding will have mass effect before showing a decrease in hemoglobin.
  - Infants with intracranial bleeding (or scalp loss) might develop decreased hemoglobin or hypotension.
- Electrolytes:
  - Sodium: Hyponatremia might cause neurologic findings in patients with decreased level of consciousness and unclear traumatic history.
- Platelets and coagulation studies:
  - Brain injury and blood loss might lead to disseminated intravascular coagulation (DIC).
  - Patient may require surgery; therefore check coagulation status, and type and cross-match the blood.

Imaging

Role of Plain Radiographs

- Except in a center where a CT-scan is unavailable, skull x-rays are not indicated.
- When no CT is available:
  - Check for linear fractures going through the temporal region (middle meningeal artery: risk of epidural bleeding).
  - 29% of linear fractures are associated with intracranial lesions.[4]
  - Check for depressed fractures.
  - Check for pneumocephalus.

Role of Computed Tomography (CT)

- Indications for CT-head[3,6,7]:
  - Any trauma with a persistent GCS below 15.
  - GCS = 15 but:
    - ▪ More than brief LOC or LOC of uncertain duration (persistent LOC is more important than a fracture for predicting intracranial hematoma).
    - ▪ Bradycardia.
    - ▪ Mechanism of injury especially concerning (fall from significant height, high-speed MVA).
    - ▪ 8.8% of patients will have positive findings on the CT scan when presenting with those criteria,[3,4] but only 1% of patients with an initial GCS of 13 to 15 will need a neurosurgical intervention.[3,8]
  - Abnormal neurologic exam.
  - LOC with lucid interval but progressive worsening headaches.
  - Signs of important local trauma or skull base fracture.
  - All penetrating injuries.
  - Skull fracture (seen on x-ray, or for infants with falls, an obvious scalp abnormality may be a clue for a skull fracture).
- What to look for on CT-head:
  - Contusions, subdural or epidural hematomas, subarachnoid blood.
  - Lesion leading to a mass effect, midline shift, herniation.

- Disappearance of basal cisterns, shape of ventricles (indirect signs of edema), loss of sulci.
- Gray/white matter differentiation.
- Skull fractures (basal skull fracture: integrity of vessels).
- Pneumocephalus.
- Petechial hemorrhages indicating diffuse axonal injury.
- Subdurals may be difficult to see; thin but diffuse subdurals can be massive.
- Indications for CT-venogram:
  - Evidence of trauma near a venous sinus (occipital fracture), to ensure patency of the sinus and rule out a tear.
- Indications for CT-arteriogram:
  - Basal skull fracture crossing the carotid canal, or evidence of blood in sphenoid sinus.
  - Any motor deficit unexplained by CT scan (suspect early infarction).
    - Beware of carotid dissection.
  - Unclear history of LOC before trauma and evidence of subarachnoid blood.
  - Crush injury to the head.
- See Chapter 4 on Diagnostic Imaging for details.

Role of Magnetic Resonance Imaging (MRI)
- MRI is not part of the primary survey.
- MRI should be reserved for the trauma center.
- Can be useful if CT does not explain a depressed consciousness level or to assess diffuse axonal injuries.
- Unexplained neurologic deficit (check for parenchymal, brainstem or spinal cord lesions).

SPECIFIC INJURIES
Skull Fractures
Linear Skull Fracture
- **Definition:** Linear fracture running through the entire thickness of bone without significant displacement.
- Simple linear fracture: Most common type of fracture, especially in children <5 years old. Linear fractures increase risk of intracranial hematoma, but risk of hematoma is less in children compared to adults.
- Basilar skull fractures represent 19% to 21% of all skull fractures.
- **Specific Types of Skull Fractures:**
  - Longitudinal temporal bone fractures:
    - Conductive deafness (ossicular chain disruption); facial palsy, nystagmus, and facial numbness.
  - Transverse temporal bone fractures:
    - Nystagmus, ataxia (labyrinth), and permanent neural hearing loss (VIII).
  - Occipital condylar fracture:
    - Rare but serious injury.[9]
    - Associated with cervical spinal injuries, lower cranial nerve injuries, and hemiplegia or quadriplegia (needs CT/MRI evaluation).
- **Mechanism:** Result from blunt trauma, usually low-energy over wide surface area.
  - Falls are more common cause than motor vehicle accidents.
- **Presentation:** No clinical signs by itself, if not associated with other injuries—except in basal skull fracture (see below) and tempoparietal fracture that involve the cochlea and labyrinth.
  - A large, boggy, scalp contusion may predict a fracture.
- **CT findings:** Linear fracture with no, or minimal, displacement (rule out epidural and subdural hematoma).
- **Management:**
  - Admit infants with simple linear fractures for **overnight observation** regardless of neurologic status.
  - Treat neurologically intact patients with linear basilar fractures conservatively, without antibiotics.

- Initially manage temporal bone skull base fractures conservatively. Tympanic membrane ruptures usually heal on their own.
- Complex linear fractures may raise suspicion for nonaccidental injury.

Depressed Skull Fracture

- **Definition:** Fracture with misalignment of the fragments, which are pushed inwards, usually caused by a greater impact injury than the linear fracture. Significant when the displacement is greater than the thickness of the skull.
- More frequently associated with intracranial findings than linear fractures.
- Depressed fractures are:
  - 75% frontoparietal.
  - 10% temporal.
  - 5% occipital.
  - 10% other.
- Most depressed fractures are open fractures (75–90%).
  - Comminuted fragments.
  - Might be opened or closed.
  - A "ping-pong" fracture can be seen in newborns (from forceps, or impingement against sacral bone during uterine contractions).
- **Mechanism:** Result from high-energy trauma, on small surface area, with relatively immobile head.
- **Presentation:** Scalp swelling/contusion/laceration.
- **CT findings:**
  - Skull fracture with displacement.
  - Look for indirect signs of dural tear (pneumocephalus).
  - Brain parenchyma underlying may have surface or intraparenchymal hemorrhage or edema.
- **Management:**
  - Can be treated conservatively or surgically depending on whether open or closed, location, extent of depression, amount of wound soiling, presence or absence of prompt careful wound cleansing.
  - Criteria for elevation of depressed skull fracture:
    - Open fracture (generally treated surgically).
    - Open with CSF leak (dural laceration).
    - Depression > thickness of skull.
    - Deficit related to underlying brain (surgery does not reduce delayed seizure risk).
    - Cosmetic area (usually on a nonurgent basis).
- Depressed fractures over a sinus require special attention (risk of blood loss, airembolism).
- Patients with contaminated open depressed skull fractures:
  - Treat surgically.
  - Tetanus toxoid and broad-spectrum antibiotics (especially in a delayed presentation).
  - Repeat CT scans over 1- to 2-month period to monitor for abscess formation.
- Follow-up is dictated by the complications associated with skull fractures:
  - Seizures, infections, extent of underlying brain parenchymal injury.

Basal Skull Fracture

- **Definition:** Fracture involving skull base (ethmoidal bone, sphenoidal bone, clivus, temporal and occipital bone, orbital roof).
- Often an extension of fractures through the cranial vault.
- Suspect a basal skull fracture with the following signs:
  - CSF rhinorrhea/otorrhea.
  - Hemotympanum.
  - Battle sign.
  - Raccoon eyes.
  - Cranial nerve injury (I, VI, VII, and VIII).

- Extensive bleeding from nose or ear may be due to carotid injury.
- **Mechanisms:** High-speed impact, MVA, television tipovers, falls, crush injury.
- **CT findings:** Fracture through the skull base (see definition).
  - Axial cuts might not show the fracture; therefore obtain reconstructions in coronal and sagittal planes.
  - Indirect signs of fracture include:
    - Pneumocranium/pneumocephalus, air–fluid levels within sinuses.
    - Fractures through carotid canal may indicate carotid injury.
- **Management:**
  - Hospitalization and observation.
  - Most are managed conservatively.
  - Most CSF leaks will cease spontaneously (otorrhea almost always stops spontaneously).
  - Massive CSF leakage may require early repair.
  - Persistent CSF leakage may require delayed repair.
  - Do NOT insert an NG tube (consult neurosurgeon).
  - Prophylactic antibiotics are not routinely recommended.
  - Look for associated injuries (post-traumatic carotid-cavernous fistula, traumatic aneurysm, LeFort fractures).

Intracranial Bleeding
Cerebral Contusion
- **Definition:** Punctuate parenchymal hemorrhage with edema, representing a region of primary neuronal and vascular injury.
  - Found on brain surface or deep.
  - Might appear in a delayed fashion.
  - Coup contusion: Direct trauma causes injury at site of impact.
  - Countercoup contusion: Deceleration causes injury at a site opposite to the site of impact.
  - Inferior frontal and temporal lobes are particularly vulnerable (especially with occipital impact).
- **Mechanism:** Contusions are formed in two ways: Direct trauma and acceleration/deceleration injury (leads to cavitation).
- **Presentation:** Focal symptoms depending on lesion size and location.
- **CT findings:** Localized contusion within specific area of gray matter.
  - Contusions may progress with time.
  - CT scans can demonstrate progression in size and number of contusions and amount of hemorrhage within contusions.
  - Most evident over the first 24 to 48 hours.
  - 25% of all trauma patients have delayed hemorrhages.[10]
- **Management:**
  - Conservative management with careful neurologic follow-up.
  - Hospitalization and rehabilitation essential for all cerebral contusions.
  - If lesion extension induces progressive loss of consciousness or neurologic deficit, surgical management might be needed.
  - Temporal lobe contusions require special consideration (restricted middle fossa space, higher risk of herniation).

Epidural Hematoma (See Fig. 4-33)
- **Definition:** Blood clots between skull's inner table and outer layer of dura.[11,12]
- More common in children than adults; possible reasons include:
  - Relatively greater dural and bone vascularization.
  - Ease with which dura strips off the skull.
  - Greater likelihood of skull fracture.
- Source of bleeding:
  - Skull fracture is most common mechanism.
  - Tear in middle meningeal artery branch (located in outer dural layer).
  - Tear in dural venous sinus.

- Delayed epidural hematoma might occur:
  - Usually in the first few hours.
  - Rare after 12 hours postinjury.
- **Mechanism:**
  - Falls most common.
  - In infants, a significant fall is more likely caused by being dropped by a caregiver than rolling off furniture.
- **Presentation:**
  - Brief loss of consciousness, then lucid interval followed by progressively increasing headaches, bradycardia, decreasing level of consciousness. Can also present with immediate and persistent decreased level of consciousness.
  - Scalp abnormality (contusion, subgaleal hematoma).
    - Be aware of boggy scalp swelling in temporoparietal area.
  - Pupillary changes (nonreactive mydriasis is sign of transtentorial herniation).
  - Motor deficit.
  - Can lead to anemia in infants.
- **CT findings:**
  - Biconvex "lens"-shaped clot.
  - Usually hyperdense, if heterogeneous might indicate active bleeding.
  - Can cause mass effect and midline shift.
- **Management:**
  - If mass effect or midline shift, should be managed surgically.
  - Small epidurals without neurologic symptoms might be managed conservatively, with repeated examination and follow-up imaging.
  - Hospitalization.
  - 10% to 12% mortality.[13]

Subdural Hematoma (See Figs. 4-30, 4-32)

- **Definition:** A rapidly clotting blood collection below the dura's inner layer but external to the brain and arachnoid membrane.
- Often associated with underlying brain injury.
- Cerebral injury results from direct pressure, increased ICP, or associated intraparenchymal insults.
- **Mechanisms:** Venous bleeding of bridging veins (between cortex and venous sinuses).
  - Classic finding of nonaccidental head injury in infants (particularly posterior inter-hemispheric in location).
- **Presentation:** Dependant on location of the subdural hematoma. Can lead to motor or sensory deficits, herniation signs, and coma.
- **CT findings:** Acute subdural hematoma appears on a noncontrast CT-head as a hyperdense crescentic lesion along the skull's inner table (tends to spread more diffusely over hemisphere than an extradural).
  - The lesion is isodense in the subacute phase (can only see mass effect on a scan).
  - The lesion becomes hypodense in the chronic phase.
  - Thin subdurals can involve a large volume because of their extent.
  - Can be difficult to see on CT because adjacent to hyperdense bone.
    - Need "blood CT windowing" for accurate visualization.
    - More often associated with cerebral contusion than an epidural hematrauma
- **Management:**
  - Depends on the patient's condition.
  - Generally, large, subdural hematomas with mass effect need surgical evacuation.
  - Smaller lesions without mass effect can be managed conservatively.
  - Hospitalization.
  - Be suspicious for nonaccidental injury if no clear mechanism, especially in young children and infants.

Subarachnoid Bleed (See Fig. 4-32)

- Very common after significant head trauma, thinly over surface of brain, in sulcal spaces.
- Can be seen with or without subdural hemorrhage or brain contusion.

- If mechanism of trauma is unclear, or large subarachnoid bleed alone, need for CT-angiogram to rule out aneurysmal bleed (rare in children, and associated with thick subarachnoid blood).

Axonal Injury
- Range from mild (concussion) to severe diffuse axonal injury.

Concussion
- Most common traumatic brain injury in children.[14]
- **Definition by Canadian Pediatric Society:** A complex pathophysiological process affecting the brain, induced by traumatic biomechanical forces. Involves a temporary alteration in mental status (confusion and amnesia) that resolves spontaneously.
- Can occur with or without LOC.
- **Mechanism:** Caused by direct blows, violent shaking, or whiplash-type injury.
- **Presentation:**
  - Cognitive features: Confusion, anterograde/retrograde amnesia, and brief LOC.
  - Symptoms: Headache, dizziness, tinnitus, loss of vision, and nausea.
  - Signs: Poor coordination or balance, vomiting, slurred speech, slow to respond to questions, and poor concentration.
- **Management:**
  - Remove from game or practice.
  - Conservative and supportive.
  - Observe for any signs of deterioration.
  - Perform baseline neurologic exam.
  - Period of rest with slow gradual return to activities.
  - If symptoms return, needs more rest.

Pediatric Sport-Related Injury—Return to Play
- Postconcussive syndrome:
  - Headaches, dizziness, nausea, fatigue, poor balance.
  - Anxiety, depression.
  - Impaired memory, poor concentration, slow processing.
- Second impact syndrome:
  - Second (even trivial) head injury during the postconcussive symptomatic period that causes increased morbidity (rarely reported in children but fear of it is the basis of return-to-play guidelines).
- Sports at risk[15,16]:
  - Boys: Football, rugby, hockey, wrestling, soccer, basketball, baseball.
  - Girls: Gymnastics, soccer, basketball, hockey, softball, volleyball.
- Return to play:
  - Depending on concussion grading (simple or complex):
    - Take a conservative approach to return to play.
    - Many schemes are described, none are universally accepted.
    - Wait until all symptoms have resolved (at rest and with exertion).
    - Progressive return to play (practice then games).
- CT abnormalities (such as contusion):
  - Out for the season, consider stopping contact sports.
  - If permanent neurologic deficit, diffuse axonal injury, or hematoma requiring surgery: No more contact sports.
  - Neuropsychological testing may be helpful.

Diffuse Axonal Injury (DAI)
- Definition: Traumatic loss of consciousness with GCS <8 and no major anomalies on CT scan.
  - Frequent cause of persistent vegetative state in patients.
  - Most significant cause of morbidity in patients with traumatic brain injury.

- Extent of axonal injury typically worse than initially visualized on CT.
- DAI is suggested in any patient demonstrating clinical symptoms disproportionate to CT findings.
- Three types depending on importance of the trauma leading to different lesion locations:
  - **Type I:** Parasagittal regions of the frontal lobes, periventricular temporal lobes (less frequent: parietal or occipital lobes, internal and external capsules, and cerebellum).
  - **Type II:** Corpus callosum (posterior body and splenium).
  - **Type III:** Brainstem involvement (superior cerebellar peduncles, medial lemnisci, and corticospinal tracts).
- **Mechanisms:** Traumatic deceleration injury such as MVAs.
  - Sudden acceleration-deceleration impact can produce rotational/shear forces.
- **CT findings:**
  - Initial CT findings may be nonspecific and subtle.
  - Multiple small petechial hemorrhages (<2 mm) located at the gray–white matter junction, within the corpus callosum, and in the brainstem.
- **MRI findings:**
  - T1-weighted: Hyper-intense punctual lesions (useful for anatomic localization; however, nonhemorrhagic lesions may be iso-intense to surrounding tissue).
  - T2-weighted sequences: Nonhemorrhagic lesions are hyper-intense.
  - Diffusion-weighted sequences: Can reveal hyperintensities in areas of axonal injury.[17]
  - Gradient-echo sequences: Demonstrate signal abnormality in areas appearing normal in T1- and T2-weighted spin-echo sequences. Abnormal signal on gradient-echo can persist years after the injury.
- **Management:**
  - Hospitalization.
  - Supportive management.
  - May require ICU ventilation and invasive ICP monitoring.
  - Rehabilitation.

Diffuse Cerebral Edema (See Fig. 4-31)

- **Definition:**
  - Increase in brain volume, developing after head injury, caused by an increase in cerebral tissue water content. (In trauma: vasogenic edema.)
  - May lead to increased (ICP), which can result in further ischemia and potential uncal herniation.
  - Blood–brain barrier injury is worsened with hypoxia, hypotension, inflammation, and oxidative stress.
- **Mechanisms:**
  - Any significant head trauma might result in blood–brain barrier disruption, osmolar changes, and edema at the cellular level.
  - Often a history of hypoxia or hypotension.
- **Presentation:** Usually in coma.
- **CT findings:** Obliteration of basal cisterns, slit ventricles, effacement of sulci.
- **Management:**
  - ABCs and supportive therapy.
  - Hyperventilate only for signs of impending herniation.
  - Mannitol (0.5–1 g/kg) or 3% NaCl (3 mL/kg) intravenously.
  - Patient may require neuromuscular blockade and paralysis.
  - Goal to keep intracranial pressure below 20 mmHg.
  - Intracranial pressure monitoring will help guide ICP management.
  - Decompressive craniectomy, for unilateral swelling, might improve the outcome.[18,19]

Penetrating Injuries
Missiles

- Handguns and shotguns fire low-velocity bullets.
- Military weapons fire high-velocity metal-jacket projectiles.

- Bullets cause damage to brain parenchyma through several mechanisms:
  - Laceration and crushing.
  - Cavitation.
  - Shock waves.
- Amount of brain damage depends on:
  - Missile trajectory.
  - Bone fragmentation.
  - Kinetic energy.
  - Intracranial pressure changes during impact.
  - Secondary mechanisms of injury (e.g., intracranial hemorrhage).
- **Management:**
  - Control bleeding from scalp and associated wounds.
  - Identify entrance and exit sites:
    - X-ray to localized metal fragment.
  - Surgical aims:
    - Debridement.
    - Evacuation of mass lesion.
    - Removal of accessible bullet.
    - Dural closure.
- Patients with poor GCS or a missile trajectory that crosses the midline have a poor prognosis.
  - Conservative nonsurgical management may be appropriate.

Nonmissile (Stab) Wounds
- Entry point may be hidden and can be difficult to assess in a nonverbal child.
- Mechanisms can be bizarre in children.
- Commonly occur in the thin bones of the skull:
  - Orbital surfaces.
  - Squamous portion of the temporal bone.
- Eyelid laceration—may be an indication for penetrating injury through orbit to intracranial space.
- Cerebral damage restricted to wound tract (except in associated vessel injury).
  - No concentric zone of coagulative necrosis as in missile injury.
  - No DAI as found in motor vehicle collisions.
- Morbidity and mortality often related to associated vascular injury.
- Can be caused by different objects:
  - Pencil, scissors, toys, spikes, forks, etc.[20]

SPECIAL CONSIDERATIONS
Head Injury in Children Under 2 Years of Age
- 10% have skull fracture associated with minor head injury.
- Impact seizure more common.
- Increased incidence of fractures if more than 3 feet fall.
- Growing skull fractures might happen in children <3 years old but usually within the first 6 months after the injury.
  - Requires significant fracture with dural disruption.
- Red flags:
  - Large, boggy hematoma suggestive of underlying skull fracture.
  - Loss of consciousness more predictive of intracranial injury than fracture.
  - Complex fractures raise suspicions of nonaccidental injury.

Neonatal Head Injury
- Incidence unknown.
- Higher morbidity and mortality.
- Usually traumatic delivery (forceps, vacuum, precipitous, C-section).

- Can cause significant blood loss.[21–24]
- Caput succedaneum:
  - Extends across sutures.
  - Pitting edema, shifts with gravity, max size, and firmness at birth.
  - Resolves in 24 to 48 hours.
- Cephalohematoma:
  - Does not cross sutures.
  - Distinct margins.
  - Firm then fluctuant.
  - Progress after birth.
  - Resolves in 2 to 4 weeks.
- Subgaleal hematoma:
  - From vacuum.
  - Can cause massive blood loss in neonate, as this is a very large potential space.
- Linear and depressed fractures:
  - Ping-pong fracture (caving of a focal area).
    - Most ping-pong fractures remodel spontaneously.
  - Facial palsy can occur.
- Posterior fossa hematomas:
  - From sinus laceration during delivery.
  - Can be treacherous to deal with surgically.

Posttraumatic Seizures and Vomiting
- Children are prone to traumatic seizures.
  - Parenchymal lesions will need prophylactic anticonvulsant therapy.
    - <2 years old: phenobarbital (load 10–20 mg/kg IV).
    - >2 years old: phenytoin (load 20 mg/kg IV).
- Children are prone to vomiting.
- Isolated vomiting episodes with a GCS of 15 and no neurologic signs are NOT associated with increased risk of intracranial lesion.[2]

GUIDELINES FOR DEFINITIVE NEUROSURGICAL MANAGEMENT
Admission Criteria
- <2 years old with fracture (complex fracture, early CT, vomiting).
- All injuries leading to neurologic deficits.
- All injuries that have a potential for progressive worsening in the next hours/days (especially epidural hematomas).
- All parenchymal injuries.

Patients to Refer to Neurosurgery
- All severe head injuries (GCS <9).
- Stabilize severely injured and refer promptly to trauma center (don't wait for CT).
- Persistent GCS <15 (>2 hr) when no CT available.
- Any child with a CT abnormality.
- Small epidural might not require surgery, but may enlarge.
- Contusions tend to enlarge in the first 72 hours and might cause mass effect and herniation, especially those in the temporal location.
- Depressed skull fractures (open or closed) may or may not require surgery.
- Penetrating trauma.
- Clinical signs of basal skull fractures.

Neurosurgical Management Considerations
- Surgery is most often required for lesions causing a mass effect or a midline shift, even if the patient has a GCS of 15.

- Large extradurals are a neurosurgical emergency.
- Surgery might be necessary:
  - To remove masses (epidural, subdural, or intracerebral hematomas).
  - To control an active hemorrhage.
  - To remove necrotic brain and prevent further swelling and ischemia.
  - To remove necrotic tissue, metal, bone fragments, or other foreign bodies to prevent infections.
  - To insert intracranial monitoring devices.
- Approach to surgery varies.
- Some surgeons are conservative, others are more aggressive.
- Exploratory burr holes are rarely, if ever, indicated.
  - Only consider rarely in desperation, in direct consultation with a neurosurgeon.

CLINICAL PEARLS

DO
- Perform quick neurologic exam after ABCs.
- Recognize the classic presentation of expanding extradural hematoma.
- Identify eyelid laceration as a sign of occult penetrating injury.
- Recogonize that sudden bradycardia in awake patient may precede herniation.
- Remember that infants with large cephalohematomas, subgaleal hematoms, or epidural hematomas can have low BP or anemia.

DON'T
- Sedate and paralyze before proper, rapid neurologic assessment.
- Treat increased intracranial pressure at the expense of ABCs.
- Remove a penetrating object without prior imaging.

REFERENCES
1. Durkin MS, Olsen S, Barlow B et al. The epidemiology of urban pediatric neurological trauma: evaluation of, and implications for, injury prevention programs. *Neurosurgery* 1998;42:300–310.
2. Da Dalt L, et al. Predictors of intracranial injuries in children after blunt head trauma. *Eur J Pediatr* 2006;165:142–148.
3. Stiell IG, et al. The Canadian CT Head Rule for patients with minor head injury. *Lancet* 2001; 357:1391–1396.
4. Boran BO, et al. Evaluation of mild head injury in a pediatric population. *Pediatr Neurosurg* 2006; 42:203–207.
5. Chung CY, et al. Critical score of Glasgow Coma Scale for pediatric traumatic brain injury. *Pediatr Neurol* 2006;34:379–387.
6. Quayle KS, et al. Diagnostic testing for acute head injury in children: when are head computed tomography and skull radiographs indicated? *Pediatrics* 1997;99:E11.
7. Simon B, et al. Pediatric minor head trauma: indications for computed tomographic scanning revisited. *J Trauma* 2001;51:231–237; discussion 237–238.
8. Wang MY, et al. A prospective population-based study of pediatric trauma patients with mild alterations in consciousness (Glasgow Coma Scale score of 13–14). *Neurosurgery* 2000;46:1093–1099.
9. Legros B, et al. Basal fracture of the skull and lower (IX, X, XI, XII) cranial nerves palsy: four case reports including two fractures of the occipital condyle—a literature review. *J Trauma* 2000;48:342–348.
10. Gudeman SK, et al. The genesis and significance of delayed traumatic intracerebral hematoma. *Neurosurgery* 1979;5:309–313.
11. Pasaoglu A, Orhon C, Koc K, et al. Traumatic extradural haematomas in pediatric age group. *Acta Neurochir (Wien)* 1990;106:136–139.
12. Pasztor A. Characteristics of the treatment of the epidural hematomas in infancy and childhood. *Zentralbl Neurochir* 1985;46:243–250.
13. Rivas JJ, et al. Extradural hematoma: analysis of factors influencing the courses of 161 patients. *Neurosurgery* 1988;23:44–51.
14. Gordon KE, Dooley JM, Wood EP. Descriptive epidemiology of concussion. *Pediatr Neurol* 2006;34:376–378.
15. Kirkwood MW, Yeates KO, Wilson PE. Pediatric sport-related concussion: a review of the clinical management of an oft-neglected population. *Pediatrics* 2006;117:1359–1371.
16. Mandel S, Maitz EA, Tracy JI, et al. Severity of sports-related concussion and neuropsychological test performance. *Neurology* 2003;61:144.

17. Kinoshita T, et al. Conspicuity of diffuse axonal injury lesions on diffusion-weighted MR imaging. *Eur J Radiol* 2005;56:5–11.
18. Aarabi B, et al. Outcome following decompressive craniectomy for malignant swelling due to severe head injury. *J Neurosurg* 2006;104:469–479.
19. Reithmeier T, Speder B, Pakos P, et al. Delayed bilateral craniectomy for treatment of traumatic brain swelling in children: case report and review of the literature. *Childs Nerv Syst* 2005;21:249–253. Discussion, 254.
20. Greenes DS, Schutzman SA. Occult intracranial injury in infants. *Ann Emerg Med* 1998;32:680–686.
21. Mohammed G, Ahmed M. Serious fetal intracranial haemorrhage associated with the vacuum extraction. *BJOG* 2003;110:1138. Letter. Author reply, 1138–1139.
22. Towner D, Castro MA, Eby-Wilkens E, et al. Effect of mode of delivery in nulliparous women on neonatal intracranial injury. *N Engl J Med* 1999;341:1709–1714.
23. Whitby EH, et al. Frequency and natural history of subdural haemorrhages in babies and relation to obstetric factors. *Lancet* 2004;363:846–851.
24. Vinchon M, Pierrat V, Tchofo PJ, et al. Traumatic intracranial hemorrhage in newborns. *Childs Nerv Syst* 2005;21:1042–1048.

SUGGESTED READINGS

1. de Guise E, Feyz M, LeBlanc J, et al. Overview of traumatic brain injury patients at a tertiary trauma centre. Can *J Neurol Sci* 2005;32:186–193.
2. Falk AC, Cederfjall C, vonWendt L, et al. Management and classification of children with head injury. *Childs Nerv Syst* 2005;21:430–436.
3. Guidelines for the acute medical management of severe traumatic brain injury in infants, children, and adolescents. *J Trauma* 2003;54(suppl):S235–S310.
4. Hahn YS, Chyung C, Barthel MJ, et al. Head injuries in children under 36 months of age. Demography and outcome. *Childs Nerv Syst* 1988;4:34–40.
5. Kim KA, Wang MY, Griffith PM, et al. Analysis of pediatric head injury from falls. *Neurosurg Focus* 2000;8:e3.
6. Kochanek PM. Pediatric traumatic brain injury: beyond the guidelines. *Curr Treat Options Neurol* 2005;7:441–450.
7. Rosman NP, Oppenheimer EY, O'Connor JF. Emergency management of pediatric head injuries. *Emerg Med Clin North Am* 1983;1:141–174.
8. Zimmerman RA, Bilaniuk LT. Pediatric head trauma. *Neuroimaging Clin N Am* 1994;4:349–366.

CHAPTER 7

Craniofacial Injury

Christopher R. Forrest, MD, MSc, FRCSC, FACS

ANATOMIC AND PHYSIOLOGIC CONSIDERATIONS IN CHILDREN

1. Cranial to facial ratio.
   - 3 months: Cranium to face = 8:1.
   - 2 years: Cranium to face = 4:1.
   - 5.5 years: Cranium to face = 2.5:1.
   - Adult: Cranium to face = 2:1.
   - Cranial-orbital injuries more common in children under age 5 years due to relative prominence of forehead (Fig. 7-1).
2. Presence of paranasal sinuses.
   - Act as "air-bags" for the vital structures and influence fracture patterns.
   - Fronto-orbital injuries more commonly associated with anterior cranial fossa fractures when frontal sinus absent or underdeveloped.
   - Radiographic evidence of paranasal sinuses:
     - Maxillary: 4 to 5 months.
     - Ethmoids: 12 months.
     - Frontal: 6 years.
3. Bone morphology.
   - Greater cancellous to cortical ratio.
   - More elastic and resistant.
   - Higher impact force per unit area needed for fracture.
   - Higher incidence of associated injuries.
4. Tooth buds and dentition.
   - Unerupted tooth buds increase strength and compliance of facial skeleton.
   - Three groups:
     - 0 to 5 years: Primary dentition.
     - 6 to 11 years: Mixed dentition.
     - 12 to 16 years: Permanent dentition (Fig. 7-2).
5. Bone metabolism.
   - Increased metabolism in children.
   - Faster healing (3 weeks).
   - Less time required for immobilization.
6. Active growth.
   - Potential for late growth disturbances after a fracture (both under and overgrowth).
   - Cranial vault.
     - Birth: 60% adult size.
     - 2 years: 80% adult size.
     - 6 years: 90% adult size.
   - Nose.
     - Maximum growth 10 to 14 years.
     - Growth complete by 16 years.
   - Orbits.
     - 90% adult size by age 7 years.

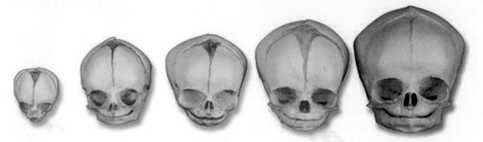

FIGURE 7-1 ● Fetal skulls from 18 weeks to 36 weeks demonstrating prevalence of frontal-orbital structures.

- Maxilla and palate.
  - 6 years: 65% adult size.
  - 10–12 years: Nearly complete.
- Mandible.
  - Last bone to grow.
  - Indicator of skeletal maturity.
    - Female: 14 to 16 years.
    - Male: 18 to 21 years.

EPIDEMIOLOGY
- Severe facial fractures in children are relatively uncommon.
- In a large series of facial fractures (adults and children)[1-5]:
  - 1.3% to 4.9% of all facial fractures occurred in <11 years old.
  - 4% to 9.2% of all facial fractures occurred in <16 years old.
- Incidence of injuries increases after age 5 years.
  - <5 years: <5% (high level of supervision).
  - >5 years: 95% due to rapid neuromotor development.
- Male:female 2 to 3:1.

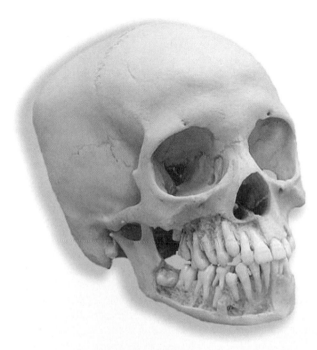

FIGURE 7-2 ● Presence of tooth buds in mixed-dentition facial skeleton.

- Causes (age dependent):
  - Falls > MVA > pedestrians > bicycles > sports.
- Distribution: >7 years—the pointy bits: Nose and mandible more common.
- Associated injuries: Present in up to 73–88% of cases of facial fractures.
  - Common:
    - Closed head injury.
    - Skull.
    - Ocular and soft tissue.
  - Uncommon:
    - C-spine.
    - Thoracic.
    - Abdominal.

HISTORY
- History of injury.
- Awareness of possible nonaccidental injury.
- Premorbid history of orthodontics important to help establish occlusion.

PHYSICAL EXAMINATION
- See specific regions.

DIAGNOSTIC IMAGING
- Key to confirm or establish diagnosis of facial fractures as children may be difficult to examine and uncooperative.
- CT scan (axial, coronal, and 3-D) first line of radiologic investigation.
- Oblique sagittal views useful to visualize orbital floor.
- Plain x-rays notoriously unreliable in establishing the diagnosis.
- Panorex—ideal in diagnosis of mandibular fractures.
- Occlusal views occasionally useful in dental-alveolar fractures.

EMERGENCY MANAGEMENT
- ABCs of trauma (See Chapter 2 on Primary Surgery for details).
- Nasal packs (anterior plus/minus posterior) important to control midface bleeding.
- Soft tissue injuries may give clues to presence of fractures.

SPECIFIC INJURIES
Cranial-Frontal Region (Fig. 7-3)
- More frequent in children <5 years of age due to prominence of forehead.
- Lack of frontal sinus until teen years predisposes to orbital roof fractures and frontal lobe injuries.
- CSF leak possible (through cribriform or orbital roof).
- Optic nerve at risk for injury with frontal trauma even in the absence of fractures.

History
- High-velocity trauma.
- Look for evidence of brain injury.
- Possibility of ocular trauma.

Physical Examination
- Forehead laceration could indicate compound skull fracture.
- Periorbital swelling and ecchymosis.
- Frontal contour depression.
- Pupil reaction—rule out relative afferent pupillary defect (RAPD) suggesting optic nerve injury.
- Change in globe position inferiorly may occur due to orbital roof fragment pushing eye downwards.
- CSF rhinorrhea.

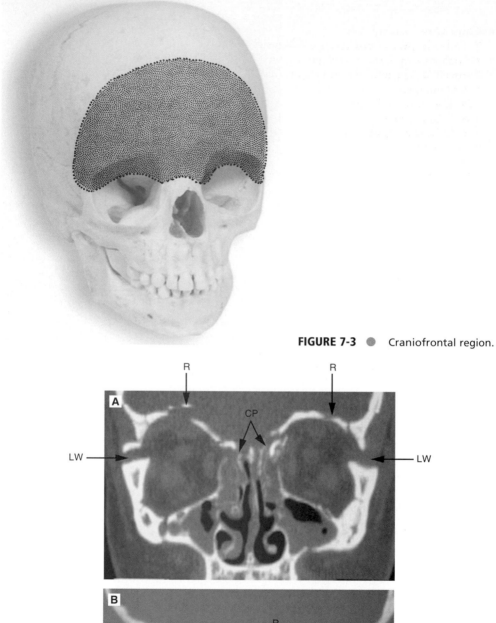

FIGURE 7-3 ● Craniofrontal region.

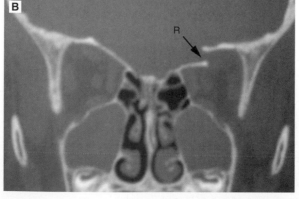

FIGURE 7-4 ● CT images showing **(A)** disruption of bilateral orbital, medial, lateral walls (LW) and roofs, (R) cribriform plate, (CP) opacification of ethmoid sinuses and anterior cranial base A (Top), and **(B)** an isolated displaced left orbital roof fracture (R) with opacification of both maxillary sinuses B (Bottom).

Investigations
- CT scan: Brain and facial bones windows.
  - Look for fracture lines: (Figs. 7-4 and 7-5)
  - Intracranial air (pneumocephalus).
    - Orbital roof.
    - Medial orbital wall.
    - Frontal bone.
    - Cribriform plate and anterior cranial base.
  - Opacification of ethmoid and sphenoid sinuses.

Management
- Consultations.
  - Neurosurgery: Rule out brain injury/CSF leak.
  - Ophthalmology: Establish visual integrity.
  - Plastic surgery:
    - Definitive management when patient stable.
    - Repair lacerations.
    - Open reduction and internal fixation displaced fractures involving frontal bone, orbital roof, nasal-orbital-ethmoid regions when patient is stable or at same time as any neurosurgical intervention.

Complications
- CSF leak (meningitis, intracranial abscess).
- Facial deformity (depression, ocular dystopia).
- Frontal sinus mucocele (in children >12 years).

Naso-Orbital Ethmoid Fractures (Fig. 7-6)
- Fracture complex involving the region of the medial orbits, nasal bones, and midline frontal areas.
- May be unilateral or bilateral.
- Classified radiologically by size of bone fragment attached to medial canthal ligament.
- Characterized by:
  - Flattened and widened nasal dorsum.
  - Acute nasofrontal angle.
  - Telecanthus—increased distance of medial canthus from midline.
  - Enophthalmos (unilateral or bilateral).

History
- High-velocity trauma.
- Look for evidence of ocular injury.
- Sensory disturbance V1 and supratrochlear nerves.
- Diplopia due to medial wall fracture.
- Epiphora.
- Epistaxis.

Physical Examination
- Swelling frontal nasal region.
- Tenderness along inferior orbital rims and nasal bones.
- Periorbital ecchymosis.
- Telecanthus.
- Enophthalmos.
- Medial rectus entrapment with diplopia.
- Flattened nasal dorsum.
- Widening of nasal base.
- Acute nasofrontal angle (with impaction of nasal bones).

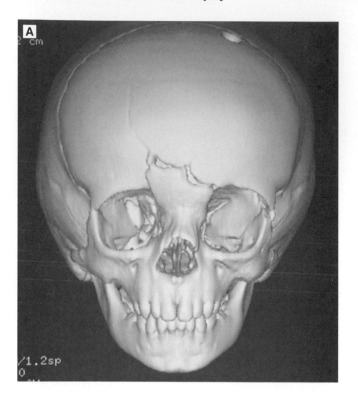

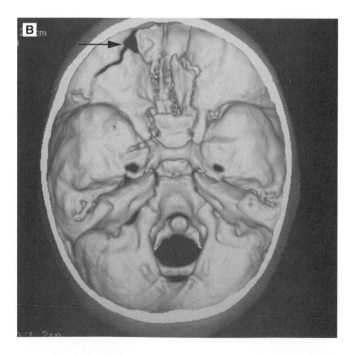

FIGURE 7-5 ● 3-D CT images showing disruption of orbital roof and anterior cranial base and left orbital roof in a 3-year-old boy.

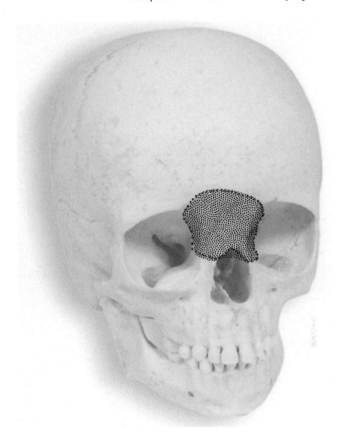

FIGURE 7-6 ● Naso-orbital-ethmoid region.

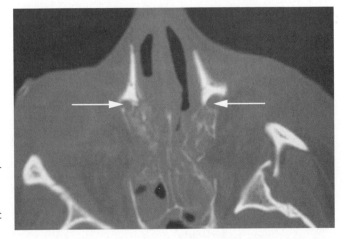

FIGURE 7-7 ● Axial CT demonstrating bilateral nasal-orbital-ethmoid fractures with comminution of both medial orbital walls, (arrows) opacification of ethmoid sinuses, and displaced fractures involving both nasolacrimal regions from the midline. There is an associated fracture of the orbital–zygomatic complex.

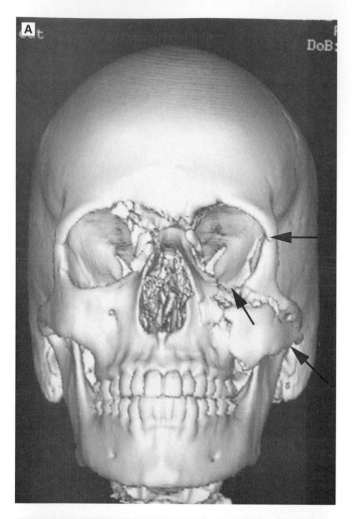

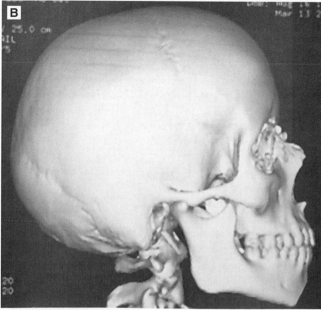

FIGURE 7-8 ● 3D CT scan demonstrating bilateral nasal-orbital-ethmoid and left lateral orbital wall fractures *(arrows)* with comminution and dis-placement of the nasal-orbital-ethmoid complex and acute nasofrontal angle on lateral view.

Investigations
- CT scan (axial, coronal, and 3-D)
- Look for: (Figs. 7-7 and 7-8)
  - Fracture lines.
  - Ethmoid sinus opacification.
  - Displacement of nasolacrimal duct from midline.
  - Medial wall fractures.
  - Pneumocephalus.
  - Splaying of nasal bones.

Management
- Consultations.
  - Neurosurgery: Rule out brain injury/CSF leak.
  - Ophthalmology: Establish visual integrity.
  - Plastic surgery:
    - Definitive management when patient stable.
    - Repair lacerations.
    - Open reduction and internal fixation of displaced fractures involving frontal bone, orbital roof, nasal-orbital-ethmoid regions with restoration of normal orbital contour and volume, reconstruction of nasal dorsum, and fixation of medial canthal tendons in appropriate position when patient is stable or at same time as any neurosurgical intervention.

Complications
- Very challenging to treat.
- Late enophthalmos.
- Residual telecanthus.
- Nasal deformity.
- Epiphora due to blocked lacrimal drainage apparatus.

Nasal Fractures (Fig. 7-9)
- Nasal fractures are the most common facial fracture in children and increase in frequency with increasing age and increasing prominence of the nose.
- Diagnosis is established clinically by assessing for nasal bone tenderness and deformity.

History
- Mechanism of injury.
- History of previous trauma.
- Epistaxis.
- Nasal obstruction.

Physical Examination
- Nasal swelling.
- Tenderness.
- Periorbital ecchymosis.
- Nasal dorsal deformity.
- Nasal pyramid deviation.
- Septal deviation.
- Rule out septal hematoma—decongest nose and if present, drain to prevent infection and late deformity.

Investigations
- Absolutely no value in radiologic imaging for nasal fractures—diagnosis based on clinical assessment.
- CT scan only if nasal-orbital-ethmoid fracture suspected (look for telecanthus).

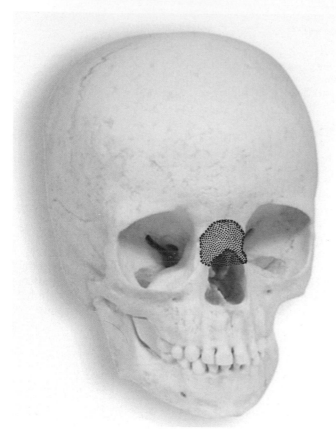

FIGURE 7-9 ● Nasal region.

Management
- Concept of nasal pyramid.
- Closed reduction within 6 hours or after swelling has peaked at 36 hours.
- Nasal splint ± nasal packing × 24 hours.
- With late presentation (>2 weeks), may need open reduction and recreation of fracture to allow reduction.

Complications
- Nasal deformity (hump).
- Nasal deviation.
- Nasal obstruction.
- Septal necrosis (due to septal hematoma).

Orbital Floor Fractures (Fig. 7-10)
- Orbital wall fractures may involve the roof or medial or lateral walls, but most commonly involve the floor, due to its thin nature and biomechanical susceptibility.
- Due to the nature of orbital anatomy, and differences in bone compliance and sinus development, children are predisposed to orbital trap-door type fractures in which the edges of the fracture snap back into position resulting in biomechanical entrapment of the periorbital tissue and inferior rectus muscle.
- CT findings may be minimal (see Fig. 7-13).
- Trap-door fractures constitute a surgical emergency and should be treated within 24 hours.

History
- Often low-velocity trauma followed by onset of diplopia, usually upgaze.
- Visual compromise may be associated with hyphema, retinal disruption.

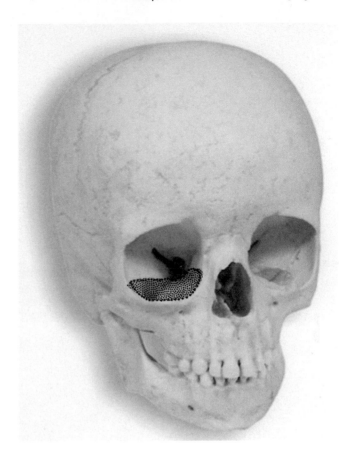

FIGURE 7-10 ● Orbital floor region.

Physical Examination
- Visual acuity.
- Change in globe position (enophthalmos, vertical dystopia).
- V2 sensory loss.
- Pain on upward gaze.
- Subconjunctival hematoma.
- Restriction of extraocular muscle range of motion.
- Positive forced duction test (not usually reliable in children unless done under general anesthesia).

Investigations
- CT scan: Axial, coronal views with reformatted sagittal oblique views useful to delineate orbital floor (Fig. 7-11).

Management
- Ophthalmologic consultation to rule out globe injury.
- Plastic surgery consultation for surgical management.
- Small blow-out fractures with no diplopia managed conservatively.
- Indications for surgical intervention:
  - Diplopia due to mechanical entrapment.
  - Enophthalmos >2 mm or vertical globe dystopia.
- Orbital floor defects greater than 1 cm × 1 cm need to be followed for development of late enophthalmos.
- Trap-door fractures represent a surgical emergency with release of the entrapped periorbital tissue and extraocular muscles ideally within 24 hours of injury.

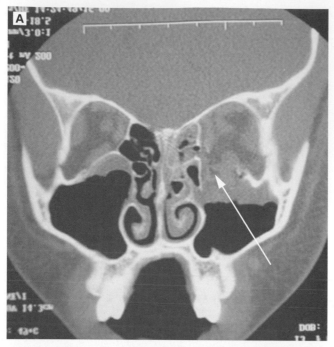

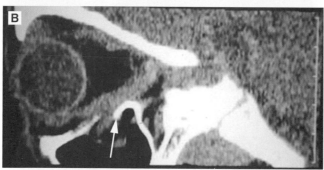

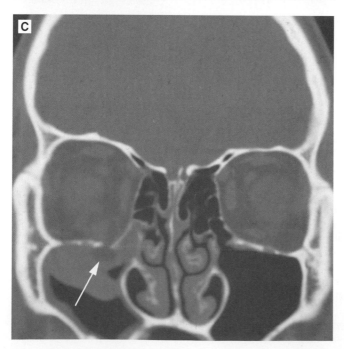

FIGURE 7-11 ● Coronal CT image **(A)** showing orbital floor fracture with herniation of periorbital contents into fracture site and reformatted oblique sagittal view, **(B)** demonstrating typical orbital floor fracture located posterior to axis of the globe and contused swollen inferior rectus muscle. A classic trap-door fracture is demonstrated with entrapment of the periorbital tissues on coronal view CT **(C)**.

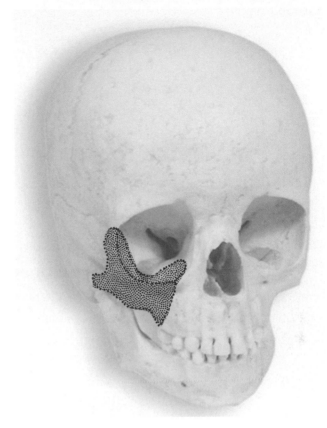

FIGURE 7-12 ● Orbitalzygo-
matic complex region.

Orbital–Zygomatic Complex (Fig. 7-12)
- Common fracture that involves the lateral orbital wall and orbital floor, mistakenly referred to as a "tripod" fracture.
- The zygoma has five articulations: The sphenoid greater wing (lateral orbital wall), maxilla (lateral zygomatico-maxillary buttress), inferior orbital rim, temporal bone (zygomatic arch), and the frontal bone (fronto-zygomatic suture).

History
- Low- or high-velocity trauma.
- Visual acuity changes.
- Diplopia.
- V2 numbness.
- Malocclusion (due to masseter spasm with mandibular deviation).
- TMJ limitation (due to coronoid impingement).

Physical Examination
- Swelling and periorbital ecchymosis.
- Specific point tenderness at fracture sites: Lateral orbit, inferior orbit, zygomatic arch, and lateral buttress of maxilla.
- Decreased sensation V2.
- Subconjunctival hematoma.
- Evidence of biomechanical entrapment.
- Depression of zygomatic high point.
- Increased transverse facial width.

Diagnosis
- CT scan: Axial, coronal, and 3D craniofacial views (Fig. 7-13).

Management
- Same as orbital floor fractures, detailed above.

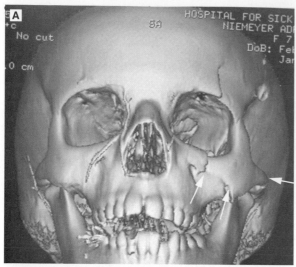

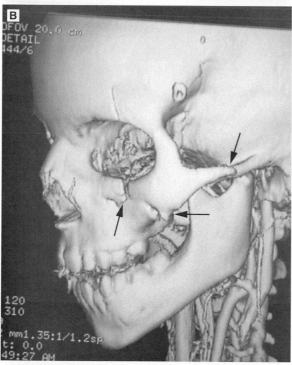

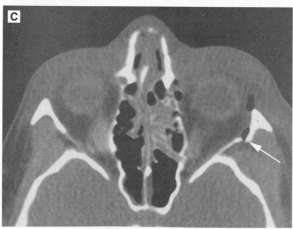

FIGURE 7-13 ● CT images (**A, B**) demonstrating typical orbital–zygomatic complex fracture with fractures through the inferior orbital rim, lateral maxillary buttress, and zygomatic arch. The fracture through the fronto-zygomatic suture is not easily visualized on 3D CT images, but the degree of displacement may be noted on the axial cut (**C**), showing a fracture through the lateral orbital wall.

- Surgical open reduction and internal fixation indicated for:
  - Displaced fractures.
  - Diplopia.
  - Enophthalmos.
  - TMJ impingement.

Complications
- Diplopia.
- Facial deformity—malar flattening, increased transverse facial width, enophthalmos.
- V2 numbness.

Maxillary/Midface (Fig. 7-14)
- Due to the unique nature of the pediatric craniofacial skeleton, true Le Fort fractures are rare in children and become more common in the teen years after development of the maxillary sinus and tooth eruption.
- Midface fractures are named after Reńe Le Fort, who investigated the biomechanics of the facial skeleton in the late 19th century.
- Hallmark of all Le Fort fractures is midface mobility.
- <10 years—dental alveolar fractures more common.
- Typical Le Fort fracture patterns not usually seen.
- Oblique fracture patterns more commonly seen.
- Designation by highest level of fracture.
- Rare to see symmetric bilateral fractures—usually combination of I and II or II and III.
- Airbags and mandatory seatbelt use reduced incidence significantly.
- Presence of Le Fort fractures indicative of high-velocity trauma.
- Airway obstruction and bleeding are primary concerns.

A

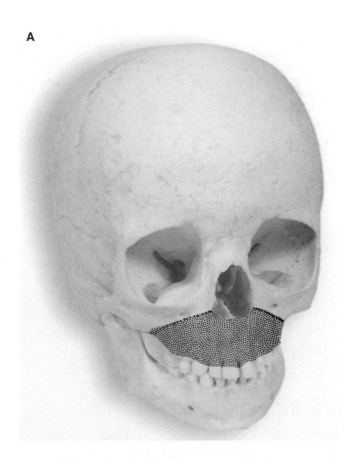

FIGURE 7-14 ● Maxillary fractures at Le Fort levels I **(A)**, II **(B)**, and III **(C)**.

B

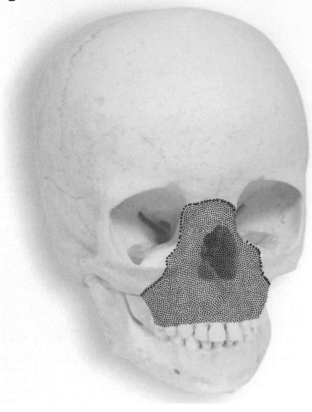

C

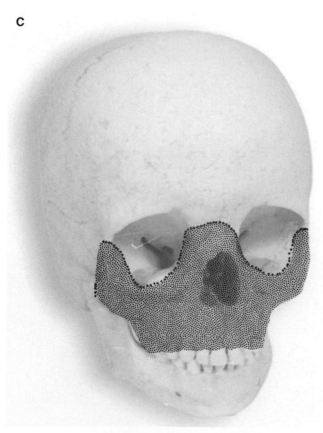

FIGURE 7-14 ● *(Continued)*

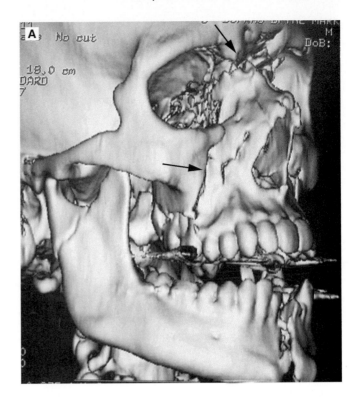

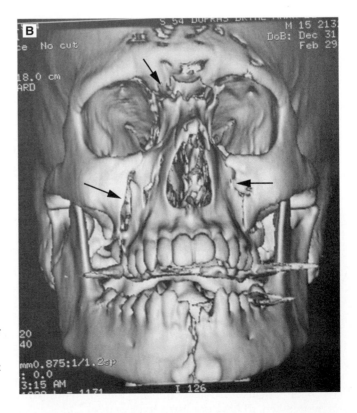

FIGURE 7-15 ● 3D CT demonstrating a pure bilateral Le Fort II fracture with posterior displacement of the midface in addition to a symphyseal mandibular fracture. Symmetric Le Fort fractures are the exception.

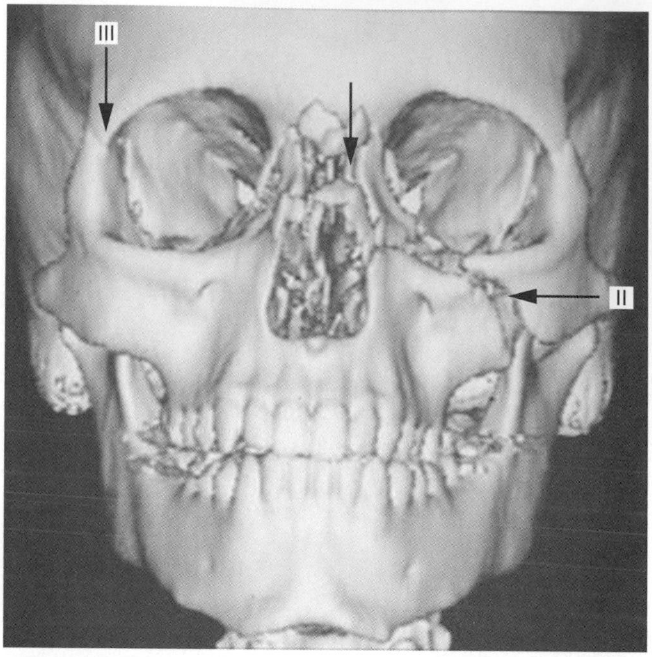

FIGURE 7-16 ●   3D CT of a left Le Fort II and right Le Fort III fracture with right side impaction and right shift of maxillary complex with resultant cross-bite.

History
- High velocity.
- Transverse impact.
- Malocclusion.
- V2 sensory disturbance.

Physical Examination
- Midface mobility.
- Swelling and ecchymosis.
- Tenderness at fracture site.
- Malocclusion.

Investigations
- CT scan: Axial, coronal, and 3D views (Figs. 7-15 and 7-16).

Management
- Airway protection.
- Control of epistaxis.
- Often poly-trauma present.
- Definitive open reduction and internal fixation of fractures when patient stable.
- Restoration of premorbid occlusal relationship.
- Restoration of facial balance (midface height and width).

Complications
- Midface growth issues.
- Malocclusion.
- Facial deformity.

Mandibular Fractures (Fig. 7-17)
- Rare under 6 years of age.
- Second most common facial fracture after nasal fractures.
- Older patients more likely to have comminuted fractures, patients in primary dentition more likely to have greenstick-type patterns.

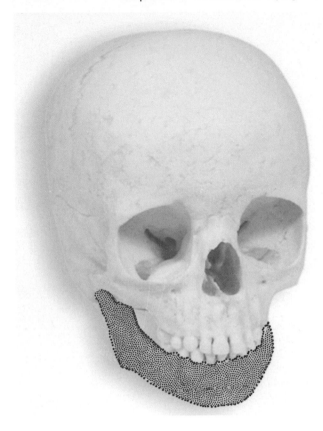

FIGURE 7-17 ● Mandible.

- Location of fracture is age dependent.
- Condyle is commonest site at any age.
- Best classified according to anatomic site (symphysis, parasymphysis, body, angle, ramus, and condyle) and degree of displacement.
- Primary deforming forces are muscles of mastication (temporalis and masseter versus floor of mouth and supra-hyoid musculature).
- Concept of closed ring—look for concomitant fractures (e.g., parasymphysis and condyle).

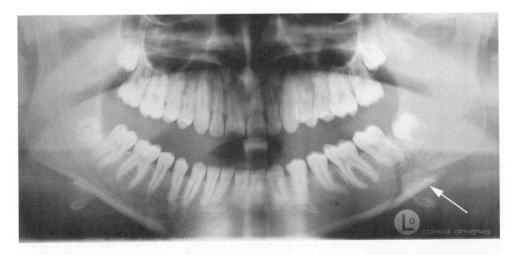

FIGURE 7-18 ● Panorex demonstrating full view of the mandible with a displaced fracture of left mandibular angle.

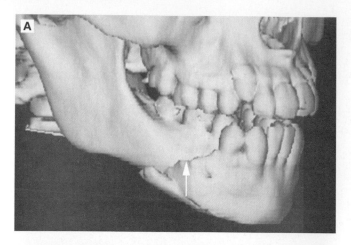

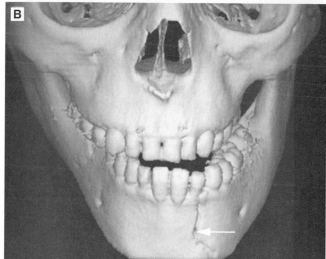

FIGURE 7-19 ● Examples of mandibular fractures. Comminuted displaced body fracture **(A)** requiring open reduction and internal fixation as compared to minimally displaced left parasymphyseal fracture **(B)** managed by a 3-week period of intermaxillary fixation.

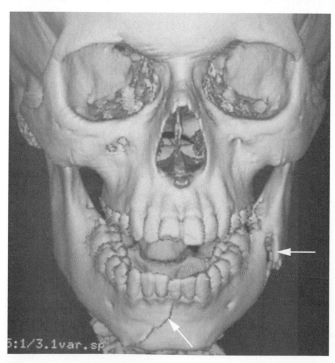

FIGURE 7-20 ● Fractures of the left angle and symphysis demonstrating closed ring concept and the need to rule out a second fracture.

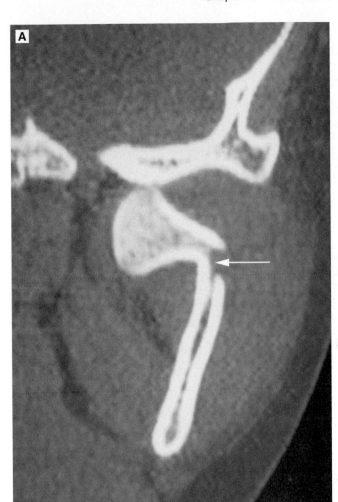

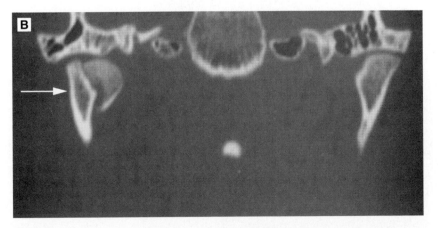

FIGURE 7-21 ● Mandibular fracture involving the mandibular condyle with typical medial displacement of the head due to pull of the lateral pterygoid muscle **(A)**. Coronal CT image of an intra-articular fracture of the mandibular condyle best managed by early range of motion **(B)**.

History

- Low or high velocity.
- Suspect mandible fracture with chin laceration following fall in young child.

Physical Examination

- Malocclusion.
- Mental nerve sensibility.
- Swelling.
- Tenderness at fracture site.
- Limited mouth opening.
- Deviation of mandible to side of condyle fracture.
- Rule out ear canal laceration with condyle fractures.

Investigations

- Panorex: Ideal.
- CT: Axial, coronal, and 3D views of mandible (Figs. 7-18 to 7-21).

Management

- Restoration of normal premorbid occlusal relationships.
- Closed reduction with intermaxillary fixation for noncomminuted fractures with minimal displacement involving tooth-bearing regions.
- Open reduction and internal fixation for comminuted, significantly displaced fractures.
- Interdental wiring: May be problematic in mixed-dentition group (ages 5 to 11 years) as primary roots partially resorbed.

Condyle Fractures

- Site of primary mandibular growth center.
- Mandibular and facial growth interlinked.
- Sequelae of condylar fracture:
  - Growth inhibition.
  - Ankylosis.
  - Rarely, overgrowth.

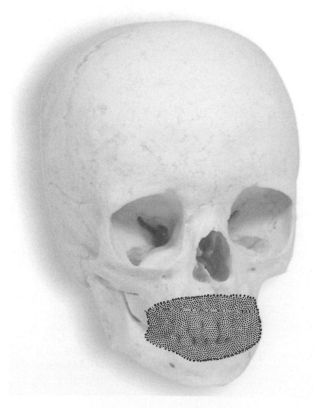

FIGURE 7-22 ● Dental–alveolar region.

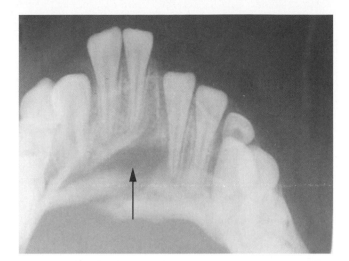

FIGURE 7-23 ● Occlusal view demonstrating comminuted displaced mandibular dental alveolar fracture in combination with symphyseal fracture.

- Ability to remodel remarkable.
- Conservative treatment usually the norm.
- Arch bars and 2- to 3-week period of intermaxillary fixation.
- Early range of motion with intra-articular fractures.

Complications
- Malunion with malocclusion.
- Nonunion—very rare.
- Mental nerve numbness.
- Dental injury with tooth loss.
- Growth anomalies—more likely with condyle fractures.
- TMJ ankylosis—with intra-articular fractures.

Dental–Alveolar Fractures (Fig. 7-22)
- More common in children due to lack of maxillary sinuses.
- Classified by age and dentition (deciduous or permanent).

History
- In children between 12 and 18 months, falls while learning how to walk may result in dental–alveolar fractures.
- Low or high velocity.

Physical Examination
- Loose or missing teeth.
- Intraoral lacerations.
- Malocclusion.

Investigations
- Panorex or CT to rule out other fractures.
- Occlusal views (Fig. 7-23).

Management
- Pediatric dental assessment to manage fractured crowns with and without pulp exposure.
- Replantation of avulsed permanent teeth with stabilization may be associated with good prognosis if done within minutes.
- Dental alveolar fragments are reduced, molded into position, and supported for several weeks with arch bars or orthodontic appliances.
- Soft tissue lacerations sutured with 4-0 or 5-0 absorbable suture.

Complications
- Trauma to deciduous teeth may also damage permanent dentition (especially if <4 years of age).
- Discoloration of teeth and enamel.
- Angulation, and partial or complete arrested root formation.

CLINICAL PEARLS

DO
1. Look for associated injury.
2. Confirm clinical diagnosis by CT scans.
3. Refer promptly for definitive treatment.
4. Note that treatment can be limited to observation or closed reduction in non-displaced or minimally displaced fractures.
5. Consult when in doubt.

DON'T
1. Overlook facial fractures—diagnosis is more difficult in children than in adults.

REFERENCES
1. Ferreira PC, Amarante JM, Silva PN, et al. Retrospective study of 1251 maxillofacial fractures in children and adolescents. *Plast Reconstr Surg* 2005;115:1500–1508.
2. Gassner R, Tuli T, Hachl O, et al. Craniomaxillofacial trauma in children: a review of 3,385 cases with 6,060 injuries in 10 years. *J Oral Maxillofac Surg* 2004;62:399–407.
3. Holland AJ, Broome C, Steinberg A, et al. Facial fractures in children. *Pediatr Emerg Care* 2001;17:157–160.
4. Posnick JC, Wells M, Pron GE. Pediatric facial fractures: evolving patterns of treatment. *J Oral Maxillofac Surg* 1993;51:836–844.
5. Zimmermann CE, Troulis MJ, Kaban LB. Pediatric facial fractures: recent advances in prevention, diagnosis and management. *Int J Oral Maxillofac Surg* 2006;35:2–13.

CHAPTER 8

Neck and Airway Injury

Paolo Campisi, MSc, MD, FRCSC, FAAP

EPIDEMIOLOGY
- Data on the epidemiology of pediatric neck and airway trauma are limited.
- In a series of 257 pediatric head and neck trauma patients admitted to an American level I pediatric trauma center[1]:
  - Male/female ratio 2.5:1.
  - Median age 9.3 years.
  - Leading major head and neck injuries were facial and skull base fractures (32.4%) and blunt and penetrating neck and laryngeal injuries (6.7%).
  - Motor vehicle trauma was the leading cause of injury in children older than 3 years, and falls the most common cause in children under 3 years.
  - Major non-head and neck trauma was present in 35% of patients.
- In a review of penetrating neck injuries in 31 children[2]:
  - This form of injury was more prevalent in males; median age was 9.5.
  - Motor vehicle trauma was the leading cause of penetrating injury (32%) followed by gunshot injury (23%).
  - Most (84%) of the penetrating neck injuries occurred in zone II of the neck (see "Classification" later in the chapter).
  - The mortality rate was 9%.

PATHOPHYSIOLOGY
- Younger children have a relatively prominent cranium and shorter neck.
  - Renders them more prone to intracranial and neurologic injury following head and neck trauma.
- Laryngeal injuries are also less frequent in the pediatric population due to:
  - A more cephalic position of the larynx that is protected by the mandible.
  - Elasticity of the pediatric laryngotracheal cartilaginous framework.
  - A narrow cricothyroid membrane that is protective against laryngotracheal separation.
- Neck and airway injuries may result from blunt or penetrating trauma.
- Blunt trauma causes both crush and shearing injuries:
  - Neck hyperextension results in crush injuries as the larynx is pressed between the offending object and the vertebral column.
  - Sudden changes in momentum also create shearing forces that may cause endolaryngeal mucosal tears, hematomas, and cartilage subluxations.
  - "Clothesline" injury: An extreme form of blunt trauma that can result in laryngeal fracture, cricotracheal separation, vascular injury, and death.
  - Examples of blunt trauma in children include motor vehicle accidents, bicycle accidents, sports-related injuries, blows from fists or feet, and falling or tripping on furniture or stair edges.
- Penetrating trauma injury is often limited to the pathway of the penetrating object.
  - Degree of injury is directly related to the object's velocity and mass.
  - Examples of penetrating trauma in children include motor vehicle crashes, gunshot wounds, animal bites, and falls onto sharp objects.

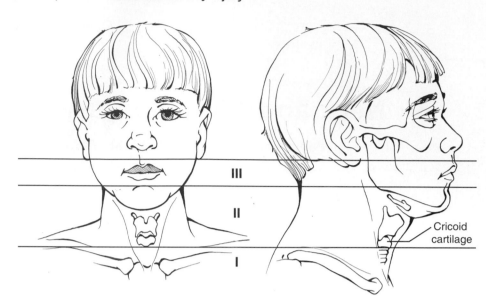

FIGURE 8-1 ● Horizontal entry zones for penetrating injuries to the neck.

CLASSIFICATION
- Neck trauma can be broadly classified into blunt trauma and penetrating trauma.
- Penetrating neck injuries are further classified in terms of their location in one of three anatomic zones (Fig. 8-1):
  - Zone I: The area between the clavicles and the inferior border of the cricoid cartilage.
  - Zone II: The area between the inferior border of the cricoid cartilage and the angle of the mandible.
  - Zone III: The area between the angle of the mandible and the skull base.
- Zone II is the most frequently injured area of the neck.[2-4]
- Zone I and III injuries have a higher mortality rate because surgical exposure is more difficult to achieve.
- The patient's stability and the penetrating injury's anatomic classification are used to determine injury management (Fig. 8-2).[4,5]

INITIAL MANAGEMENT
- Evaluate according to Advanced Trauma Life Support protocol.
- Promptly initiate a directed primary survey of airway, breathing, and circulation.
- Assume that every neck trauma patient has both an airway and cervical spine injury until proven otherwise.
- Establishing a secure airway in a child with neck trauma presents several challenges:
  - Potential concomitant cervical spine injury.
  - An attempt at intubation may further compromise an unstable airway.
  - Any form of surgical airway under local anesthesia may not be well tolerated by the conscious pediatric patient.
- Urgent involvement of anesthesia and otolaryngology services is recommended to establish a surgical airway.
- See Chapter 3 on Airway Management and Chapter 21 on Procedures for further details.

EVALUATION
- History
  - Use all available information sources (patient, parent, witnesses) to determine mechanism of injury.

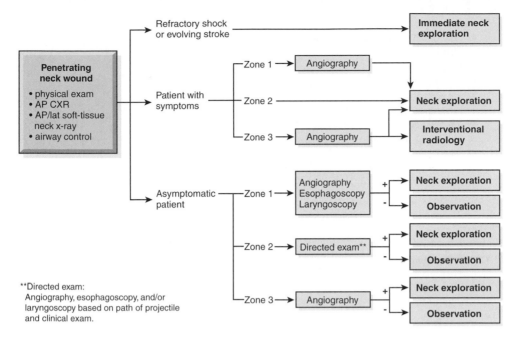

FIGURE 8-2 ● Algorithm for the initial management of patients with penetrating injuries to the neck. (Modified from Bailey BJ, ed. *Head and neck surgery—otolaryngology.* 2nd ed. Lippincott-Raven; 1998, chapter 73.)

- • Establish the amount of time elapsed from the time of injury.
  - • If a penetrating neck injury, determine the type of penetrating object. This includes the size of a knife or the caliber of a gun causing the injury.
  - • Patient symptoms related to the injury: Pain, dyspnea, dysphagia, dysphonia (hoarseness), drooling.
- • Physical Examination
  - • Vital signs and oxygen saturation.
  - • Signs of airway distress:
    - ▪ Nasal flaring.
    - ▪ Subcostal indrawing.
    - ▪ Tracheal tug.
    - ▪ Stridor.
    - ▪ Cyanosis.
  - • Signs of laryngeal injury:
    - ▪ Dysphonia (hoarseness).
    - ▪ Subcutaneous emphysema or crepitus.
    - ▪ Hemoptysis.
    - ▪ Laryngeal tenderness.
    - ▪ Loss of thyroid cartilage prominence.
    - ▪ Air emanating from the neck wound.
    - ▪ Tracheal deviation.
  - • Signs of vascular injury:
    - ▪ Hypotension.
    - ▪ External hemorrhage.
    - ▪ Breach of the platysma.
    - ▪ Expanding hematoma.
    - ▪ Vascular bruits on auscultation.
    - ▪ Asymmetry of arterial pulses.
    - ▪ Contralateral hemiparesis.
    - ▪ Decreased level of consciousness.

- Signs of neurologic injury:
  - Asymmetry of the lower face (facial nerve).
  - Diminished gag reflex (glossopharyngeal nerve).
  - Weak, breathy voice and cough (vagus nerve).
  - Inability to shrug shoulder (accessory nerve).
  - Deviation of tongue on protrusion (hypoglossal nerve).
  - Horner syndrome (sympathetic chain).
  - Motor weakness of arm (brachial plexus).
  - Hypoxia and hypoventilation (phrenic nerve).
  - Abnormal reflexes, lower limb weakness (spinal cord).
- If patient is stable, a flexible nasolaryngoscopy may be performed by the otolaryngologist to assess the upper airway. This may reveal airway edema, mucosal lacerations, hematomas, and vocal fold paralysis.

IMAGING
- Requesting imaging may result in delaying definitive patient management.
  - Avoid imaging studies that will not alter management approach.
  - Ensure airway patency prior to transport for imaging.
- Cervical x-rays:
  - Three views of the entire cervical spine are required to rule out a spinal injury.
  - Also inspect views for airway patency, subcutaneous air, and foreign bodies.
  - See Chapter 9 on Cervical Spine Injury for details.
- Chest x-rays:
  - Required in the setting of thoracic trauma and injury to zone I of the neck.
  - The views are inspected for pneumothorax, hemothorax, widened mediastinum, pneumomediastinum, and foreign bodies.
- Computed tomography (CT) scan of the neck:
  - This imaging modality is useful when a laryngeal fracture is suspected but not readily apparent on plain radiography.
  - CT scanning provides a detailed view of the bony, soft tissue, and airway anatomy.
  - CT scan should be deferred in an unstable patient.
- Four-vessel angiography:
  - Angiography is recommended in stable patients with zone I and III penetrating injuries (see Fig. 8-2).[5]
  - Allows for therapeutic intervention such as embolization and balloon occlusion when surgical exposure to injured vessels is difficult and associated with high morbidity.
  - Angiography should be deferred in an unstable patient.
- Barium or Gastrografin swallow study:
  - Swallow study is used in stable patients to identify esophageal perforation.
  - Gastrografin produces a milder inflammatory response in comparison to barium when it leaks into surrounding tissue.
  - Barium induces less lung inflammation when aspirated. It should be preferentially used when there is a risk of aspiration.

SPECIFIC INJURIES
Laryngeal Injuries[6]
- Any blunt trauma to the larynx should be observed for at least 24 hours.
- The presence of hoarseness, stridor, hemoptysis, and loss of anatomical landmarks is highly suggestive of laryngeal injury.
- A stable patient with minor trauma can be successfully managed with head of bed elevation, voice rest, and humidified air. Intravenous corticosteroids may prevent laryngeal edema that may develop in the hours following the injury.
- An unstable patient or evidence of significant laryngeal injury should be managed urgently in conjunction with the anesthesia and otolaryngology services.
- Endotracheal intubation should be performed in a patient with an expanding hematoma, a diminishing level of consciousness, or cardiorespiratory collapse.

- In severe laryngotracheal injuries, a surgical airway may be required.
- Figure 8-3: A plain x-ray of severe blunt trauma to the larynx. Laryngeal landmarks are obscured by edema and major subcutaneous emphysema.

Esophageal Perforation[7]

- Patients with a suspected or confirmed esophageal injury should not be given anything by mouth.
- The injury may be confirmed with a barium or Gastrografin swallow study.
- The injury may be managed conservatively or by surgical exploration and repair.
- Prophylactic antibiotics are recommended: Clindamycin 10 mg/kg IV q8h.

Cervical Vascular Injuries[5]

- Do not blindly clamp blood vessels. Other vital structures may be damaged.
- Direct pressure is usually sufficient to control bleeding.
- The stable patient may be investigated by angiography.
- The unstable patient requires urgent neck exploration.

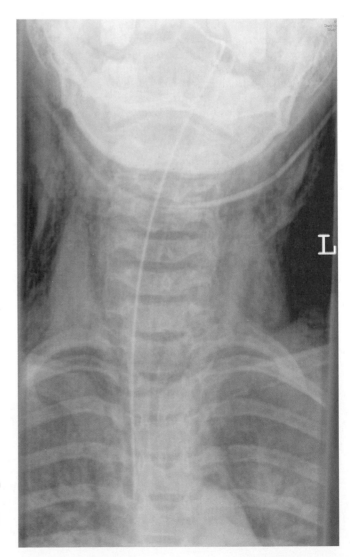

FIGURE 8-3 ● A plain neck x-ray of a child who suffered a severe blunt trauma to the larynx. The radiograph demonstrates loss of laryngeal landmarks and the presence of subcutaneous air.

Burn and Inhalational Injuries[8]

- Assume airway is injured if there is evidence of burns in head and neck areas. Singed nasal hairs, smoke stains, and erythema of the nasal and oral mucosa suggest airway burn.
- Airway edema may develop following the injury. If an airway burn is suspected, intubate the patient prior to the onset of airway edema.

Caustic Ingestions[9,10]

- Airway injury can be caused by alkaline and acidic substances.
- Determine the type and amount of substance ingested.
- Obtain substance information from the local poison control center.
- Copiously irrigate all affected skin and mucosal surfaces.
- Never induce emesis. The regurgitated substance may further injure the airway and/or digestive mucosa.
- Endotracheal intubation may be required with significant airway edema or respiratory compromise.

DEFINITIVE MANAGEMENT

- See Figure 8-2 for managing penetrating neck wounds.
- Main objectives for any neck trauma are airway stabilization, cervical spine protection, and management of concomitant visceral and vascular injuries.
- Achieve airway stabilization with endotracheal intubation or by surgical airway.
- Definitive management of an injured airway depends on injury type and severity.
  - This may involve laryngobronchoscopy and open exploration.
  - In severe laryngeal injuries, airway stenting and tracheostomy may be required.
- Open neck explorations are required to repair visceral and vascular injuries.

CLINICAL PEARLS

DO
- Maintain effective communication with anesthesiology and otolaryngology services.
- Always consider a cervical spine injury with neck trauma.
- Look for other head and neck injuries that may need immediate attention (epistaxis, septal hematoma, cerebrospinal fluid leak, etc.).
- Position the patient's head down to prevent an air embolus from entering the venous system, if an injury to the jugular vein is suspected.
- Always consider the possibility of child abuse with any type of injury.

DON'T
- Delay management of an unstable patient with imaging studies.
- Remove an impaled object in the emergency department, as it may precipitate a severe hemorrhage.
- Intubate a patient if you suspect a laryngeal fracture or laryngotracheal separation.
- Blindly clamp blood vessels because other vital structures may be damaged. Direct pressure is usually sufficient to control bleeding.
- Perform cricothyroidotomy in young children as they have overlapping laryngeal cartilages.

REFERENCES

1. Lim LHY, Kumar M, Myer CM III. Head and neck trauma in hospitalized pediatric patients. *Otolaryngol Head Neck Surg* 2004;130:255–261.
2. Abujamra L, Joseph MM. Penetrating neck injuries in children: a retrospective review. *Pediatr Emerg Care* 2003;19:308–313.
3. Kim MK, Buckman R, Szeremeta W. Penetrating neck trauma in children: an urban hospital's experience. *Otolaryngol Head Neck Surg* 2000;123:439–443.

4. Mutabagani KH, Beaver BL, Cooney DR, et al. Penetrating neck trauma in children: a reappraisal. *J Pediatr Surg* 1995;30:341–344.
5. Mansour MA, Moore EE, Moore FA, et al. Validating the selective management of penetrating neck wounds. *Am J Surg* 1991;162:517–521.
6. Ford HR, Gardner MJ, Lynch JM. Laryngotracheal disruption from blunt pediatric neck injuries: impact of early recognition and intervention on outcome. *J Pediatr Surg* 1995;30:331–335.
7. Dimirbag S, Tiryaki T, Atabek C, et al. Conservative approach to the mediastinitis in childhood secondary to esophageal perforation. *Clin Pediatr (Phila)* 2005;44:131–134.
8. Whitelock-Jones L, Bass DH, Millar AJW, et al. Inhalation burns in children. *Pediatr Surg Int* 1999;15:50–55.
9. Baskm D, Urganci N, Abbasoglu L, et al. A standardized protocol for the acute management of corrosive ingestion in children. *Pediatr Surg Int* 2004;20:824–828.
10. de Jong AL, Macdonald R, Ein S, et al. Corrosive esophagitis in children: a 30-year review. *Int J Pediatr Otorhinolaryngol* 2001;57:203–211.

CHAPTER 9

Pediatric Cervical Spine Injuries

Shauna Jain, MD, FRCPC

INTRODUCTION
- Maintain a high index of suspicion for spinal cord injuries.
  - Especially important in multiply injured patient.
- Hemodynamic and other life-threatening injuries take priority.
- Avoid unnecessary manipulation of the spine.
- Children are a challenge to assess and treat as they are:
  - Not able to communicate location of pain or neurologic symptoms.
  - Difficult to restrain if agitated or frightened.
  - Immobilize and limit movement by:
    - Having parent at their side.
    - Using distraction techniques.
    - Removing the hard board as soon as possible.
    - Administering adequate analgesia.
- Investigation of cord injuries in children requires knowledge of:
  - Specific differences between the adult and pediatric spine.
  - Differences in injury patterns.
  - Anatomic variants and radiographic characteristics.

EPIDEMIOLOGY OF PEDIATRIC C-SPINE INJURIES
- The incidence of spinal cord injury is 1% to 2% of the pediatric trauma population.[2,7]
- The majority of spinal injury (60–80%) occurs in the cervical spine.[1]
- The major cause for pediatric spinal injuries is motor vehicle accidents, followed by falls and child abuse.[2]
- Goals of spinal injury treatment are to prevent secondary injury by[3]:
  - Maintaining a high index of suspicion.
  - Immobilization of the C-spine.
  - Minimizing spinal manipulation.
  - Ensuring the patient's hemodynamic stability and oxygenation.

ANATOMIC CONSIDERATIONS
- By 8 years of age the spine becomes anatomically similar to the adult spinal column.
  - Adult-type fracture patterns are not seen until early adolescence.[1,2]
- Age differences of C-spine injury location and type:
  - Children <14 years tend to have higher C-spine injuries (C1-C4).
  - Children >14 years tend to have lower C-spine injures (C5-C7).[1,12]
    - The fulcrum of the immature spine is C2-C3, leading to higher injuries; whereas the fulcrum of the adolescent spine is lower at C5-C6.[4,5]

- Children <10 years tend to have dislocations and Spinal Cord Injury without Radiologic Abnormality-type (SCIWORA)-type injuries and injury patterns.
- Children >10 years tend to have fractures.[1]
  - Children are prone to dislocation and SCIWORA injuries because of the pediatric spine's greater mobility from weaker neck musculature, larger head-body ratio, greater ligament and joint capsule laxity, anterior vertebral wedging, underdeveloped uncinate processes, and horizontal articulating facet joints.[1,4]
- Congenital spinal abnormalities, such as atlantoaxial instability in trisomy 21 and Klippel–Feil syndrome, and bony weaknesses such as os odontoideum and block vertebra, place these children at greater risk for spinal injury.[4]

SPINAL STABILIZATION
Indications for C-Spine Stabilization
- A high index of suspicion for spinal cord injury is always necessary.
- When in doubt, immobilization is always the appropriate choice.
- Historical risk factors for spinal injury include:[7,21]
  - Pedestrian or cyclist hit by a vehicle at >30 km/hr.
  - Passengers in motor vehicle collisions occurring at >60 km/hr.
  - Serious injury of other occupants of the vehicle.
  - Patient thrown from a vehicle.
  - Fall from more than 3 meters.
  - Patient kicked by a horse or a fall from a horse.
  - Being backed over by a car.
  - Being thrown over the handlebars of a bicycle.
  - Thrown by electric shock.
  - Neck pain or neurologic symptoms at any time after the injury.
- Indicators of spinal injury on examination include:[7,21]
  - Neck tenderness.
  - Neurologic deficit.
  - Unexplained hypotension or bradycardia.
  - Acute torticollis after trauma.
  - Evidence of major trauma from other significant injuries.

Keys to Immobilization of Children:
- Proper immobilization involves:
  - A fitting semirigid cervical collar and fixation to a spinal board.
  - Ensuring the collar is appropriately and properly fitted.
  - Children <3 years of age: May use sandbags on either side of the child's head.
- Fixation to the spinal boards:[15]
  - Children have large heads relative to their bodies, causing their heads to flex.
  - For neutral alignment: Elevate the torso with padding or recess the occiput through a hole in the spinal board (Fig. 9-1).
  - Proper alignment is when the external auditory canal is in line with the shoulders.
  - Use tape straps across the forehead, shoulders, pelvis, and thighs (Fig. 9-2).
  - Do not tape across the chest as this may restrict respiratory movement.
  - Ensure patient is off backboard within 2 hours to prevent pressure sores.

THE C-SPINE AND THE AIRWAY
- See Chapter 3 on Airway Management for details.
- Proper airway alignment MUST be maintained at all times.
  - During intubation ONE person must maintain the cervical spine in neutral alignment.

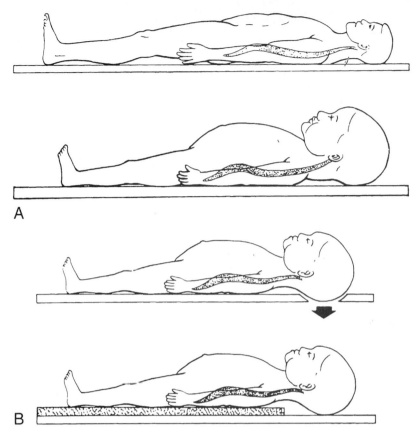

FIGURE 9-1 ● Effects of backboard on cervical spine position. **A.** Adult and child immobilized on standard backboard. **B.** Backboards modified with occipital recess and mattress pad to allow neutral positioning of the cervical spine in a young child. (Reprinted with permission from Herzenberg J, Hensinger R, Dedrick D, et al. Emergency transport and positioning of young children who have an injury of the cervical spine: the standard backboard may be hazardous. *J Bone Joint Surg* 1989;71-A:15–21.)

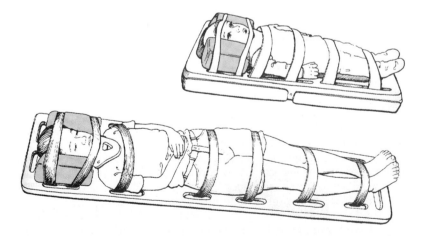

FIGURE 9-2 ● Cervical spine immobilization should not place the patient at an increased risk for morbidity. Securing straps should be placed around bony prominences, and strap location reassessed after any movement of the patient. A neutral position of the neck should be ensured, and if necessary (younger child), a spacer can be placed underneath the child's torso and lower extremities to achieve the desired position. (From Woodward GA. Neck trauma. In: Fleisher GR, Ludwig S, eds. *Textbook of pediatric emergency medicine.* 4th ed. Philadelphia: Lippincott Williams & Wilkins; 2000, with permission.)

- When intubation is difficult, bagging with 100% oxygen is an acceptable and preferred alternative.
- It may be necessary to use a jaw thrust or an oral airway to ensure airway patency.
- Never force the neck out of neutral alignment.
- A high C-spine injury may result in diaphragmatic (C3-C5) or intercostal muscle paralysis leading to respiratory failure.
  - These patients require intubation to provide adequate respirations.

CLINICAL ASSESSMENT FOR SPINAL INJURY

- Ensure a complete neurologic exam.
- Look for evidence of spinal cord injury, including an exam of the spinal cord tracts:
  - Corticospinal tract:
    - Lies posterolaterally in the cord.
    - Controls ipsilateral motor function.
    - Tested by examination of muscle strength (voluntary or involuntary to a painful stimulus).
  - Spinothalamic tract:
    - Lies anterolaterally in the cord.
    - Responsible for contralateral pain and temperature sensation.
    - Test by checking sensation to pinprick, temperature, and light touch in all dermatomes.
  - Posterior columns:
    - Lie posterior in the cord.
    - Control proprioception and vibration sense.
    - Tested by position sense and vibration of fingers and toes.
- Clinically, the neurologic level is determined from the major dermatomes and myotomes (Fig. 9-3).
- Complete versus incomplete lesions:
  - A complete spinal injury implies no motor or sensory function below a certain level.
  - With an incomplete spinal injury, some motor or sensory function is preserved with possible sacral sparing (loss of all motor and sensory function below a certain nerve root level but sensation persists perianally).
- Spinal shock occurs when injury to the spinal cord causes it to temporarily lose function below the level of injury.
  - Results in flaccidity and areflexia.
  - Return of the bulbocavernous reflex signals resolution of the spinal shock state, patients generally recover within 24 hours.[21]
- Incomplete spinal cord lesions:
  - Spinal cord injury may follow certain clinical patterns that may be useful in identifying the type and location of injury.
  1 Central cord syndrome:
    - Typically after hyperextension injury.
    - Injury to anterior spinal artery which supplies the central cord.
    - Clinically see motor loss greater in upper extremities than lower extremities.
  2 Anterior cord syndrome:
    - Anterior spinal injury causing anterior cord infarction.
    - Paraplegia and loss of pain and temperature sense below affected sensory level but preserved posterior column function (position and vibration sense).
  3 Brown-Séquard syndrome:
    - Hemisection injury to the cord.
    - Ipsilateral corticospinal and posterior column loss (motor, vibration, and proprioception) and contralateral spinothalamic (pain and temperature) injury one to two levels below the motor loss.

Sensory dermatomes

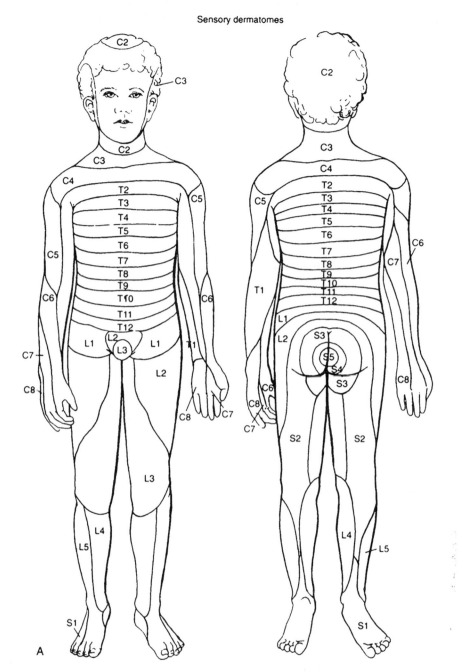

FIGURE 9-3 ● **A.** Sensory dermatomes. **B.** Motor dermatomes. Knowledge of sensory and motor dermatomes can be invaluable in description of neurologic findings during initial and subsequent evaluations. (From Woodward GA. Neck trauma. In: Fleisher GR, Ludwig S, eds. *Textbook of pediatric emergency medicine.* 4th ed. Philadelphia: Lippincott Williams & Wilkins; 2000, with permission.)

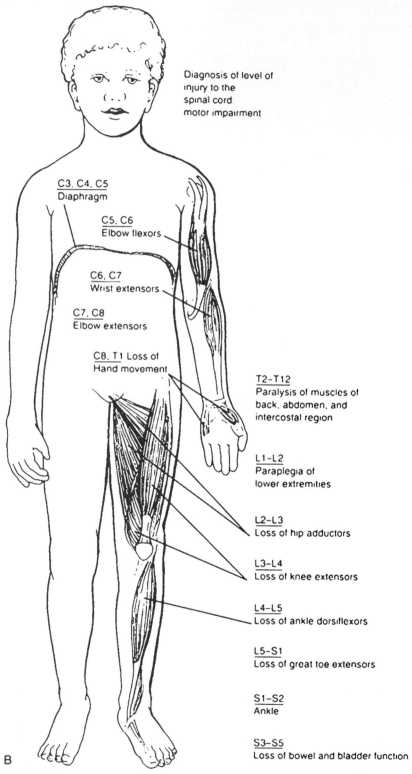

Diagnosis of level of
injury to the
spinal cord:
motor impairment

C3, C4, C5
Diaphragm

C5, C6
Elbow flexors

C6, C7
Wrist extensors

C7, C8
Elbow extensors

C8, T1 Loss of
Hand movement

T2–T12
Paralysis of muscles of
back, abdomen, and
intercostal region

L1–L2
Paraplegia of
lower extremities

L2–L3
Loss of hip adductors

L3–L4
Loss of knee extensors

L4–L5
Loss of ankle dorsiflexors

L5–S1
Loss of great toe extensors

S1–S2
Ankle

S3–S5
Loss of bowel and bladder function

B

FIGURE 9-3 ● *(Continued)*

SPECIFIC PEDIATRIC SPINAL INJURIES
SCIWORA (Spinal Cord Injury Without Radiologic Abnormality)
- Particularly seen in younger children and cervical spine injuries.[6]
  - Bony radiologic imaging is normal but underlying cord injury may have occurred.[1]
  - Pediatric spinal column can stretch more than the spinal cord.
    - In cadaver neonates, the spinal column would stretch by 2 cm but the cervical cord would only stretch by ¼ inch before there was spinal injury.[4]
  - Other possible causes include ischemia of the cord from direct vascular injury or hypoperfusion.
- SCIWORA injuries require a high index of suspicion and careful history-taking.
  - Patients may report transient neurologic symptoms (paresthesia, numbness, weakness, or shock-like sensations in their extremities) at the time of or shortly after the trauma.[15,18, 21]
- Maintain spinal immobilization and obtain additional radiologic imaging including CT and MRI of the spinal cord.
- Outcome correlates with the degree of neurologic symptoms at the time of presentation and degree of injury seen on MRI.
  - Poor outcome is associated with major hemorrhage and edema of the spinal cord, conversely if no more cord abnormalities are seen there is generally full recovery.[15,18]
- Management involves consultation with a neurosurgeon and proper immobilization.
- Transient quadraparesis may be a subset of SCIWORA injury.
  - Classic picture of transient paralysis after a sports injury with full recovery within 24 hours.
  - CT and MRI are normal.
  - Represents a spinal cord concussion and deserves rest from contact activities for at least 6 weeks.

Atlas Fractures
- Uncommon pediatric fracture.
- Difficult to identify because:
  - Need good odontoid views.
  - Younger children have an incompletely ossified odontoid.
  - If suspected, a CT of C1-C2 should be obtained.

Jefferson or Burst Fracture
- Seen in adolescents after an axial compression injury (diving or a fall on the head).
- Odontoid view demonstrates displacement of the axis' lateral masses with respect to the odontoid by >6 mm or asymmetry of the lateral masses with respect to the odontoid.

Atlanto-Occipital Dislocation
- More common in pediatric population because:
  - Smaller occipital condyles.
  - More horizontal orientation of the atlanto-occipital joint leading to easier slippage.
- Injury often leads to cardiorespiratory arrest at the scene of the accident.
  - Survivors generally suffer significant neurologic sequelae.
- Apparent on the lateral cervical spine radiograph as a misalignment of the normal basion–odontoid relationship. (See the "Imaging in Suspected Spinal Injury" section below for specific measurement guidelines.)

Atlantoaxial Subluxation (AAS)
- Children are at particular risk for AAS because of their:
  - Disproportionately large heads.
  - Weak cervical muscles.
- Subsets of children are particularly prone.
  - Trisomy 21.
  - Skeletal dysplasia.

- Juvenile rheumatoid arthritis.
- Infections of the pharynx.
- Hypoplastic odontoid.
- Children may present with painful torticollis.
- Injury carries high risk of neurologic sequelae depending on the degree of subluxation.
- A certain amount of subluxation permitted at this level without neurologic damage as the spinal cord is at its widest at C1-C2 and narrows further down the cervical canal.
- AAS is seen on lateral spine radiographs as forward subluxation of the atlas on the axis by >5 mm (measurement from the anterior arch of the atlas to the odontoid).[4]

Atlantoaxial Rotatory Subluxation (AARS) or Fixation

- Children are more prone to this problem because of their anatomy, which allows greater movement of the atlas and axis.
- Presents as torticollis and must be distinguished from benign torticollis (secondary to contraction of the sternocleidomastoid [SCM] muscle).
  - Benign torticollis:
    - SCM is shortened on the opposite side to which the head is tilted (chin points opposite to contracted muscle).
    - Causes include benign paroxysmal torticollis, fibrosis of the SCM, inflammation or infection in the region of the SCM or neck.
    - Managed by identifying and treating the underlying cause and a soft neck collar and analgesics.
  - AARS:
    - Rare, but requires prompt recognition as early treatment improves outcome.
    - Causes include minor trauma, infection, or surgery of the head or neck (Grisel syndrome) or may be associated with rheumatoid arthritis.
    - Chin is tilted toward the SCM muscle in spasm because the muscle is trying to correct the abnormality (head rotated in one direction but tilted to the other side, often described as a "cock robin" or a bird that is listening for a worm).
    - Strongly suspect in a child with >1 week history of torticollis that has not responded to conservative treatment (analgesics and soft collar).
    - Difficult to identify with plain films because the head tilt obscures landmarks, but can be appreciated with dynamic CT scanning and 3D reconstruction.

C2 (Axis) Fractures

Odontoid Fractures

- In children <7 years of age there is a cartilaginous synchondrosis between the odontoid and body of the axis that is susceptible to fracture.
- In older children, fractures tend to occur at the base of the odontoid.
- Odontoid fractures are of three types and may be seen on plain films:
  - Type 1 fractures extend through the tip of the odontoid.
  - Type 2 fractures extend through the base of the dens, and are the most frequent of the odontoid fractures.
  - Type 3 fractures are the most unstable and originate at the base of the dens through the body of the axis.

C2 Posterior Element Fractures (Hangman's Fracture)

- A bilateral pars interarticularis break, which is a result of a hyperextension injury.
- Seen on the lateral C-spine radiograph and may appear as subluxation of C2 on C3.
- May be confused with normal radiographic finding of pseudosubluxation of C2 on C3.
  - Line of Swischuck is helpful to differentiate from pseudosubluxation (Fig. 9-4).

Injuries from C3 to C7

- Injuries at these levels usually follow an adult pattern.
- Laxity of the ligaments may result in facet dislocation without associated fracture.

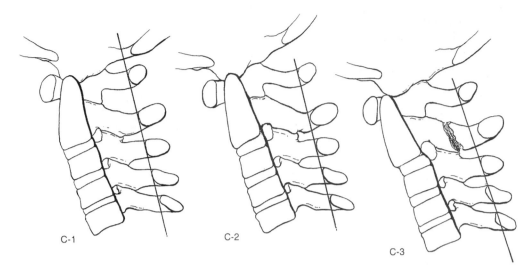

FIGURE 9-4 ● Posterior cervical line of Swischuk. Line is drawn from the cortex of the spinous process of C1 to the cortex of the spinous process of C3. Relationship of the line to cortex of the spinous process of C2 is noted. If the line is situated more than 2.0 mm anterior to the cortex of the spinous process of C2, underlying cervical pathology should be present. This line should only be used with anterior displacement of C2 on C3. (From Woodward GA. Neck trauma. In: Fleisher GR, Ludwig S, eds. *Textbook of pediatric emergency medicine.* 4th ed. Philadelphia: Lippincott Williams & Wilkins; 2000, with permission.)

CLINICALLY CLEARING THE PEDIATRIC C-SPINE

- Clearing the cervical spine may be challenging in children who may not be developmentally able to communicate spinal pain or tenderness, one of the key components to evaluating patients for spinal injury.
- There are established guidelines for clinically clearing the C-spine based on a large, multicenter study, the National Emergency X-Radiography Utilization Study (NEXUS).[8,16]
- In this study, of 3,065 children <18 years of age who suffered blunt trauma, there were 30 children with cervical spine injury.
- The study found that there was 100% sensitivity and 100% negative predictive value for excluding cervical spine injury if the following five criteria were met, which can be remembered by the acronym NSAID:
  - **N**eurologically intact (no evidence of neurologic deficit).
  - **S**pinal tenderness absent (no midline cervical tenderness).
  - **A**lert (the patient is fully alert with Glasgow Coma Scale score 15/15).
  - **I**ntoxication absent (no history or physical evidence of intoxication).
  - **D**istracting injuries absent (definition of distracting injury up to discretion of physician but patient must be able to fully focus on answering questions about the cervical spine exam).
- If children do not meet the above five criteria they should undergo radiologic imaging to clear the cervical spine; this includes children not able to communicate spinal tenderness.
- The study included only 4 children <9 years; therefore, the above guidelines cannot guarantee 100% sensitivity in children <9 years of age; in this age group there should be a lower threshold for radiologic imaging.

IMAGING IN SUSPECTED SPINAL INJURY
Plain Film Imaging
- If a fracture is seen at one vertebral level, the entire spine should be imaged, as there is a 10% to 16% chance of multiple-level injuries.[4]
- Indications for plain films:
  - Patient does not meet criteria for clinical clearance and a spinal injury is suspected.

Plain Film Imaging for the Cervical Spine
- Cervical spine imaging begins with three plain film views:
  - Anterioposterior (AP).
  - Lateral.
  - Odontoid (open mouth) view.
- The lateral plain film has a fracture detection sensitivity of 79%, which increases to 94% with the AP and odontoid views.[13, 22]
- Always ensure that the following are included and present in the lateral film:
  - Base of the skull.
  - All seven cervical vertebrae.
  - T1.
  - A swimmer's view or a shoulder pull down may be required to visualize C7-T1, the most frequently obscured area.
- **Note:** Congenital bony abnormalities tend to be smooth and sclerotic and fracture edges tend to be jagged.[19]

AP View
- Ensure parallel alignment and equal spacing of all spinous processes and facets.
- Check that interpedicular distances are symmetrical. (Fig. 9-5).
  - For thoracic vertebra, make sure that it is possible to see all the spinous processes through the vertebral bodies.
  - Evidence of new scoliosis from muscle spasm may suggest spinal injury.

Odontoid View
- Children <8 years may have normal overhang of the lateral masses of C1 with respect to C2 of up to 6 mm.[4]
  - Symmetry of distance between C1 and C2 is more important than bony congruity.[9,17]
- Ensure bony integrity of the odontoid.
  - In children <8 years the odontoid view is often technically difficult to obtain.
  - CT is imaging of choice if there is clinical suspicion of injury.

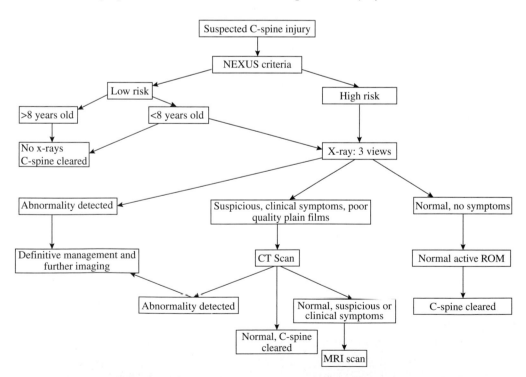

FIGURE 9-5 ● Algorithm for radiographic evaluation.

- Most fractures of the odontoid occur at the base or at the synchondrosis.
  - Both fracture types are seen on the lateral or AP view.[19]

Lateral View
- For the cervical projection, make sure that all seven vertebra and the cervicothoracic junction are clearly visualized.
  - Trace lines for proper vertebral alignment (Fig. 9-8):
  - Anterior vertebral line.
  - Posterior vertebral line.
  - Spinolaminar line.
  - Posterior spinous line.
  - Trace each vertebral body and make certain that all contours are even.
  - Make sure that intervertebral spaces are equal.
  - All the facets should lie in a parallel line.
  - Check that the distances between spinous processes show no evidence of widening.
- Check specific measurements:
  - Atlanto-dental distance should be less than or equal to 5 mm.[19]
  - Soft-tissue measurements should not exceed ¾ vertebral body width or 7 mm at C2 and the width of the vertebral body or 14 mm at C6.[19]
  - The anterior height of the vertebral body should not differ by more than 3 mm when compared to the posterior vertebral body height.[4]
- Atlanto-occipital dislocation suggested by (Fig 9-6)[4]
  1. Distance between the basion and tip of dens >10 mm.
  2. Wackenheim clivus line (line along posterior aspect of clivus to odontoid) should intersect or be tangential to the odontoid.
  3. Powers ratio of BC/AO, >0.9 where B = basion, C = spinolaminar line of atlas, A = anterior tubercle of atlas, and O = opisthion (Fig 9-6).
  4. Harris methods: posterior axial line drawn tangentially along the posterior cortex of axis body should lie within 12 mm of the basion or the gap between the basion and the odontoid tip should be less than 12 mm.[19]
     - **Note:** Some of these tests may not be possible in children <12 years of age who have an unossified odontoid process, in which case tests 1 and 4 are the most useful.
- The pediatric spine has numerous normal variants:[21,4]
  - Children may not have cervical lordosis.

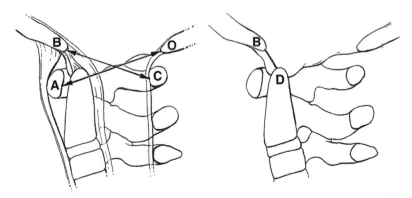

FIGURE 9-6 ● Examples of methods to assess occipatal/C1 relationships. *A:* Cl anterior arch; *B:* basion (anterior margin of foramen magnum); *C:* anterior portion of the posterior ring of Cl; *O:* opisthion (posterior margin of foramen magnum); *D:* tip of the dens (odontoid process). These landmarks may not be easily visible on all radiographs. A ratio of BC to AO greater than 0.9 to 1.0 suggests anterior dislocation or subluxation of the atlanto-occipital joint. A BD distance greater than 10 to 12.5 mm should be viewed as suspicious for atlanto-occipital dislocation. (From Woodward GA. Neck trauma. In: Fleisher GR, Ludwig S, eds. *Textbook of pediatric emergency medicine.* 4th ed. Philadelphia: Lippincott Williams & Wilkins; 2000, with permission.)

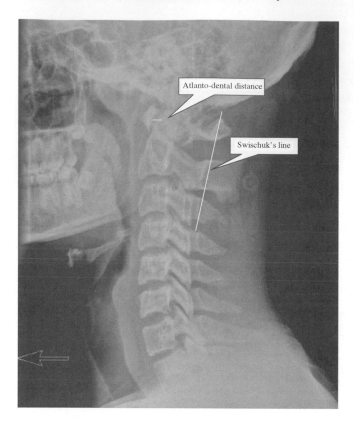

FIGURE 9-7 ● Plain film imaging of the thoracic and lumbar spine.

- Children tend to have wedge-shaped vertebrae (abnormal when anterior and posterior heights differ by more than 3 mm).[4]
- Synchondrosis of the odontoid may be radiolucent up to 16 years.[4]
- Pseudosubluxation of C2 on C3 (and less commonly C3 on C4) will change the alignment of the normal spinal lines. Differentiated from a fracture by Swischuk's line (Fig. 9-7).

Flexion/Extension Plain Films
- Often not useful in acute trauma assement[10,11]

CT Imaging for Suspected Spinal Injury
- The sensitivity of CT for fracture detection is up to 93% and better with image reconstruction.[4,22]
- Indications for CT imaging:
  - Injury is seen on plain films with need to further delineate the bony injury.
  - There is a clinical suspicion of injury not seen on plain films.
  - The entire cervical spine cannot be properly visualized.
- CT is great for bony injury but ligamentous injury is not well assessed; delayed flexion/extension plain films, dynamic flexion/extension studies, or MRI are better diagnostic studies.[10,11]

MRI for Suspected Spinal Injury
- Indications MRI imaging:[14]
  - Suspected cases of SCIWORA.
  - Patients with altered levels of consciousness to clear the C-spine.[14]
  - For immediate evaluation of ligamentous injuries instead of waiting one week postinjury for proper flexion/extension views.

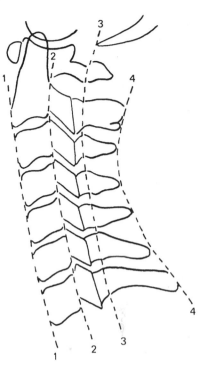

FIGURE 9-8 ● Four contour lines of alignment with normal cervical spine lordosis: 1. Anterior vertebral bodies. 2. Posterior vertebral bodies (anterior spinal canal). 3. Spinolaminal line (posterior spinal canal). 4. Spinous process tips. (Reprinted with permission from Gerlock A, Kirchner S, Heller R, et al. *Advanced exercises in diagnostic radiology: the cervical spine in trauma.* Philadelphia: Saunders; 1978: 6.)

- Prognostic information regarding spinal injury.
- Patients with an equivocal CT.
- Look for evidence of spinal hematoma that may require decompression.

SPINAL INJURY AND ASSOCIATED INJURIES
- Ensure prompt transport of child with spinal injury to closest pediatric trauma center.
- C-spine injuries carry an associated risk of other injuries to the neck as well, such as carotid artery dissection.
  - Ensure complete evaluation of patient and consider other injures.
- If one spinal injury is found, risk for another injury of the spine, therefore should image entire spine.

MANAGEMENT OF SPINAL CORD INJURY
- Prepare to transport patients with suspected spinal cord injury to a tertiary care facility experienced in pediatric trauma.
- Avoid unnecessary delay.
- Secure patient's airway as needed, to ensure oxygenation and ventilation.
  - If a skilled physician is not available for intubation, then mask ventilation is the best alternative to preserve spinal stability.
- Maintain hemodynamic stability.
  - Aggressive fluid resuscitation is an important component of spinal cord injury management to prevent secondary injury.
- Patients may be hypotensive from other traumatic injuries or rarely from neurogenic shock.
  - Neurogenic shock results in autonomic dysregulation (loss of normal sympathetic response to shock), so patients present with hypotension and bradycardia.
  - In addition to fluid resuscitation, patients may need vasopressors to maintain normotension and atropine may be required for clinically significant bradycardia.
- Spinal hematomas causing cord compression as seen on MRI require rapid diagnosis and surgical evacuation.

- Steroid controversy:
  - Contact neurosurgical service before initiating treatment to determine practice at the receiving site.
  - Recommendations are based on studies by Bracken and associates which notably excluded patients <13 years).[20] Bracken steroids showed some promise in limited neurologic improvement in nonpenetrating spinal cord injury if reported **within 8 hours** of injury.
  - Studied methylprednisolone dose of 30 mg/kg over 15 minutes and then 5.4 mg/kg/hr for 23 hours if started within 3 hours of injury, and if started within 3 to 8 hours to be continued for 48 hours.[5]
  - Current recommendations by the Congress of Neurologic Surgeons and American Association of Neurologic Surgeons:
    - Methylprednisolone for either 24 or 48 hours is recommended as an option in the treatment of patients with acute spinal cord injuries that should be undertaken only with the knowledge that the evidence suggesting harmful side effects is more consistent than any suggestion of clinical benefit.[23]
- Consult neurosurgery and/or orthopedic surgery for all suspected or detected spinal injury.

CLINICAL PEARLS

DO
- Prevent secondary injury through proper spinal immobilization and systemic stabilization.
- Make certain that the C-spine is always in neutral alignment.
- Consider that children have different injury patterns than adults.
- Consider that children have different radiologic variants and normal measurements than adults.
- Use NEXUS criteria to clear C-spines in children >8 years of age.
- Image the entire spinal column if a fracture is seen at one level, as the patient is at high risk for other fractures.
- Involve the neurosurgical or orthopedic service in all suspected spinal injury.

DON'T
- Skip a complete neurologic exam because a child is uncooperative; instead, use distractors or parents as aids.
- Skip immobilization because the mechanism of injury is unknown or unclear; instead, always immobilize when in doubt.
- Disregard NEXUS criteria because a child is <8 years; do utilize with caution and logic.
- Ignore seemingly benign findings such as history of transient neurologic symptoms or torticollis after trauma, which may suggest C-spine injury.

REFERENCES

1. Kokoska E, Keller M, Rallo M, et al. Characteristics of pediatric cervical spine injuries. *J Pediatr Surg* 2001;36:100–105.
2. Brown R, Brunn M, Garcia V. Cervical spine injuries: a review of 103 patients treated consecutively at a level 1 pediatric trauma center. *J Pediatr Surg* 2001;36:1107–1114.
3. American College of Surgeons Committee on Trauma. *Advanced trauma life support.* American College of Surgeons, St. Clair St. Chicago, IL; 6th ed. 1997.
4. Roche C, Carty H. Spinal trauma in children. *Pediatr Radiol* 2001;31:677–700.
5. Proctor M. Spinal cord injury. *Crit Care Med* 2002;30:S489–S499
6. Hadley MN. Management of pediatric cervical spine and spinal cord injuries. *Neurosurgery* 2002;50:S85–99.
7. Brown GJ, Cheng NG, McCaskill ME, et al. An approach to pediatric cervical spine injury. Pediatric Emergency Medicine Database. The Children's Hospital at Westmead, Paramatta, Austrailia.
8. Viccellio P, Simon H, Pressman BD, et al. A prospective multicenter study of cervical spine injury in children. *Pediatrics* 2001;108:e20–e31.
9. Buhs C, Cullen M, Klein M, et al. The pediatric trauma C-spine: is the odontoid view necessary? *J Pediatr Surg* 2000;35:994–997.
10. Dwek JR, Chung CB. Radiography of cervical spine in children: are flexion-extension radiographs useful for acute trauma? *AJR* 2000;174:1617–1619.

11. Pollack CV, Hendey GW, Martin DR, et al. Use of flexion-extension radiographs of the cervical spine in blunt trauma. *Ann Emerg Med* 2001;38:8–11.
12. Patel JC, Tepas JJ, Mollitt DL, et al. Pediatric cervical spine injuries: defining the disease. *J Pediatr Surg* 2001;36:373–376.
13. Reynolds R. Pediatric spinal injury. *Curr Opin Pediatr* 2000;12:67–71.
14. Flynn JM, Closkey RF, Mahboubi S, et al. Role of magnetic resonance imaging in the assessment of pediatric cervical spine injuries. *J Pediatr Orthop* 2002;22:573–577.
15. Hadley MN. Spinal cord injury without radiographic abnormalitiy. *Neurosurgery* 2002;50:S100–S104.
16. Hoffman JR, Wolfson AB, Todd K, et al. Selective cervical spine radiography in blunt trauma: methodology of the NEXUS. *Ann Emerg Med* 1998;32:461–469.
17. Swischuk LE, John SD, Hendrick EP. Is the open mouth odontoid view necessary in children under 5 years? *Pediatr Radiol* 2002;30:186–189.
18. Pang D, Pollack IF. Spinal cord injury without radiographic abnormality in children—the SCIWORA syndrome. *J Trauma* 1989;29:654–664.
19. Swischuk LE. *Emergency radiology of the acutely ill or injured child: the spine and spinal cord.* 4th ed. Philadelphia: Lippincott Williams & Wilkins; 2000:532–591.
20. Bracken MB, Shepard MJ, Holford TR, et al. Administration of methylprednisolone for 24 or 48 hours or tirilazad mesylate for 48 hours in the treatment of acute spinal cord injury. Results of the third national acute spinal cord injury randomized controlled trial. National acute spinal cord injury study. *JAMA* 1997;277:1597–1604.
21. Hall DE, Boydston W. Pediatric neck injuries. *Pediatr Rev* 1999;20:13–20.
22. Baker C, Kadish H, Schunk JE. Evaluation of pediatric cervical spine injuries. *Am J Emerg Med* 1999;17:230–234.
23. Guidelines for the management of acute cervical spine and spinal cord injuries: Guidelines committee of the section on disorders of the spine and peripheral nerves of the American Association of Neurological Surgeons/Congress of Neurological Surgeons. *Neurosurgery* 2002;50:S67–72.

CHAPTER 10

Thoracic Trauma in Children

Patricio Herrera, MD
Jacob C. Langer, MD, FRCSC

EPIDEMIOLOGY

- Thoracic trauma accounts for between 4.5% and 8% of the patients seen in a pediatric trauma center (Tables 10-1 and 10-2).[1,2]
- Next to head injury, it is the second most common cause of mortality in pediatric trauma (Table 10-3).[3]
- In multi-injured children, thoracic trauma increases mortality 20-fold.
- When combined with head trauma, blunt chest injury has mortality of 40–70%.
- Most common causes of thoracic trauma in children:
  - Motor vehicle accidents (MVAs).
  - Pedestrians.
  - Unrestrained passengers.
  - Bicycle riders.
  - Falls.
- Thoracic trauma epidemiology varies according to social, economic, cultural, and geographic characteristics.
  - Frequency of highway car accidents, car–pedestrian accidents, extreme outdoors activities, socioeconomic status, and degree of unsupervised activities all determine incidence of thoracic trauma.
- Trauma pattern among infants and teens differs:
  - Teens: more penetrating injury and more front seat injuries.
  - Resembles adult pattern.[4]
- Thoracic trauma injuries will often result in abnormal ABCs, requiring:
  - Intubation.
  - Chest tube insertion.
  - Fluid and possible blood administration.
- 10% will need emergency surgery to control bleeding or air leak from lung.

PATHOPHYSIOLOGY

- Compliant chest wall results in more forces transmitted to internal organs, rather than rib fractures.
- The increased tissue elasticity results in increased mediastinal mobility.
- Therefore, tension pneumothorax requires lower pressures and develops more rapidly.[5]
- More prone to hypoxia due to:
  - Higher metabolic rate.
  - Increased oxygen consumption per kilogram of body mass.
  - Reduced functional residual capacity.
- Reduced cardiac capacity for compensation of hypovolemia because of two mechanisms:
  - Stiffness of ventricular wall.
  - Limited improvement by increasing heart rate from tachycardia.
- Children at greater risk for rapid decompensation when exposed to trauma to the chest or trauma with hypovolemia.

TABLE 10-1

Frequency of Injury Among Blunt Thoracic Trauma Pediatric Victims[2,13]

Type of Injury	Relative Frequency[2] (%) (N = 80)	Relative Frequency[13] (%) (N = 137)
Pulmonary contusion	71	27
Rib fracture	35	24.8
Pneumothorax	25	13.1
Isolated rib fracture	11	
Hemothorax	11	18.2
Cardiac	6	2.2
Diaphragmatic rupture	1	2.9

TABLE 10-2

Epidemiology of Chest Injury Regarding Mechanism of Injury[4,8]

	Frequency (%)	Mortality (%)
Blunt	60–80	4–5
MVA	75	
Pedestrian	33	
Occupant	41	
Penetrating	20–40	15–20
Knife	30	
Gun	60	

TABLE 10-3

Mortality Associated with Thoracic Injuries, Overall and Stratified by Diagnosis

Diagnosis	Mortality (%)
Overall	7–15
Isolated chest injury	5
Chest + abdomen	20
Chest + head	35
Blunt + rib fractures[a]	42
Lung laceration	43
Hemothorax	53
Heart/great vessels	75

[a]Blunt chest trauma plus rib fractures, not isolated rib fracture from blunt mechanism.

CLASSIFICATION

- Chest injuries are divided according to mechanism of injury, (e.g., blunt versus penetrating).

Blunt Trauma

- Accounts for over 70–80% of injuries in children with thoracic trauma.[3,4]
- Round or plain surface impacts or holds the chest, transferring energy to the chest wall and internal organs.
- Chest wall's elastic deformation delivers energy directly to internal organs, while deceleration mechanisms tend to hurt the mediastinal structures instead.

Penetrating Trauma

- Object or fragment intrudes the rib cage, directly damaging or disrupting internal organs.
- Position and orientation of the wound tract determine which organs will be injured.
- Most frequent causes are gunshot wounds, stabbing, and impalement.
- Mortality of gunshot injuries is up to 17%.[6]
- Impalement is infrequent. Mainly from falls or falling objects, usually around the house or going over fences.
- Do not remove penetrating objects either on the scene or in the ED. Must be removed in the operating room in a controlled setting.

INITIAL STEPS IN EVALUATION AND MANAGEMENT OF THORACIC TRAUMA

- Patient evaluation follows ATLS/PALS principles.
- ABCs with assessment of airway, breathing, and cervical spine stabilization.
- See Chapter 2 on Primary and Secondary Survey for details.
- Primary survey of chest focused on detecting and treating major life-threatening injuries (mnemonic ATOMCF):
  - Airway obstruction.
  - Tension pneumothorax.
  - Open pneumothorax.
  - Massive hemothorax.
  - Cardiac tamponade.
  - Flail chest.
- Two broad groups of patients:
  - Awake and crying.
  - Unconscious.
- A small, crying patient should be approached in a comforting manner.
  - Assess airway.
  - Give oxygen by face mask.
- Assess breath sounds for symmetry.
  - Decreased breath sounds and hyperresonance suggest pneumothorax.
- In an unconscious or comatose patient (GCS < 8):
  - Secure airway.
  - Assist breathing.
  - Maintain cervical spine immobilization.
  - Assess air entry by auscultation, and order CXR to ensure proper endotracheal tube placement.
  - Assess perfusion by palpating pulses and obtaining blood pressure.
- Whether awake or unconscious, suspicion of a tension pneumothorax should be managed with immediate needle decompression.[5]
  - Do not delay intervention for CXR.
- Suspect hypovolemia and give a normal saline bolus of 20 mL/kg to any patient with multiple or high-energy trauma.

- Re-evaluate need for repeat boluses until improvement in hemodynamic profile is seen and adequate, age-matched urine output is obtained.
- Expose chest completely and palpate gently looking for wounds, deformities, seatbelt or tire markings, crepitations, or tenderness.
  - Paradoxical movement of any segment of the chest wall should be documented and investigated.
- Gunshot wounds should have a surface marker placed prior to obtaining chest x-ray.

HISTORY
- Important features are:
  - Where was the child?
  - Was he or she wearing a seatbelt or in a car seat?
  - How was the child positioned after the accident?
  - Was it a prolonged extrication?
  - What is the clinical status of other members in the vehicle?
  - How much damage was there to the vehicle/bicycle?
- Cars hit on the side carry a higher incidence of head and thoracic trauma, compared to front/rear impacts.[7]

PHYSICAL EXAM
- Ensure complete exposure during primary survey.
- Look for wounds in the axilla, perineum, back, or other hidden areas.
- Main cause of cardiac tamponade is a small stab wound to one of the ventricles.
- Three entities present with the following features:
  - Unstable patient, both hypotensive and hypoxemic.
  - Unresponsive to supplementary oxygen, with respiratory difficulty.
  - A patent airway.
- Tension pneumothorax:
  - Absent or diminished breath sounds on one side.
  - Hyper-resonant on chest percussion.
  - Distended neck veins (unless hypovolemic).
  - A gush of air and immediate improvement should be experienced after needle decompression.
- Massive hemothorax:
  - Absent or diminished breath sounds on affected side.
  - Dullness on chest percussion.
  - Jugular veins are flat because of hypovolemia.
- Cardiac tamponade:
  - Normal or unremarkable auscultation and percussion.
  - Muffled heart sounds.
  - Distended neck veins (extremely rare in pediatric trauma as usually related to penetrating injury).
  - Pulsus paradoxus.

IMAGING
- Obtain AP chest film and if there is high-energy trauma, obtain C-spine and pelvis films to complete primary survey.
- Radiologic evaluation with chest CT should only be done when the patient is hemodynamically stable (Table 10-4).
- Gunshot wounds need CXR with surface markers on any wound to evaluate trajectories.
  - If any trajectories go across thorax (transmediastinal), surgical exploration is indicated.
- Multiply injured patients may benefit from FAST (focused assessment sonography for trauma) to rule out massive intra-abdominal or thoracic hemorrhage and cardiac tamponade. See Chapter 4 on Diagnostic Imaging for details.

TABLE 10-4

Indications for Additional Studies

CT of the Chest	Angiography	Bronchoscopy
Diagnosis MVA related blunt trauma, falls higher than 10 feet, any penetrating trauma	Widened mediastinum, high-energy mechanism	Suspicion or certainty of central airway lesions secondary to blunt or penetrating trauma to the neck or chest
Suspicion Lung contusion, mediastinal widening, hemothorax		*Has to be done by the* **most** *experienced person available*

EMERGENCY DEPARTMENT THORACOTOMY
- Extremely rare.
- Emergency room thoracotomy should be limited to:
  - Patients who arrive in the emergency room with vital signs and subsequently suffer a witnessed cardiac arrest.
  - Patients with penetrating injuries who arrive pulseless but with electric myocardial activity.
    - Survival in this scenario is 50%, compared to 2.3% published for overall emergency room thoracotomy survival in pediatric patients.[8]

INDICATIONS FOR CHEST TUBE INSERTION
- Partially decompressed tension pneumothorax.
- Confirmed and clinically significant pneumothorax.
- Small pneumothorax considering road or air transport risks.
- Hemothorax of any magnitude (Table 10-5).

DEFINITIVE MANAGEMENT OF THORACIC TRAUMA
- See Figure 10-1.
- ABCs take priority, along with C-spine precautions.
- Rule out tension pneumothorax, hemothorax, and cardiac tamponade.
- Persistent tachycardia without an obvious cause may indicate internal thoracic or abdominal organ injury.

TABLE 10-5

Chest Tube Size by Patient Weight[4]

Weight (kg)	Chest Tube Size
3–5	10–12 FR
6–9	12–16 FR
10–11	16–20 FR
12–14	20–22 FR
15–18	22–24 FR
19–22	24–28 FR
23–30	24–32 FR
>32	32–40 FR

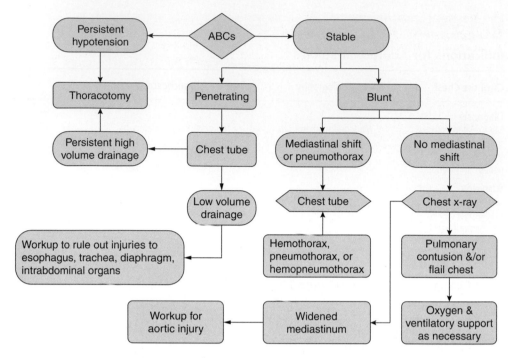

FIGURE 10-1 ● Management of thoracic injuries.

- Up to 8% of thoracic trauma patients require surgery.
  - Immediate versus delayed thoracotomy should be decided (Table 10-6).
- Several approaches exist for repairing lung, heart, or great vessel lacerations.[14,15]

SPECIFIC BLUNT INJURIES
Rib Cage and Diaphragm:
- Rib fractures.
- Sternal fracture.
- Scapular fracture.
- Flail chest.
- Hemothorax.
- Diaphragmatic rupture.

TABLE 10-6

Emergency Versus Delayed Indications for Thoracostomy[8]

Immediate	Delayed
Massive hemothorax[a]	Clotted hemothorax
Massive continuous bronchopleural fistula	Persistent chylothorax
Cardiac tamponade	Traumatic intracardiac defects
Esophageal injury	Chronic atelectasis
Diaphragmatic injury	Foreign body removal
Aortic injury	
Penetrating trauma to main airway	
Open pneumothorax	

[a]Massive hemothorax: 20–25% of estimated blood volume (EBV) being recovered at the moment of chest tube placement, or persistent hemorrhage, with a rate of bleeding that exceeds 2 mL/kg/hr.

Rib Fracture
- Usually older children and teenagers.
- Infrequent in children under 10 because of thoracic elasticity.
  - If present in this age group, should raise concern about the amount of energy involved in the accident.
  - In children under 3 years of age, suspect child abuse.
- If four or more fractured ribs, always suspect that another intrathoracic organ may be injured.[3]
- Watch for subsequent pain with movement and deep breathing.
- If not accompanied by pneumothorax, rib fracture rarely produces tachypnea, but shortness of breath could be produced by pain.
- Treatment:
  - Rest and analgesia.
  - Immobilize under special circumstances, with duct-taping of the entire rib from spine to sternum.
  - May relieve pain.

Sternal Fracture
- Caused by significant amount of energy applied to one spot.
  - Usually a weight-bearing knee or shoulder against the sternum.
- History of pain only when holding deep breath or lifting heavy objects.
- Single-point pain triggered by palm pressure on the different segments of sternum.
- Radiologic confirmation usually very difficult.
- Diagnosis relies on high index of suspicion because of the mechanism and location of pain.
- If MVA related, suspect cardiac contusion.
- Treatment:
  - Rest and avoiding possibly risky activities (sports, bicycle, skates, etc.).
  - Nonsteroidal anti-inflammatory agents (NSAIDs) first 24 to 48 hrs.

Scapular Fracture
- Rare.
- High-energy impact on upper chest.
- Should search for specific vascular or lung complications.
- Radiologic evaluation of the scapula with axial views.
- Treatment:
  - May require surgical correction.
  - Orthopedic surgery consultation needed, after patient has been stabilized following ABC prioritization.
  - Rest and analgesia.

Flail Chest
- Segment of one or more ribs fractured in two different points.
  - Generates unstable "soft" area experiencing paradoxical movement with respiratory pressure changes.
- Diagnosis mainly clinical, confirmed radiologically.
- High-energy mechanism needed.
  - Rare in pediatrics due to elasticity of chest wall.
- The important feature is not the mechanical abnormality of the chest wall, but the underlying pulmonary contusion that produces hypoxemia despite high inhaled oxygen concentration (V/Q mismatch).
- Consolidation of the affected lung is seen on chest x-ray and CT scan.
- Treatment:
  - May need mechanical ventilation (admit patient likely to the intensive-care unit).

Hemothorax (Due to Chest Wall Bleeding) Figure 10-2
- Blood in the pleural space due to rupture of intercostal vessels or to bone bleeding from a fractured rib.

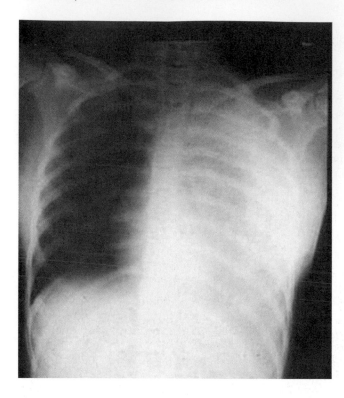

FIGURE 10-2 ● Left hemo-thorax. There is diffuse opacity of the left chest due to blood, which may arise from the lung, chest wall, or vascular structures within the chest.

- Can be severe enough to produce hypotension.
- Clinical signs: Dullness on percussion and asymmetric air entry on auscultation, both in the more dependant areas of the chest.
- Treatment:
  - Chest tube insertion.
  - Need for surgical intervention determined by amount of blood recovered, and rate of bleeding (see Table 10-6).

Diaphragmatic Rupture
- Usually result of blunt abdominal trauma.
  - Acute high pressure in abdominal compartment produces shearing of the diaphragm with herniation of abdominal viscera into the chest.
  - More frequent in the left hemi-diaphragm.
  - CXR may show:
    - "Large aerated cysts" near base of left lung.
    - NG tube going into left hemithorax can confirm diagnosis, or a contrast study through the NG tube if there are any doubts.
- Treatment:
  - Prompt surgical management because hernia incarceration likely.

Specific Injuries to the Lungs, Airway, and Esophagus
- Pneumothorax, hemopneumothorax, lung contusion, pneumatocele, bronchial or tracheal tear, and esophageal rupture.

Pneumothorax (Figure 10-3)
- Air presence in pleural space.
  - Air can come from the airway, lung, or from outside the chest wall through an open wound or a leaking chest tube system.

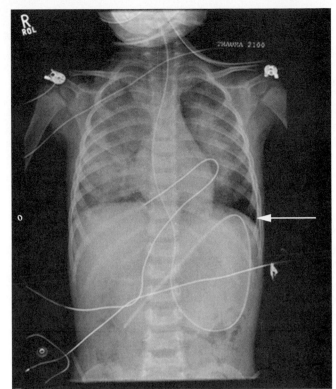

FIGURE 10-3 ● Left pneumothorax *(arrow)*. There is partial collapse of the left lung, with associated bilateral pulmonary contusion. There is no shift of the mediastinum, indicating that this is *not* a tension pneumothorax.

- Clinical signs:
  - Tachypnea.
  - Shortness of breath.
  - Hyper-resonance on percussion.
  - Diminished breath sounds on auscultation of the affected side.
- Signs can be subtle or obvious depending on size of pneumothorax and respiratory baseline condition.
- Large pneumothorax can present with subcutaneous emphysema.
- Treatment:
  - Chest tube insertion.
  - See Table 10-5 for chest tube sizes.
  - See Chapter 21 on Procedures for details.

Tension Pneumothorax (Figure 10-4)
- Air in the pleural space is under pressure because of a one-way valve mechanism.
- Impairs venous return to the heart due to mediastinal shift away from affected side.
- Clinical signs:
  - Hypotension.
  - Distended jugular veins.
  - Shifted heart sounds.
  - Hyper-resonance.
- Treatment:
  - Immediate needle decompression, followed by chest tube insertion.

Hemopneumothorax
- Blood and air present in pleural space.
  - Usually secondary to the same parenchymal lung injury.
- Management principles are the same as for isolated pneumothorax or hemothorax.

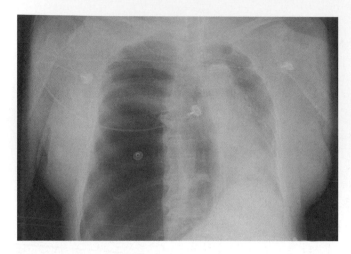

FIGURE 10-4 ● Tension pneumothorax. The lung is collapsed with mediastinal shift to the opposite side, indicating a tension pneumothorax. This is a life-threatening emergency and must be immediately treated with needle decompression, followed by tube thoracostomy. Ideally, this diagnosis should be made and treated before an x-ray like this is taken. (Courtesy of Fred Brenneman, MD.)

Pulmonary Contusion (Figure 10-5)

- Pulmonary consolidation due to hemorrhage and swelling secondary to direct mechanical injury to the lung parenchyma.
- Seen on initial chest films.
  - Can become evident within 6 to 8 hours after trauma and resuscitation.[3]
- Usually stable from third day on.
- Most will only need some supplementary oxygen, but depending on extent of contusion, some will need full support for acute respiratory distress syndrome.[3]
- Usually after consolidation comes contamination.
  - Some administer initial brochial-alveolar lavage and culture to rationalize antibiotic treatment.
- Full functional recovery occurs, but sometimes may take several months.[9]

Pneumatocele

- Usually seen after pneumonia, but can also infrequently occur from blunt trauma with acute high pressure inside the airway.[9]
- Diagnosis can be made on CXR or CT.
- Usually resolves on its own within 2 months.
- Surgery recommended if pneumatocele increases in size or produce respiratory difficulty.
- When rapid growth of the pneumatocele is seen, early formal lobectomy is recommended.[9]

Bronchial or Tracheal Tears

- Infrequent, usually small tears close to carina, in posterior membranous wall of trachea and bronchi.
- Usual presentation is:
  - Dyspnea.
  - Subcutaneous emphysema of the neck or chest wall (present in 85% of patients).
  - Possible hemoptysis.
- Usually the CXR shows subcutaneous emphysema, pneumothorax, and/or pneumomediastinum with some degree of atelectasis that does not completely resolve with a chest tube.
- Persistent, continuous air leak (inspiratory and expiratory).
- Treatment:
  - Antibiotic therapy (first-generation cephalosporin).
  - Early bronchoscopy.
  - Medical treatment should be sufficient for most tears up to one-third of the circumference and should include gentle respiratory physiotherapy and frequent CXR to assess complete lung re-expansion.

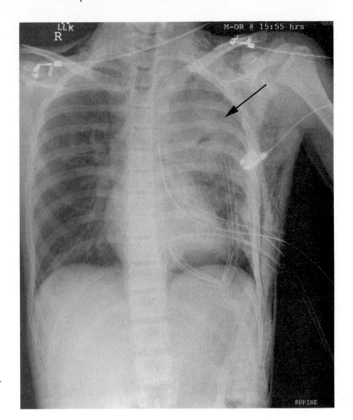

FIGURE 10-5 ● Left pulmonary contusion *(arrow)*. The upper lung is opacified, suggesting direct trauma to the parenchyma.

- Indications for surgery:
  - Incomplete re-expansion.
  - Signs of pleural empyema.
  - Respiratory embarrassment because of bronchopleural fistula formation.
  - Delay will only increase the probability of stenosis, chronic atelectasis, chronic bronchopleural fistula, empyema, or recurrence.

Esophageal Rupture

- Usual mechanism from blunt trauma is sudden increase in pressure.
- Rupture can occur proximally at the end of the pyriform sinus or in distal part of esophagus.
- Cervical esophagus rupture associated with abrupt hyperextension of the neck (boxing injury).[10]
- Classic presentation is mild pneumomediastinum that can compromise base of neck and supraclavicular spaces.
- Pleural effusion (on either side) can be present.
- Esophagography and endoscopy to establish definite diagnosis.
- NG tube should only be placed under endoscopic visualization.
- Treatment:
  - Usually medical (broad-spectrum antibiotics and NPO) with or without thoracostomy tubes.
  - If significant signs of mediastinitis are present, a surgical approach can be taken, consisting of esophageal repair, wide drainage of mediastinal pleura, and possible exclusion of the esophagus with a proximal esophagostomy.

Specific Injuries to the Heart and Great Vessels

- Cardiac tamponade, cardiac contusion, blunt cardiac rupture, blunt aortic injury, and commotio cordis.

Cardiac Tamponade
- Blood present in potential space of pericardium.
- Restricts passive filling of myocardium, creating a preload impairment and subsequently shock that only responds to liberating the pressure and surgically addressing intrapericardial bleeding's origin.
- Penetrating trauma is the most frequent cause.
- Clinical picture:
  - Muffled heart sounds.
  - Low blood pressure.
  - Tachycardia.
  - Jugular vein distension.
  - **Normal** breath sounds (helps distinguish it from tension pneumothorax).
- Diagnosis can be confirmed by FAST if available.
- Treatment:
  - Pericardiocentesis (which at the same time confirms the diagnosis if no ultrasound is available).
  - Definitive treatment is operative exploration of the pericardium.
- Air from tracheobronchial injuries can rarely also produce cardiac tamponade.
- Watch for pneumopericardium on CXR!

Cardiac Contusion
- Clinical presentation: Child with A-P chest wall compression or high-energy accident, possibility of other systems and organs injured.
  - Partial or no response to volume resuscitation, possibility of development of repolarization anomalies or wide-complex arrhythmias.[1,8]
- Myocardium bruising and swelling due to direct compression between the sternum and the thoracic vertebrae.
- A young child may have cardiac contusion without a sternal fracture.
- Echocardiogram may reveal dyskinetic areas.
- Vasoactive drugs could be gently used in resuscitation, but increasing metabolic stress into the myocardial wall could negatively affect myocardial function.
- If suspected, obtain and follow CPK, CPK-MB, and troponin I levels, along with follow-up and imaging before definite discharge. (Echocardiogram within 2 weeks after trauma.)
- There are some reports of delayed spontaneous rupture of pseudoaneurysm secondary to cardiac contusion and silent myocardial necrosis up to 2 months after trauma.[11,12]

Blunt Cardiac Rupture
- Results from high-energy MVA or very high falls.
- Patients present in a variety of forms:
  - Sudden death episode just seconds or minutes after the traumatic event (ventricular wall rupture) with cardiovascular collapse because of either exsanguination or cardiac tamponade.
  - Acute heart failure of rapid onset because of the rupture of a tendinous cord, with a heart murmur and valvular dysfunction, and delayed diagnosis; same as VSD secondary to trauma.

Blunt Aortic Injury
- Uncommon in pediatrics.
- Usually seen in MVA ejection victims over 7 years old.
- Aortic wall ruptures because of deceleration forces.
- Occurs around the ligamentum arteriosum, at the junction between the fixed and mobile portions of the aorta.
- Mortality at the scene of injury up to 85%.

- No specific sign or pain pattern, therefore maintain a high index of suspicion.
- Suspect if:
  - First rib and sternal fractures.
  - Transient hypotension.
  - Paraplegia.
  - Hypertension in upper extremities.
  - Weak pulses in lower limbs.
- CXR may show:
  - Mediastinal widening.
  - Loss of normal aortic knob.
  - Deviation of the mediastinum and mainstem bronchus.
  - Apical cap.
  - Fractured rib 1 or 2.
  - Hemothorax.
- If suspected, CT angiography of the chest or conventional angiography of the arch to confirm diagnosis.
- Same mechanism is responsible for carotid disruption from innominate truncus, in severe head and neck trauma leading to an intrathoracic lesion (high speed MVA, snowboard jumping).
- Treatment:
  - Medical: Keep blood pressure under control using beta-blockers.
  - Surgical treatment for repair.
- Growth must be kept in mind if any repair shall consider graft interposition, in order to avoid pseudo-coarctation over time.

Commotio Cordis
- Extremely rare occurrence.
- Sudden cardiac death from a blow to the precordium at vulnerable period (15 to 30 ms before the peak of the T-wave).
  - Impact during the vulnerable period results in ventricular fibrillation and sudden death.
  - Dependent on:
    - Location of impact.
    - Timing of impact.
    - Force of impact.
- Treatment:
  - Prompt defibrillation could be lifesaving.[3]

Indirect Trauma–Pulmonary Blast Injury
- Suspect blast injury regardless of:
  - Distance between patient and the blast center.
  - The absence of injuries in other people at the scene.
- Eardrums are the first injured tissues after a blast.
  - Of those severely injured in the 2004 Madrid bombing, 67% had eardrum injuries, mostly bilateral.
- Lungs are the next target for blast injuries.
  - Frothy oral secretions with pulmonary edema of rapid onset carries a poor prognosis.
  - Expanding wave of pressure/underpressure expands into the airway and produces capillary disruption within the alveoli.
  - Followed by edema, hemorrhage, and systemic gas embolism that can affect brain and spine.
  - Israeli experience suggests that after successful management of initial respiratory failure with mechanical ventilation and support, long-term respiratory function is very good in most cases.

CLINICAL PEARLS

DO

- Expose the chest completely and palpate for wounds, deformities, crepitations, or tenderness.
- Consider tension pneumothorax and cardiac tamponade if patient has distended neck veins.
- Remember that pulmonary contusions may not be seen on the initial chest x-ray. Clinical suspicion and repeat imaging are required for recognition.
- Consider bronchial or tracheal tears in the presence of persistent inspiratory and expiratory air leak.

DON'T

- Delay intervention when suspecting tension pneumothorax. A chest x-ray should NOT be done before needle decompression.
- Miss any wounds in the axilla, perineum, back, or hidden areas. Always expose the patient completely.
- Place NG tube blindly when you suspect esophageal rupture. This needs to be done under endoscopic visualization.

REFERENCES

1. Eichelberger MR. *Pediatric trauma: prevention, acute care, rehabilitation.* St. Louis: Mosby Year Book; 1993.
2. Holmes JF. A clinical decision rule for identifying children with thoracic injuries after blunt trauma. *Ann Emerg Med* 2002;39:492–499.
3. Sartorelli KH, Vane DW. The diagnosis and management of children with blunt injury of the chest. *Semin Pediatr Surg* 2004;13:98–105.
4. Bliss D, Silen M. Pediatric thoracic trauma. *Crit Care Med* 2002;30(suppl):409–415.
5. American College of Surgeons Committee on Trauma. *ATLS student course manual.* 7th ed. Chicago: American College of Surgeons; 1997.
6. Cotton BA, Nance ML. Penetrating trauma in children. *Semin Pediatr Surg* 2004;13:87–97.
7. Orzechowski KM, Edgerton EA, Bulas DI, et al. Patterns of injury to restrained children in side impact motor vehicle crashes: the side impact syndrome. *J Trauma* 2003;54:1094–1101.
8. O'Neil J. *Principles of pediatric surgery.* 2nd ed. St. Louis: Mosby Year Book; 2003.
9. Haxhija EQ, Nores H, Schober P, Hollwarth ME. Lung contusion-lacerations after blunt thoracic trauma in children. *Pediatr Surg Int* 2004;20:412–414.
10. Pearson FG, Cooper JD, Deslauriers J, et al. *Thoracic surgery.* 2nd ed. Churchill Livingstone. Elsevier; 2002:1845.
11. RuDusky BM. Myocardial contusion culminating in a ruptured pseudoaneurysm of the left ventricle—a case report. *Angiology* 2003;54:359–362.
12. Pollak S, Stellwag-Carion C. Delayed cardiac rupture due to blunt chest trauma. *Am J Forensic Med Pathol* 1991;12:153–156.
13. Balci AE, Kazez A, Eren S, et al. Blunt thoracic trauma in children: review of 137 cases. *Eur J Cardiothorac Surg* 2004;26:387–392.
14. Gasparri M, Karmy-Jones R, Kralovich KA, et al. Pulmonary tractotomy versus lung resection: viable options in penetrating lung injury. *J Trauma* 2001;51:1092–1097.
15. Cothren C, Moore EE, Biffl WL, et al. Lung sparing techniques are associated with improved outcome compared with anatomic resection for severe lung injuries. *J Trauma* 2002;53:483–487.

CHAPTER 11

Abdominal and Pelvic Trauma

Mohammed Zamakhshary, MD, MEd, FRCSC
Paul W. Wales, MD, MSc, FRCSC, FACS

EPIDEMIOLOGY

- Blunt trauma accounts for >90% of injuries in children.
- 8–12% of blunt trauma victims will have abdominal injuries.
- Penetrating injuries account for less than 10% of all abdominal injuries.
- Although more common than thoracic injuries, abdominal injuries are 40% less fatal.[1]
- Mortality from solid organ injuries is typically determined by the degree of injury.[2,3]

PATHOPHYSIOLOGY

- Motor vehicle crashes (MVCs), pedestrian collisions, and falls are the most common mechanisms of pediatric abdominal trauma.[4]
- Be suspicious of possible abdominal injuries in seatbelt injuries, handlebar injuries, nonaccidental injuries, and snowboarding and all-terrain vehicle accidents.[4]
- There are important anatomic differences between children and adults:
  - Children are smaller, transferring kinetic energy over a smaller area.[4]
  - Ribs are less calcified and more pliable, resulting in more force transmitted to thoracic and upper abdominal organs.[4]
  - Thinner abdominal wall and weaker musculature provide less protection to intra-abdominal organs.[4]
  - Infants and young children are at higher risk for multiple organ injuries due to the close proximity of intra-abdominal organs.[4]

INITIAL EVALUATION

- See Chapter 2 on Primary and Secondary Survey for details.
- Resuscitate by following Advanced Trauma Life Support (ATLS) guidelines.
- Maintain a high index of suspicion for abdominal injuries in children.
- **Most solid organ abdominal injuries are treated nonoperatively.**
- Nonoperative treatment requires an accurate diagnosis and evaluation of injuries.
- Decision to manage abdominal injuries nonoperatively should be reserved for centers experienced in this approach.
- The appropriate expertise (surgical, critical care, anesthesia, nursing, and blood bank) is required to enable rapid operative treatment in case of complications.

HISTORY

- Acquire an "AMPLE" history: Allergies, Medications, Past medical history, Last meal, and Events (mechanism).
- Acquire a detailed history of the mechanism of injury.
- Unclear mechanism or repeated visits to the emergency room should raise suspicion for nonaccidental injuries.
- Certain traumatic mechanisms indicate patterns of injury.[5] For example, handlebar, seatbelt, and nonaccidental injuries are associated with pancreatic and duodenal injuries.[6,7]

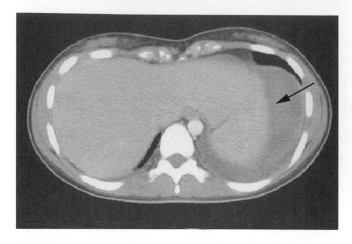

FIGURE 11-1 ● Adolescent female with mononucleosis presented with splenic rupture after a trivial fall. CT scan shows free fluid *(arrow)* in left upper quadrant.

- Children with bleeding disorders are at high risk from solid organ injuries even with minor injury mechanisms.[4,8–9]
- Epstein–Barr virus (EBV) infection with splenomegaly places children at high risk of splenic rupture from trivial trauma mechanisms (Fig. 11-1).[4]

PHYSICAL EXAMINATION

- Physical signs indicative of possible abdominal injuries include:
  - Abdominal tenderness.
  - Distension.
  - Abrasions.
  - Ecchymosis.
- Cotton and associates documented the predictive value of these physical examination abnormalities (tenderness Odds Ratio (OR) 40.7, ecchymosis OR 15.8, and abrasions OR 16.8).[10]
- Accurately examining a small child with trauma can be challenging due to age, limited verbal ability, and distraction from painful injuries.[11]
- Repeated physical examination improves accuracy and confidence.
- Presence of the seatbelt sign (ecchymosis across the abdomen caused by wearing a lapbelt) should raise suspicion of intra-abdominal injuries (Fig. 11-2).
- Due to aerophagia, abdominal distension in children is commonly from gastric distension (Fig. 11-3).
  - Early placement of nasogastric or orogastric tubes along with Foley catheterization allows for more accurate abdominal physical exam.

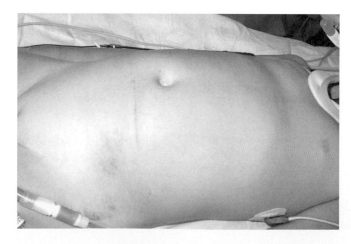

FIGURE 11-2 ● Seatbelt sign. This patient has classic abdominal wall contusion and abrasions.

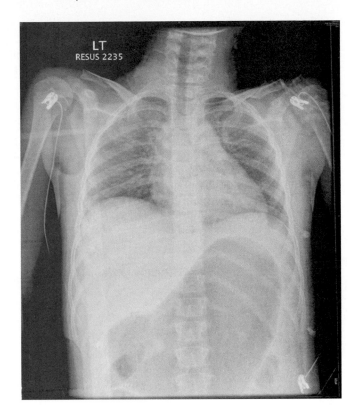

FIGURE 11-3 ● Gastric distension. Significant abdominal distension in children may be caused by gastric distension from aerophagia.

LABORATORY INVESTIGATIONS

- Laboratory tests in pediatric trauma should include:
  - Complete blood count (CBC).
  - Blood type and screen.
  - Serum electrolytes and glucose.
  - Venous blood gas and renal function.
  - Liver transaminases (ALT, AST).
  - Amylase and/or lipase.
  - Coagulation profile (INR, PTT).
  - Urinalysis (UA).
  - Beta-HCG (if a female is more than 10 years of age).
  - Toxicology screen as indicated.
- Laboratory investigations are a *screening* tool for intra-abdominal injuries.
- Their true utility is uncertain.
- Results may suggest an injury and call for definitive imaging.
- Amylase:
  - Often initially normal in pancreatic injuries.
  - Can be abnormal with no pancreatic injury.
  - Elevation may reflect:
    - Salivary amylase from head and neck injury.
    - Bowel obstruction.
    - Small bowel injury.
  - Elevated amylase <500 μ/L in the short-term should raise suspicion of hollow viscous injury.
- Holmes and associates performed a prospective, nonrandomized study examining the utility of laboratory testing in pediatric abdominal trauma while adjusting for physical examination findings.[12]

- 1,095 injured children presented to an American level 1 trauma center.
- 107 of 1,095 (10%) had abdominal injuries.
- Using a logistic regression model and internally validating the model, the independent predictors of abdominal injuries were found to be: **Predictor OR (95% CI)**.
  - Low blood pressure, 4.1 (1.1, 15.2).
  - Abdominal tenderness, 5.8 (3.2, 10.4).
  - ALT >125 or AST >200, 17.4 (9.4, 32.1).
  - UA showing >5 RBC/hpf, 4.8 (2.7, 8.4).

IMAGING
- Diagnosis of intra-abdominal injuries relies on diagnostic imaging modalities.
- History, physical exam, and laboratory investigations are important *screening* tools for abdominal injuries but have limited sensitivity and specificity.
- Radiologic modalities used are as follows:

X-Rays
- Pediatric trauma patients should receive the standard:
  - Lateral C-spine.
  - AP chest.
  - Pelvic x-rays.
  - See Chapter 4 on Diagnostic Imaging for details.

Plain Abdominal X-Rays
- Abdominal series have no role in investigating acutely injured children.

Computed Tomography (CT)
- Intravenous contrast-enhanced CT is the gold standard for diagnosing and evaluating intra-abdominal injuries.
- CT evaluates solid organs, hollow viscera, free air, and the retroperitoneum.
- Hemodynamic stability is a prerequisite to acquiring a CT scan.
- The need for oral contrast is controversial.
  - Proponents argue oral contrast may enhance diagnostic utility of CT in hollow viscus injuries.
  - Opponents of oral contrast stress:
    - The risks of vomiting and aspiration, especially in children with both torso and head injuries.
    - It does not have time to opacify the distal bowel, and therefore does not fully rule out a perforated viscus.
    - Delaying CT until full bowel opacification is achieved is unacceptable for trauma patients.
- In a recent prospective adult study, 500 patients in a level 1 trauma center underwent IV contrast-enhanced CT without oral contrast:[13]
  - Sensitivity and specificity of CT for detecting blunt bowel injuries were 90.5 and 99.6, respectively.
  - At the Hospital for Sick Children, oral contrast is used selectively, reserving it for patients with a high pretest likelihood of having a duodenal injury.

Focused Assessment Sonogram for Trauma (FAST)[5]
- To rapidly assess for free fluid in the abdomen or in the pericardial sac.
- Widely accepted in the initial workup of adult trauma patients.
- Created to replace diagnostic peritoneal lavage (DPL), *not* CT scan.
- FAST is reliable in detecting abdominal free fluid in pediatric patients.[5]
- Utility of FAST in children is questionable.
  - Hemoperitoneum alone is NOT an indication for surgery in children.
  - Almost all solid organ injuries (liver/spleen) are managed nonoperatively.

- FAST may play a role in very specific clinical scenarios:
  - A hemodynamically unstable child who requires emergency surgery (e.g., craniotomy), to rule out the abdomen as the source of hemorrhagic shock.
  - To triage patients for CT scans of the abdomen, as 41% to 75% of scans performed for trauma are normal (e.g., FAST could act as a screening tool for the need for CT scan).
- Maintenance of FAST skills can be challenging with low volumes of pediatric trauma.
- Use of FAST in pediatric trauma should be determined on an institution-specific basis.

MRI
- MRI is not needed for managing pediatric abdominal or pelvic trauma.
- May be beneficial for certain disease processes.

GI Studies
- UGI series, small bowel follow-through, and contrast enemas have no role in workup of an acutely injured child.

Diagnostic Peritoneal Lavage (DPL)
- CT scan availability has eliminated need for DPL in traumatized children.
- A positive DPL is NOT an indication for abdominal surgery in hemodynamically stable patients.
- DPL provides no information about retroperitoneal injuries.
- Performed by infusing 10 mL/kg normal saline into peritoneal cavity followed by gravity drainage of fluids and examination (gross and microscopic) of the fluids.
- The criteria for a positive DPL are as follows:
  - 10 mL of gross blood return.
  - >100,000 RBCs/mm^3.
  - >500 WBCs/mm^3.
  - Amylase >175 IU/dL.
  - Bile, bacteria, or vegetable matter on microscopy.

SPECIFIC ORGAN INJURY
Spleen
- Most injured abdominal organ in children.
- Mostly blunt mechanism, with MVCs and falls being most common.
- History and physical signs in patients with splenic injury:
  - Left shoulder pain (Kehr sign).
  - Abrasions to left upper quadrant.
  - Tenderness in left upper quadrant.
  - Abdominal distension.
  - Signs and symptoms of hypovolemic shock.
  - Recent history of EBV infection (Fig. 11-1).
- Diagnosed with IV enhanced CT scan.
- Missed injuries are rare.
- The degree of splenic injury is graded by CT scan (Table 11-1).
- CT grade of injury does NOT correlate with need for operative intervention.
- **Hemodynamic condition is most important in making treatment decisions.**
- Nonoperative treatment in *hemodynamically stable children.*
- Adequate fluid and blood administration is required to achieve hemodynamic stability.

Nonoperative Management of Splenic Injuries
- Successful in **97%** of cases.
- Is more successful in pediatric trauma centers compared to adult centers.
- Requires aggressive and adequate fluid and blood resuscitation.
- Initial admission to ICU or close observation unit.
- Complete bed rest initially.
- Close observation when reinstating mobilization.

TABLE 11-1

AAST Splenic Injury Scale

Grade	Inquiry Description
I. Hematoma	Subcapsular, nonexpanding, <10% of surface area
Laceration	Capsular tear, nonbleeding, <1 cm of parenchymal depth
II. Hematoma	Subcapsular, nonexpanding, 10–50% of surface area; intraparenchymal, nonexpanding, <2 cm in diameter
Laceration	Capsular tear, active bleeding, 1–3 cm of parenchymal depth that does not involve a trabecular vessel
III. Hematoma	Subcapsular, >50% of surface area or expanding, ruptured subcapsular hematoma with active bleeding, intraparenchymal hematoma, >2 cm or expanding
Laceration	>3 cm or parenchymal depth or involving trabecular vessels
IV. Hematoma	Ruptured intraparenchymal hematoma with active bleeding
Laceration	Laceration involving segmental or hilar vessel producing major devascularization (>25% of spleen)
V. Laceration	Completely shattered spleen
Vascular	Hilar vascular injury that devascularizes spleen

Adapted from the American Association for the Surgery of Trauma (AAST).
Moore EE, Shackford SR, Pachter HG, et al. Organ injury scaling: spleen, liver and kindly 1989 (29):1664–66.

- Restriction of activity postdischarge (Table 11-2).
- Requires high level of expertise in nonoperative treatment.
- Results in fewer transfusions compared to operative treatment.
- American Pediatric Surgery Association (APSA) used injury grade to stratify patients and provide evidence-based guidelines for nonoperative treatment and resource utilization in children with liver and spleen injuries (Table 11-2).[14]
  - APSA guidelines were developed retrospectively and then validated prospectively.
  - Reviewed 832 pediatric splenic/liver trauma patients, the use of ICU beds, length of stay, need for transfusion, laparotomy, and post-injury imaging utilization were recorded.
  - The guidelines were based on injury grade and evaluated prospectively in 16 centers over a 2-year period.
  - Using the guidelines resulted in a statistically significant shift toward more optimal use of resources, as evidenced by fewer ICU stays ($p <0.0001$), decreased length of stay ($p <0.0006$), and less follow-up imaging ($p <0.0001$) in each injury grade.
  - This improvement was not associated with any adverse events.

TABLE 11-2

APSA Guideline to Optimize Utilization of Resources in Splenic Injuries

Injury Grade	I	II	III	IV
ICU stay (days)	None	None	None	1
LOS (days)	2	3	4	5
Predischarge imaging	None	None	None	None
Postdischarge imaging	None	None	None	None
Activity restriction (wk)	3	4	5	6

From Stylianos S. Evidence-based guidelines for resource utilization in children with isolated spleen or liver injury. J Pediatr Surg 2000;35:164–169.

- Indications for operative treatment:
  - Persistent hypotension, despite ongoing aggressive resuscitation (>50% of blood volume transfused within first 24 hours—e.g., 40 mL/kg of blood).
  - Other indication for laparotomy (e.g., pneumoperitoneum).
  - Clinical deterioration despite active nonoperative treatment.
- Operative treatment:
  - Initial attempts are to preserve the spleen.
  - Angiographic embolization may have role if evidence of contrast extravasation "blush" on CT scan.
  - Main advantage of splenorrhaphy or partial splenectomy is to preserve the spleen's immunologic function, to prevent overwhelming postsplenectomy infections (OPSI).
  - Splenectomy is indicated in the unstable patient.
- All splenectomized patients require vaccination prior to discharge to protect against the following encapsulated organisms:
  - *Streptococcus pneumoniae.*
  - *Haemophilus influenzae* type B.
  - *Neisseria meningitides.*
- Penicillin prophylaxis is also required, the duration of which is uncertain.
  - Recommendations vary from as short as 2 years to lifelong prophylaxis.
- OPSI risk is 0.23% to 0.42%/yr, and lifetime risk is 3.2% to 5%.
  - The greatest risk is in children under the age of 5 years.[15]
  - Mortality from OPSI is 38% to 69%.[16]

Liver

- Second most injured abdominal organ in pediatric blunt trauma.
- Right lobe is injured more often than left lobe.
- History and physical signs seen in patients with liver injury include:
  - Abdominal pain and/or distension.
  - Right shoulder pain from diaphragmatic irritation.
  - Abrasions to right side of the abdomen.
  - Tachycardia and hypotension.
- Associated injuries are common in children with liver trauma.
- Elevated transaminases on initial blood work raise suspicion for liver injury.
- CT for diagnosing and grading liver injuries (Table 11-3).

TABLE 11-3

AAST Liver Injury Scale

Grade	Injury Description
I. Hematoma	Subcapsular, nonexpanding, <10% of surface area
Laceration	Capsular tear, nonbleeding, <1 cm deep parenchymal disruption
II. Hematoma	Subcapsular, nonexpanding, hematoma 10–50%, intraparenchymal, nonexpanding, <2 cm in diameter
Laceration	<3 cm of parenchymal depth, <10 cm in length
III. Hematoma	Subcapsular, >50% of surface area or expanding, ruptured subcapsular hematoma with active bleeding, intraparenchymal hematoma, >2 cm
Laceration	>3 cm or parenchymal depth
IV. Hematoma	Ruptured central hematoma
Laceration	Parenchymal destruction involving 25–75% of hepatic lobe
V. Laceration	Parenchymal destruction >75% of hepatic lobe
Vascular	Juxtahepatic venous injuries (retrohepatic cava/major hepatic veins)
VI. Vascular	Hepatic avulsion

Adapted from the American Association for the Surgery of Trauma (AAST).
Moore EE, Shackford SR, Pachter HG, et al. Organ injury scaling: spleen, liver and kindly 1989 (29):1664–66.

- CT grade of liver injury does not predict need for operative intervention.[17]
- Nonoperative management:
  - Mainstay of treatment.
  - Follows the same principles observed in splenic injuries (see above).
  - **90% to 95%** of liver injuries can be treated nonoperatively.
  - Liver injuries require more blood transfusions than do splenic injuries.
- Interventions available to the surgeon treating liver injuries are:
  - Angiographic embolization of ongoing bleeding or hemobilia.
  - Endoscopic retrograde cholangiopancreatography (ERCP).
  - Percutaneous drainage of biloma and fluid collections.
- Indications for operative intervention are similar to splenic trauma.
- Operative treatment:
  - The principle operative approach is that of "damage control."
  - Definitive repair or formal resection is rarely indicated.
  - Ongoing resuscitation and correction of coexistent hypothermia or coagulopathy.
  - Complications of operative treatment include:
    - Rebleeding.
    - Infection.
    - Biloma.
    - Biliary obstruction.
    - Hemobilia.
- Activity restriction and postdischarge investigations should follow the American Association of Pediatric Surgeons recommendations (Table 11-2).

Small Bowel
- Small bowel injury is less common than spleen and liver trauma.
- Diagnosis can be difficult and requires a high index of suspicion.
- Diagnosis usually requires serial physical examinations and may require serial imaging studies. Therefore, diagnosis of small bowel injuries can be delayed.
- In a recent review of GI injuries in 11,592 children over 12 years:[18]
  - The incidence of small bowel injury was <1%.
  - The mechanism of injury was most likely related to specific point of energy transfer (seatbelt 19%, handlebar 13%, and abuse 9%).
- Bowel injury occurs at fixation points (e.g., Ligament of Trietz) or ileocecal valve.
- Consider nonaccidental trauma in patients with small bowel injury and an unclear mechanism.
- Symptoms and signs of possible small bowel injury:
  - A mechanism associated with high incidence (see above).
  - Abdominal pain or back pain.
  - Abdominal tenderness and peritonitis.
    - Peritonitis, despite careful examination, was present in less than 50% of small bowel injury in one review.[19]
- Linear ecchymosis, "seatbelt sign," has a high association with intra-abdominal and spine injuries.
  - In a recent study[20] of 61 children with ecchymosis, 21% had lumbar spine injuries, 23% had a hollow viscus injury, and 8% had both.
- CT is unreliable in the diagnosis of hollow viscus injuries.
- CT signs suggestive of bowel injury:
  - Pneumoperitoneum—an absolute indication for surgery.
  - Bowel wall thickening.
  - Bowel wall enhancement.
  - Free fluid in the absence of solid organ injury.
  - Mesenteric stranding.
  - Chance fractures (CT is also unreliable in diagnosing these fractures unless coronal reconstructions are acquired).

- Serial physical examinations are the cornerstone of diagnosis.
- Indications for diagnostic laparoscopy:
  - Physical signs and/or CT signs of small bowel injury.
  - Patient with distracting injuries that render physical examination unreliable.
- Diagnosed small bowel injury mandates operative treatment.
  - Limited segmental resection of affected area and primary anastomosis.
  - Stomas rarely needed in managing small bowel injuries.
- Children treated nonoperatively should be followed closely for delayed presentation with an ischemic stricture.
- Ischemic strictures usually present 3 to 8 weeks post-injury.

Duodenum
- Duodenal injuries occur in two forms: *hematoma or perforation.*
- Duodenal injuries are associated with high mortality, especially in delayed diagnosis.
- Duodenal injuries usually present with abdominal pain and tenderness.
- Mechanism is usually blunt (seatbelt, handlebar with compression of duodenum against spine).
- Duodenal obstruction could produce bilious vomiting.
- CT is diagnostic in only 60% of cases.
  - Diagnostic findings include extravasation or retroperitoneal air or foregut obstruction from a hematoma.
- Upper GI series may be useful for diagnosis.
- Duodenal injury raises suspicion of associated pancreatic, biliary, or spinal injuries (Chance fracture).
- Duodenal hematomas result from blunt force to the abdomen.
  - Hematoma results from shearing injury to submucosal vessels.
  - Usually cause obstructive symptoms with bilious emesis.

Treatment of Duodenal Hematoma
- Nonoperatively with bowel rest, nasogastric tube decompression, and parenteral nutrition.
- May take more than 4 weeks to resolve.
- Surgery is almost **never** necessary.
- Avoid nasoduodenal and nasojejunal feeding tubes due to high risk of perforation.

Treatment of Duodenal Perforation
- Operative treatment is indicated.
- Extent of repair dependent on:
  - Degree of injury.
  - Associated injuries.
  - Degree of retroperitoneal contamination.
- Relatively small, fresh injuries are treated by primary closure and drainage.
- Larger perforations or gross contamination may require pyloric exclusion with gastric and biliary drainage, gastrojejunostomy, and a feeding jejunostomy.

Pancreas
- Relatively protected from injury due to retroperitoneal location.
- Pancreatic injuries are uncommon, occurring in <5% of all abdominal injuries.
- Pancreatic trauma is most common cause of pancreatitis in children.
- Child abuse, handlebar injuries, and seatbelt injuries are frequently associated with pancreatic injuries (Fig. 11-4).
- The pancreas is compressed between the intruding object and the spine.
- Diagnosis of pancreatic injuries is difficult and often delayed.
- Associated injuries are common.
- Hyperamylasemia is usually seen in pancreatic injuries, but may be delayed.
  - Absence of hyperamylasemia does not rule out a pancreatic injury.
- Degree of elevation of serum amylase does not correlate with degree of injury.

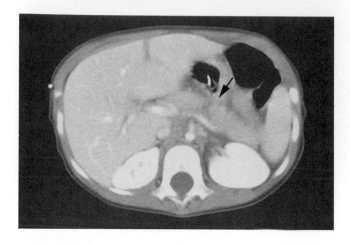

FIGURE 11-4 ● Blunt traumatic pancreatic transaction. CT scan shows the low attenuation linear line across the body of the pancreas *(arrow)* where it was compressed between a seatbelt and the spinal column.

- Abdominal CT with IV and oral contrast may help make the diagnosis.
- CT is only 60–70% accurate in making the diagnosis.
- Initial CT is often negative due to small amount of retroperitoneal fat in children.
- Initial biochemical tests and CT may be falsely negative.
- If highly suspicious of pancreatic injury, repeat CT and blood work are indicated.
- Pancreatic injury may not be evident until peripancreatic edema sets in.
- CT signs suggestive of pancreatic injury include:
  - Peripancreatic inflammation.
  - Stranding in root of mesentery.
  - Low attenuation linear transection of pancreas in region of body of gland (Fig. 11-4).
  - Free fluid in the lesser sac.
  - Duodenal injury.
- ERCP may aid in diagnosing pancreatic ductal injury, thus determining need for surgical treatment.
- The degree of the pancreatic trauma is determined by severity of the injury and the presence or absence of ductal disruption (Table 11-4).

Treatment
- Pancreatic contusions *without* ductal disruption are treated nonoperatively.
  - Nonoperative treatment entails bowel rest and total parenteral nutrition (TPN).
  - Percutaneous drainage may be required for fluid collections.
  - Once pain, tenderness, and hyperamylasemia resolve, oral fluids are introduced.

TABLE 11-4

Pancreatic Injury Severity Scale

Grade	Injury Description
I. Hematoma	Minor contusion without duct injury
Laceration	Superficial laceration without duct injury
II. Hematoma	Major contusion without duct injury or tissue loss
Laceration	Major laceration without duct injury or tissue loss
III. Laceration	Distal transection or parenchymal injury with duct injury
IV. Laceration	Proximal (to the right of the superior mesenteric vessels) transection or parenchymal injury involving the ampulla
V. Laceration	Massive disruption of pancreatic head

Moore EE, Shackford SR, Pachter HG, et al. Organ injury scaling: spleen, liver and kindly 1989 (29):1664–66.

- Ductal injuries usually require operative treatment.
  - Ductal injuries distal to superior mesenteric vein are treated by a spleen-preserving distal pancreatectomy.
  - Ductal injuries in region of pancreatic head are challenging to treat and may require pancreaticoduodenectomy.
- Nonoperative management has a role in patients with delayed diagnosis where operative risk is increased. Such patients require aggressive percutaneous drainage and supportive care.
- ERCP may play a role in treating these injuries.
- Pseudocyst is most common complication of nonoperative treatment of pancreatic injuries, occurring in approximately 10% of patients.
- Pseudocysts cause pain, nausea, obstructive symptoms, and elevated serum amylase levels.
- Treatment of traumatic pseudocysts:
  - Smaller pseudocysts resolve with bowel rest and TPN.
  - Octreotide as an adjunct to nonoperative treatment or as treatment of complications remains controversial.
  - Pseudocysts that persist beyond 4 to 6 weeks require intervention.
  - Intervention options include percutaneous drainage, endoscopic or operative internal drainage.
  - Choice of drainage technique is based on location of pseudocyst and local expertise.
  - Treatment in children is internal drainage.
- Outcomes of pancreatic injuries in children are favorable.

PENETRATING ABDOMINAL INJURIES
- Penetrating injuries are uncommon in children.
- Almost always require operative exploration and treatment.
- The gastrointestinal tract is more frequently injured than solid organs.
- Table 11-5 provides the frequency of intra-abdominal organ injury.

GENITOURINARY TRAUMA
Kidney
- Kidney is the third most common intra-abdominal organ injured from blunt trauma in childhood (28%) and less commonly injured in penetrating trauma (10%).[21,22]
- Associated injuries are common in 40% to 50% of renal injuries.

TABLE 11-5

Frequency of Organ Injury in Penetrating Abdominal Trauma

Organ	Frequency (%)
GI Tract	70
Stomach	13
Duodenum	4
Jejunum/ileum	24
Colon/rectum	27
Liver	27
Vascular	19
Kidney	10
Spleen	9
Genitourinary tract	8
Pancreas	6

Adapted from Cotton BA, Nance ML Penetrating trauma in children. *Semin Pediatr Surg* 2004;13:87–97.

- Renal injuries are not usually life-threatening.
- Kidneys with preexisting disease, such as tumors or hydronephrosis, are susceptible to injury and may be first diagnosed by hematuria following a relatively mild injury.
- Most injuries result from direct parenchymal trauma resulting in contusion, intracapsular hematoma, or fracture.
- Pediatric kidney is at increased risk of injury compared to adults because:
  - Relative large size of kidneys.
  - Pliable ribcage does not provide as much protection.
  - Weaker abdominal musculature.
  - Less cushioning from lack of perinephric fat.
- Microscopic hematuria is usually present.
- CT scan with IV contrast is imaging modality of choice.
- CT is indicated in children with:
  - Gross hematuria.
  - Microscopic hematuria >50 RBC/hpf.
- In unstable patients requiring emergency surgery, a one-shot IVP shows a functioning contralateral kidney. In general, use of IVP is decreasing.
- Grading of renal injuries is based on AAST classification (Table 11-6).

Treatment

- Stable patients with minor or major injuries are placed on bed rest with daily clinical examinations and urinalysis to monitor the degree of hematuria.
  - When hematuria clears, patient may be discharged on restricted activity.
- Patients with extravasation of urine, but no expanding flank mass, may also be observed.
  - Expansion of extravasation, continued hemorrhage, or evidence of infection are all indications for delayed surgery.
- Nonoperative treatment results in a renal salvage rate >90%.
- Immediate surgery may be necessary for a shattered kidney, renal pedicle avulsion, continued hemorrhage, or a penetrating injury.
  - At laparotomy, the renal pedicle is controlled before opening Gerota's fascia or encountered bleeding may lead to nephrectomy.
  - Partial nephrectomy may be possible if only a portion of the kidney is injured because of the segmental vascular anatomy.
  - Repair to the collecting system is done with absorbable suture. Wide drainage is used to prevent accumulation of blood or urine.

TABLE 11-6

Renal Injury Grading

Grade	Injury Description
I	Renal contusion with microscopic or gross hematuria and no renal injury on radiographic studies Nonexpanding subcapsular hematoma without parenchymal laceration
II	Nonexpanding perirenal hematoma confined to the renal retroperitoneum Renal cortex laceration <1 cm with no urinary extravasation
III	Renal cortex laceration >1 cm with no urinary extravasation
IV	Renal laceration extending through renal cortex into medulla and collecting system with positive urinary extravasation on renal imaging Segmental renal artery or vein injury indicated by a segmental parenchymal infarct on renal imaging Renal artery or vein injury with a contained hematoma Thrombosis of the main renal artery
V	Completely shattered kidney Avulsion of the renal pedicle

Adapted from Moore EE, Shackford SR, Pachter HG, et al. Organ injury scaling: spleen, liver and kindly 1989 (29):1664–66.

- Late complications occur in major injuries and include infection, urinoma, renal dysfunction, and hypertension.
- Follow-up imaging study should be done in 6 weeks.

Urinary Bladder

- Extraperitoneal bladder injuries are usually caused by extensive pelvic fractures. Penetrating injuries are rare. Bursting injuries may occur if the bladder is full.
- Children may present with abdominal pain, tenderness, and hematuria (gross or microscopic).
- Bladder injuries may be intraperitoneal, extraperitoneal, or combined.
- Cystography is indicated for pelvic fractures, significant hematuria, and blood at the urethral meatus. Cystography is best as some intraperitoneal injuries may be missed without full bladder distension with contrast.
- CT cystogram is performed at the time of CT for evaluation of abdominal trauma. A Foley catheter should be present and clamped during the CT. Delayed images of the pelvis 5 minutes after contrast injection may show bladder injuries.
- CT cystogram will show "flame"-shaped extravasation in extraperitoneal injuries, while in intraperitoneal injuries there will be contrast around loops of bowel (Fig. 11-5).

Treatment

- Extraperitoneal: Nonoperative treatment is appropriate (Foley, and a repeat cystogram in 1–2 weeks).
- Intraperitoneal: Two-layer repair with absorbable sutures and drainage of prevesical space. A suprapubic catheter may be placed. Shards of bone from a pelvic fracture must be removed.
- Penetrating: All treated by surgical repair.
- Complications include stone formation, fistulas, and stenosis of ureters or urethra.

Urethral Injuries

- Most common mechanism is a pelvic fracture or straddle injury.
- In the male, most are at the membranous urethra.
- Classic sign is blood at the urethral meatus or a perineal hematoma. The patient may have difficulty voiding.
- A hematoma confined to Buck's fascia involves the penis. If the fascia is breached, the hematoma spreads along Colle's fascia over the scrotum, perineum, lower abdomen, and inguinal ligaments.

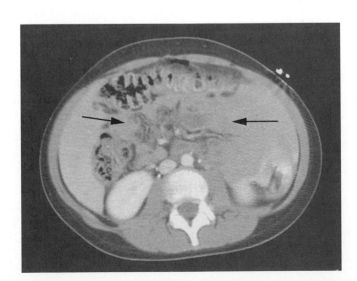

FIGURE 11-5 ● Bladder rupture. CT scan demonstrates extravasation of contrast between loops of intestine *(arrows)* in a patient with an intraperi-toneal bladder rupture.

- Retrograde urethrogram is performed if urethral injury is suspected.
- A Foley may be passed if the urethra is intact to the bladder neck. Do not insert a urethral catheter if the urethra is injured on urethrogram or if there is resistance to insertion of a Foley. Insert a suprapubic catheter instead.
- Urethral injuries associated with pelvic fractures involve the posterior urethra. Associated bladder injuries are common. These injuries require a retrograde urethrogram, followed by cystography.

Treatment

- Anterior urethra: Partial injuries can be splinted over a silastic catheter for 14 days. For more extensive injuries, most should be treated with a suprapubic catheter and delayed repair over a stent 3 to 6 months later.
- Posterior urethra: Suprapubic catheter with placement of a silastic catheter as for anterior injuries. Primary repair converts a closed pelvic fracture to an open one, with a higher infection risk.
- Urethral injuries in females usually treated by direct repair, stenting, and suprapubic vesicostomy.

Genital Injuries

Males

- Most blunt injuries involve the penis.
- Rupture to the corpus cavernosum causes hemorrhage into the surrounding tissues.
- Urinary catheter stents the urethra open.
- Surgery is indicated to evacuate the hematoma, repair the corpus, and repair the urethra.
- Partial amputations should be reattached.
- Scrotal injuries may be observed if mild.
  - Exploration may be safest to evacuate hematoma, control bleeding, and repair a ruptured testicle.

Females

- Almost all from straddle injuries.
- Sexual assault is important to recognize.
- Examination usually requires general anesthetic. Urethroscopy, cystoscopy, vaginoscopy, and proctoscopy may be required.
- Repair of lacerations runs the risk of fistula formation.

CLINICAL PEARLS

DO
- Look for patterns of injury based on mechanism of injury.
- Adequately resuscitate patients with appropriate volumes of isotonic fluid and blood.
- Insert NG and Foley in children with abdominal injury to increase sensitivity of physical examination.
- Transfer patient if your facility lacks surgical, anesthetic, and transfusion service expertise to manage patients nonoperatively.
- Maintain high index of suspicion and perform serial examinations and imaging studies for the detection of hollow viscus injuries.

DON'T
- Under-resuscitate bleeding patients. They need isotonic saline and/or blood.
- Delay referral to a trauma center for children with abdominal trauma.
- Forget that positive FAST is not an indication for operation in children. Resuscitate first.
- Perform a CT in a hemodynamically unstable patient.
- Insert a Foley catheter if blood at urethral meatus.

REFERENCES

1. Cooper A, Barlow B, Discala C, et al. Mortality and truncal injury: the pediatric perspective. *J Pediatr Surg* 1994;29:33–38.
2. Fact Sheet 2. The National Pediatric Trauma Registry, October 1993. Available at http://www.nptr.org.
3. *Childhood injury: Cost and Prevention Facts.* CSN Economics and Insurance Resource Center. National Public Services Research Institute; 1996.
4. Wegner S, Colletti TJ, Van Wie D. Pediatric blunt abdominal trauma. *Pediatr Clin North Am* 2006; 53:243–256.
5. Keller MM. Blunt injury to solid abdominal organs. *Semin Pediatr Surg* 2004;13:106–111.
6. Arkovitz MS, Johnson N, Garcia VF. Pancreatic trauma in children: mechanism of injury. *J Trauma* 1997;42:49–53.
7. Rance CH, Singh SJ, Kimble R. Blunt abdominal trauma in children. *J Paediatr Child Health* 2000; 36:2–6.
8. Fort DW, Bemini JC, Johnson A, et al. Splenic rupture in hemophilia. *Am J Pediatr Hematol Oncol* 2003;16:225–229.
9. Jona JZ, Cox-Gill J. Nonsurgical therapy of splenic rupture in a hemophiliac. *J Pediatr Surg* 1992; 27:523–524.
10. Cotton BA, Beckert BW, Monica K, et al. The utility of clinical and laboratory data for predicting intra-abdominal injury among children. *J Trauma* 2004;56:1068–1075.
11. Moss RL, Musemeche CA. Clinical judgment is superior to diagnostic tests in the management of pediatric small bowel injury. *J Pediatr Surg* 1996;31:1178–1182.
12. Holmes JF, Sokolove PE, Land C, et al. Identification of intra-abdominal injuries in children hospitalized following blunt torso trauma. *Acad Emerg Med* 1999;6:799–806.
13. Allen TL, Mueller MT, Bonk RT, et al. CT scanning without oral contrast solution for blunt bowel and mesenteric injuries in abdominal trauma. *J Trauma* 2004;56:314–322.
14. Stylianos S. Evidence-based guidelines for resource utilization in children with isolated spleen or liver injury. *J Pediatr Surg* 2000;35:164–169.
15. Davidson RN, Wall RA. Prevention and management of infections in patients without a spleen. *Clin Microbiol Infect Dis* 2001;7:657–660.
16. Waghorn DJ. Overwhelming infection in asplenic patients: current best practice preventive measures are not being followed. *J Clin Pathol* 2001;54.214–218.
17. Miller K, Kou D, Sivit C, et al. Pediatric hepatic trauma: does clinical course support intensive care unit stay? *J Pediatr Surg* 1998;33:1459–1462.
18. Canty TG Sr, Canty TG Jr, Brown C. Injuries of the gastrointestinal tract from blunt trauma in children: a 12-year experience at a designated pediatric trauma center. *J Trauma* 1999;46:234–240.
19. Bruny JL, Bensard DD. Hollow viscus injury in the pediatric patient. *Semin Pediatr Surg* 2004;13: 112–118.
20. Sivit CJ, Taylor EA, Newman KD, et al. Safety belt injuries in children with lap belt ecchymosis: CT findings in 61 patients *AJR Am J Roentagenol* 1991 (157):111–114.
21. Cooper A, Barlow B, DiScala C, et al. Mortality and truncal injury: the pediatric perspective. *J Pediatr Surg* 1994;29:33–38.
22. Tarman GJ, Kaplan GW, Lerman SL, et al. Lower genitourinary injury and pelvic fractures in pediatric patients. *Urology* 2002:59:123–126.

CHAPTER 12

Orthopedic Trauma

Andrew Howard, MD, MSc, FRCS(C)

EPIDEMIOLOGY
- Fractures are common in childhood.
- Approximately 2% to 3% of children suffer a fracture treated in the emergency room within a given year.
- Many isolated fractures heal readily with simple or no treatment.
- Multiple fractures during childhood are common.

ANATOMY AND PATHOPHYSIOLOGY
Growth Plates
- Cartilagenous growth plates persist in the growing skeleton as soon as secondary centers of ossification form at the ends of the long bones.
- Average ages at which secondary centers of ossification appear and fuse to the skeleton are shown in Figure 12-1.
- Growth plates account for the longitudinal growth of bones.
- Growth plates are weaker in tension than the nearby bone and are commonly involved in fractures.
- Most growth plate injuries heal rapidly and do not cause permanent alterations in longitudinal or angular growth.
- Injuries with the potential to cause permanent growth arrests are:
  - Higher-energy injuries.
  - Injuries to the distal femoral physis.
  - Injuries with higher numerical classification in the Salter–Harris scheme (Fig. 12-2).
- Radiographic interpretation of the growing skeleton can be difficult due to:
  - Presence of growth plates.
  - Variations in the appearance of secondary ossification centers.
    - For example, the elbow has six secondary ossification centers.
- Radiographic interpretation can be assisted by:
  - Referring to normal radiographs.
  - Taking comparison x-rays of the contralateral uninjured limb.[1]

Periosteum
- Periosteum around children's bones is much thicker, tougher, and more active than that around adult bones, because it is continually contributing to bone circumferential appositional growth.
- Periosteum is often torn on the side of the bone that failed in tension (usually the direction the apex of angulation points) and is often intact on the opposite, compression side.
- Intact periosteum confers stability after fracture reduction, but must be accommodated in performing the reduction maneuver.

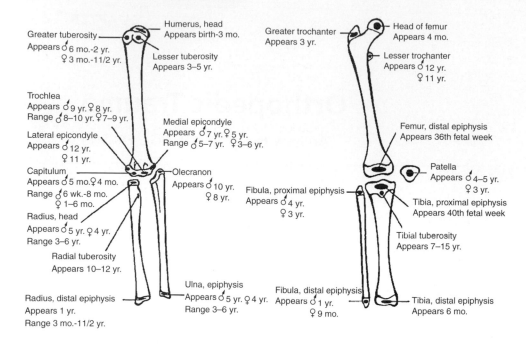

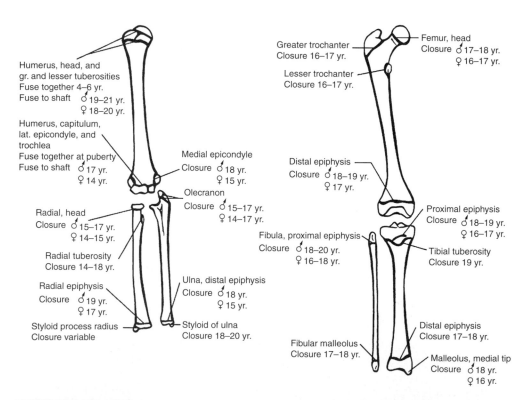

FIGURE 12-1 ● *Above.* Average age of appearance of secondary centers of ossification for girls and boys. *Below.* Average age of closure of growth plates and fusion of secondary centers to primary centers for girls and boys. (From Beaty JH, Kasser JR. *Rockwood and Wilkins' fractures in children.* 6th ed. Philadelphia: Lippincott Williams & Wilkins; 2006.)

RISK FACTORS AND CLASSIFICATION

Inflicted Injury

- Have a high index of suspicion for inflicted injury as the risk for re-injury and fatality is high.
- The diagnosis remains a clinical one, using all information from history, physical findings, and radiographic and ancillary tests.[2,3]
- Risk factors include:
  - Injuries inappropriate to the child's developmental level (e.g., long bone fractures prior to walking age).
  - Delayed presentation.
  - Inconsistent history.
  - Unwitnessed injuries.
  - Multiple injuries.
  - Injuries at different stages of healing.
  - Inappropriate parent—child dynamics.
- Specialized pediatric services or teams exist to provide comprehensive medical assessment in cases where inflicted injury is a possibility.
- The legal responsibility to report suspected child abuse to governmental authorities (Children's Aid Society) rests with the primary physician.
- See Chapter 19 on Nonaccidental Injury for further details.

Unintentional Injury

- **High—energy fractures are associated with more:**
  - Nerve injuries.
  - Vascular injuries.
  - Skin injuries or open fractures.
  - Swelling or compartment syndromes.
  - Growth plate damage.
  - Delayed healing.
  - Permanent disability.
  - Additional fractures in the same limb or elsewhere.
  - Systemic injuries.
  - Central nervous system injuries.
  - Requirement for operative reduction and stabilization.
- **High-energy mechanisms include:**
  - Motor vehicle occupant.
  - Pedestrian struck by motor vehicle.
  - Cyclist struck by motor vehicle.
  - Falls from heights (more than twice the child's standing height).
  - Motorized sports and recreation.
  - High-speed activities (e.g., skiing, snowboarding).
- **Low-energy mechanisms include:**
  - Sports and leisure injuries.
  - Team sports, field sports.
  - Playground injuries.
  - Falls.

Location of the Fracture

- Fractures can occur in the:
  - Diaphysis (shaft).
  - Metaphysis (flare).
  - Physis (growth plate).
  - Epiphysis (secondary center of ossification).
- Metaphyseal and growth plate fractures heal in half the time of diaphyseal fractures of the same bone.

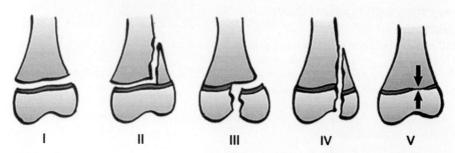

I   II   III   IV   V

FIGURE 12-2 ● Salter–Harris classification of growth plate injuries. Type I crosses the growth plate completely, type II crosses the growth plate and a portion of metaphysis. Risk of subsequent growth disturbance is low after either of these types, except for high-energy injuries in the lower extremity (e.g., distal femur). Type I and II injuries are the most common varieties seen. Type III injury extends across part of the growth plate then across the epiphysis and into the joint, and type IV injury occurs through the metaphysis, across the growth plate and the epiphysis, and then into the joint. Type III and IV injuries need accurate reduction and stabilization because the joint surface is involved, and carry a higher risk of growth disturbance because the fracture line crosses the progenitor cells, which are on the epiphyseal side of the growth plate. Type V injuries are crushing injuries to the growth plate—they may be difficult or impossible to diagnose on an initial radiograph but can cause growth disturbance later. Type V injuries are very uncommon. (From Beaty JH, Kasser JR. *Rockwood and Wilkins' fractures in children.* 6th ed. Philadelphia: Lippincott Williams & Wilkins; 2006.)

- Intra-articular fractures are often accompanied by growth plate fractures in children (see the description of the Salter–Harris classification below).
  - Require accurate reduction and stabilization to prevent posttraumatic arthritis.

Pattern of the Fracture
- Fracture pattern reveals the type and direction of force.
  - Spiral fracture = twisting around long axis of bone.
  - Transverse fracture = bending force.
  - Transverse fracture with butterfly fragment = higher peak bending force, butterfly fragment is on concave (compression) side of the bent bone.
  - Oblique fracture = bending in compression.
  - Avulsion fracture = tensile force.

Growth Plate Fractures: Salter–Harris Classification (Fig. 12-2)
- Five different anatomic patterns of growth plate injury.[4]
- Risk of permanent damage to the growth plate is determined by:
  - The energy of the fracture.
  - The specific growth plate involved.
  - The fracture pattern.
- Upper-extremity growth plates commonly have low-energy injuries.
  - Results in type I and II fracture patterns.
  - Almost never have permanent problems.
- Lower-extremity growth plates are much stronger.
  - Even type I or II injury of the distal femur has a high risk of growth arrest.
- Early orthopedic consultation is suggested for all growth plate injuries in the lower extremity, and for high-grade (Salter–Harris III or IV) or high-energy and displaced injuries in the upper extremity.

Open Fractures: Gustillo Classification (Table 12-1)
- The Gustillo classification: Extent of soft tissue injury associated with fracture.[5,6]
- Risk factors for infection include:
  - High-energy trauma.
  - More extensive soft-tissue damage.
  - Contamination.
  - Circulatory impairment.
  - Delay prior to surgical debridement.

TABLE 12-1

Gustillo Classification of Open Fractures

Gustillo Grade	Soft Tissue Injury	Antibiotic Prophylaxis
I	Small laceration ≤1 cm, often inside to out	Cefazolin 40 mg/kg IV
II	Laceration 1–10 cm, grafts or flaps will not be needed for coverage	Alternative if pen/ceph allergy: clindamycin 10 mg/kg IV
IIIa	Large laceration >10 cm, or extensive soft-tissue degloving irrespective of wound size, but bone can be covered	Cefazolin 40 mg/kg IV *plus* gentamicin 2.5 mg/kg IV. Add metronidazole 10 mg/kg IV if grossly contaminated (fecal, barnyard, soil) or extensive devitalized tissue for anaerobic coverage
IIIb	Large laceration, bone cannot be covered, often extensive contamination	Alternative if pen/ceph allergy: clindamycin 10 mg/kg IV
IIIc	Open fracture with arterial injury in same limb	

- Antibiotic and tetanus administration depend on extent of injury and contamination.
  - Grade I and clean grade II injuries require gram-positive coverage.
  - Contaminated grade II and all grade III injuries require:
    - Gram-positive and gram-negative coverage.
    - May require anaerobic coverage if:
      - Gross amounts of soil or fecal material are present.
      - A lot of dead or devitalized tissue is present.
      - Tetanus toxoid and/or immune globulin may be indicated for patients whose immunity is not up to date (Table 12-2).

INITIAL MANAGEMENT
Resuscitation Priorities
Airway and Cervical Spine
- *Cervical spine protection* must be maintained until bony or ligamentous injury has been excluded.
- See Chapter 9 on C-spine Injuries.
- Cervical spine held in neutral position with combination of:
  - Appropriately sized cervical collar.
  - Sandbags or rolled towels secured against the side of the head.
- In infants, the larger head flexes the neck if supine on a flat surface. (Fig. 12-3)
  - For children <4 years, maintain the neck in neutral position with one of the following:
    - A hollow beneath the head.
    - A folded towel or small blanket under the shoulders.
- Consider cervical spine injury:
  - In all cases of head injury.
  - If patient complains of neck pain.
  - Patients with any neurologic deficit.

Circulation
- *Pelvic fractures* can cause exsanguinating hemorrhage.[7–9]
- Bind the pelvis circumferentially with a sheet to decrease its internal volume.

TABLE 12-2

Guide to Tetanus Prophylaxis in Routine Wound Management in Children and Adolescents

History of Absorbed Tetanus Toxoid (Doses)	Clean, Minor Wounds		All Other Wounds[a]	
	Td or Tdap[b]	TIG[3]	Td or Tdap[b]	TIG[c]
<3 or unknown	Yes	No	Yes	Yes
≥3[d]	No[e]	No	No[f]	No

Td, adult-type diphtheria and tetanus toxoids vaccine; TIG, tetanus immune globulin (human); Tdap, booster tetanus toxoid, reduced diphtheria toxoid, and acellular pertussis.

[a] Such as, but not limited to, wounds contaminated with dirt, feces, soil, and saliva; puncture wounds; avulsions; and wounds resulting from missiles, crushing, burns, and frostbite.

[b] Tdap is preferred to Td for adolescents who never have received Tdap. Td is preferred to tetanus toxoid (TT) for adolescents who received Tdap previously or when Tdap is not available.

[c] Immune globulin IV should be used when TIG is not available.

[d] If only 3 doses of fluid toxoid have been received, a fourth dose of toxoid, preferably an adsorbed toxoid, should be given. Although licensed, fluid tetanus toxoid rarely is used.

[e] Yes, if ≥10 years since last tetanus-containing vaccine dose.

[f] Yes, if ≥5 years since last tetanus-containing vaccine dose. More frequent boosters are not needed and can accentuate adverse effects.

(Reproduced from *AAP Red Book 2006 Report of the Committee on Infectious Diseases.* 27th ed. Copyright © 2006 by the American Academy of Pediatrics. All rights reserved)

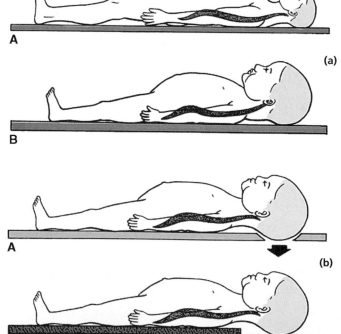

(a)

(b)

FIGURE 12-3 ● The child's neck is flexed on a level back-board because of the large head **(a)**. To keep the cervical spine in neutral alignment, the spine board must have a hollow for the head, or the body must be elevated on firm blankets **(b)**. (From Herzenberg JE, Hensinger RN, Dedrick DK, et al. Emergency transport and positioning of young children who have an injury of the cervical spine: The standard backboard may be hazardous. *J Bone Joint Surg [Am]* 1989;71:15–22, with permission.)

- Prompt orthopedic consultation is required, as external fixation of the pelvis is part of the resuscitation for patients with pelvic fracture and excessive blood loss.
- Concomitant abdominal injury may require laparotomy.
  - Can be performed at the same operative session as pelvic stabilization.
- There is little proven role for angiographic embolization of pelvic bleeding in children until pelvic stabilization has been achieved.
- *Femoral fractures* can contribute to blood loss (500 mL to 1 L per femoral fracture, or 20% of blood volume), but an isolated femoral fracture is unlikely the cause of hemodynamic instability, so other causes should be sought.[1]
- *Open wounds* with ongoing visible blood loss are best managed by direct pressure over the bleeding point. Avoid attempts to clamp vessels blindly.
- *Intravenous lines* placed peripherally should be put into uninjured or less injured limbs to ensure that infused fluids and drug reach the central circulation.
- *Impaired circulation* in a deformed limb can be substantially improved by realigning and splinting the limb in near-anatomic position.

Disability
- Assessment of gross motor function and circulation at each extremity is performed and documented early in the primary survey.

Exposure
- Expose all limbs for a detailed secondary survey.
- Ensure complete exposure to assess for musculoskeletal injuries.
- Maintain core body temperature.

Evaluation
History
- AMPLE history for possible surgical intervention.
- Allergies, medications, past history, last meal, events surrounding injury.
- Mechanism of injury is important.
  - High energy versus low energy (see above).
- Mechanism determines likely or associated injuries, severity and risk of complications, and long-term outcome.

Likely or Associated Injuries
- *Seatbelt injury* from a frontal collision with flexion around seatbelt.
  - Transverse abdominal bruising.
  - Abdominal visceral injury.
  - Lumbar spine flexion—distraction injury (Chance fracture).
  - Head injury from striking vehicle interior.
- *Pedestrian injury.*
  - Ipsilateral lower extremity fracture from bumper (tibia and or femur depending on child's height).
  - Chest injury and head injury from contact with hood.
- *Child occupant* injured in side-impact crash.
  - Ipsilateral head, chest, abdomen, and limb injury.
- *Fall from a height* onto legs.
  - Calcaneal or tibial plateau fractures plus lumbar spine injury.

Severity and Risk of Complications
- A distal tibial fracture from a motorized mechanism (e.g., motorbike, snowmobile, ATV) may appear similar radiographically to a low-velocity sports injury.
- Higher-energy mechanism means greater energy transfer to leg.
  - Greater displacement at time of injury, more stretching, tearing, or crushing of soft tissues.
  - Greater likelihood of compartment syndrome, vascular damage, or nerve damage.

Long-Term Outcome
- High-energy (motorized) mechanisms have higher likelihood of residual functional deficits at 6 months for a given level of anatomic injury.[10]

Mechanism of Injury
- Mechanism of injury can be elicited from:
  - Patients.
  - Adult caregivers.
  - Witnesses and bystanders.
  - EMS personnel—first responders.

Physical Examination—Secondary Survey

Comfort
- Ensure child's comfort during exposure and examination.
- Move obviously deformed limbs as little as possible.
- Do not elicit fracture crepitus as a physical sign.
- Splint fractures as early as possible—splinting is an excellent analgesic.
- Remove spine board after spine has been properly examined and it is no longer needed for transfers.

Look, Feel, Move
- Expose all limbs.
- Look, feel, move.
  - From sternum and scapula to fingertips.
  - From ASIS to toes.
- Examine pelvis for shape, tenderness, and horizontal/vertical stability.
- Horizontal stability best assessed by medial then lateral pressure on both ASISs.
- Vertical stability best assessed by traction on one leg at a time with pelvis stabilized.
- Only examine an unstable pelvis once!
  - Repeated motion can disrupt a clot and lead to extra blood loss.
  - Bind unstable pelvis with sheet to reduce volume and motion.
- Palpate cervical spine for tenderness.
  - A fully awake and cooperative child can put the neck through a range of motion with collar briefly removed (see Chapter 9 on C-spine Injuries for details).
- Log-roll the child and inspect and palpate the thoracic and lumbar spine, to the sacrum.
  - Signs of injury include:
    - Tenderness.
    - Bruising.
    - Swelling.
    - Deformity.
- Boggy swelling over the lumbar spinous processes in conjunction with an abdominal belt bruise denotes a seatbelt injury to the spine.
- Multiple injuries are difficult to diagnose in the presence of pain or in a child who is not fully alert due to injury or medication.
- Careful initial examination, and a *repeated physical examination at 24 hours* until the child is fully alert, minimizes the chance of missing injuries.
- Commonly missed fractures include:
  - Metatarsal, tarsal, metacarpal, and carpal fractures.
  - Look for signs of bruising or pain on palpation.

Vascular Exam
- Document a distal neurologic and vascular exam on all four limbs, injured or not.
- Document presence or absence of pulses.
  - Radial, ulnar, anterior tibial (dorsalis pedis), and posterior tibial pulses.
- Use Doppler to detect pulses and measure occlusion pressures in injured limbs with nonpalpable pulse.
- Document color, temperature, and motor function as important signs of circulatory integrity in limbs with absent pulses.

TABLE 12-3

Upper and Lower Extremity Nerve Motor and Sensory Exam

Nerve	Sensory	Motor
Radial Nerve	First dorsal web space	Thumb extension, extension across MCP joints
Median Nerve	Ulnar border of the index finger	Thumb opposition
Ulnar Nerve	Tip of small finger	Abduction of index finger
Anterior Interosseous Nerve	N/A	Flexion of DIP joint of index finger and thumb
Peroneal Nerve	Deep branch—first dorsal web space	Great toe dorsiflexion
Tibial Nerve	Sole of foot at metatarsal heads	Ankle and toe plantar flexion

Neurologic Exam
- Record objective function of a distal innervated muscle for all major nerves in all extremities.
  - Establishes that the nerve is intact along its course.
- Record the power of each muscle according to the Medical Research Council (MRC) system.
  - 0 = No movement.
  - 1 = Flicker.
  - 2 = Moves without gravity.
  - 3 = Moves against gravity.
  - 4 = Weaker than full strength.
  - 5 = Full strength.
- In the presence of a neurologic injury, complete the examination by examining all movements across all joints and grading them.
- The screening sensory exam includes areas of sole innervation (Table 12-3).
- Recording of peripheral nerve function should be objective (e.g., record muscle power), repeated as necessary if there is injury, and age appropriate.
- Observe and give toys to younger children who cannot cooperate with exam to determine overall function of the extremities.
  - Parents are useful examiners of frightened younger children.

Imaging
Ordering Radiographs
- Plain radiographs of the initial trauma survey:
  - Lateral C-spine.
  - Chest.
  - Pelvis.
- No further radiographs required if patient is being transferred to a trauma center.
- Do not delay transport to obtain more radiographs.
- If undertaking further investigation of a stable patient in a community setting:
  - Complete secondary survey.
  - Order plain radiographs on all regions suspicious for fracture or dislocation.
- Two views at 90 degrees for injured limb segments and the spine.
- AP pelvis, inlet view, and outlet view for pelvic ring disruption.
- 45-degree obliques internal and external rotation for acetabular fractures.
- Include the joint above and below an injured segment.
- Take initial radiographs with splint in place.
  - More comfortable for child and adequate for gross assessment.

Interpreting Radiographs

- A systematic approach to include all abnormal and normal structures is important.
  - Bone: Trace all cortical outlines looking for fractures.
  - Joints: Ensure joint alignment.
    - A line through the radius should point at the center of the capitellum on all views.
  - Soft tissues: Swelling indicates injury, air in soft tissues indicates open fracture, "fat pad" signs in elbow indicate radiographically occult fractures.
- Radiographs of the noninjured side are useful for comparison.
  - Clinicians unfamiliar with appearance of secondary ossification centers (Fig. 12-1).
- Clinical correlation of radiographs and clinical findings is necessary for diagnosing minimally displaced or undisplaced fractures.
- See Chapter 4 on Diagnostic Imaging for further details.

CT Scans

- These images will be used by the hospital/team/surgeon performing definitive fracture management.
  - **Do not obtain orthopedic CT images prior to stabilization and transfer.**
- Complex flat bone trauma—cervical spine, thoracolumbar spine, pelvis—useful for anatomic detail of fractures.
- Intraarticular fractures—useful for anatomic detail and operative planning of joint and growth plate fractures.
- CT angiography—allows rapid assessment of vascular injury.
  - Faster than conventional angiography with some potential loss of detail.

MRI Scans

- Indicated to image the spinal cord when clinical signs of injury are present.
- Do not play a major role in management of orthopedic injuries.
- See Chapter 13 on Thoracic and Lumbar Spine Injuries for further details.

SPECIFIC INJURIES
Life-Threatening Injuries: Pelvic Fractures
Hemodynamic Considerations

- Major pelvic fractures are less common in children than in adults because of the more pliable skeleton and less exposure to dangerous activities.
- Pelvic ring disruption can produce life-threatening bleeding.
- Initial stabilization for hemodynamic instability includes a sheet or binder to close down the pelvic volume, as well as fluid and blood resuscitation.
- Prompt general surgical and orthopedic referral is necessary for definitive management of bleeding, which may be from both the pelvis and an intraabdominal source.[11]
- Laparotomy treats abdominal bleeding, and external fixation treats pelvic bleeding. Both can be performed at the same operating session.
- Preoperative CT scanning can provide additional information about both abdominal and pelvic injuries, but may, in some cases, be deferred until a resuscitative laparotomy and external fixation of the pelvis have been performed.
- Embolization of vessels in the angiography suite is rarely used in children and can be reserved for bleeding unresponsive to external fixation.
- As with all circumstances where major transfusion is required, avoid hypothermia and give platelets and clotting factors as necessary to ensure adequate coagulation.

Urologic Injury

- Urethral or bladder injury occurs in 9–24% of pelvic trauma.[7–9,11]
- Signs of urethral injury:
  - Blood at penile meatus.
  - Perineal bruising or swelling.
  - High-riding prostate.

- If any of above signs are present, do NOT insert a Foley catheter.
- A retrograde urethrogram MUST be performed.

Bowel Injury
- Suspect bowel injury if:
  - Evidence of blood on digital rectal examination.
  - Palpable bony fragments on digital rectal examination.
  - Evidence of gas in soft tissue on radiography.
- MUST perform sigmoidoscopy under general anesthesia to rule out an open pelvic fracture involving the rectum or sigmoid colon.
  - Diverting colostomy needed to minimize risks of infection.

Perineal Injury
- Deep perineal lacerations may communicate with pelvic fractures.
  - May require diverting colostomy during fracture irrigation and debridement.

Soft-Tissue Degloving
- Crush injuries (e.g., vehicle runovers) may result in massive degloving of skin and soft tissues over the pelvis and upper thighs.
- Massive soft-tissue injuries create dead space with fat necrosis and hematoma, which may require operative drainage or debridement.

Neurologic and Vascular Injury
- If significantly displaced pelvic fracture, consider possible injury to:
  - The lumbosacral plexus.
  - The common, internal, and external iliac vessels.

Rare Severe Injuries
Amputations and Near Amputations
- An amputated distal part that could be replanted should be:
  - Carefully wrapped in sterile dressings and towel.
  - Cooled (not frozen).
  - Transported with the patient.
- Radiographs of the amputated part aid in planning operative reconstruction.
- Replantation is more likely to be successful if:
  - Done quickly after injury.
  - The injury is a clean, sharp wound.
  - There is minimal crushing, contamination, or soft-tissue loss.
- Digits have longer ischemic time because they lack muscle.
- Near amputations, and limb injuries with high-grade open fractures involving vessel and/or nerve damage, require careful and repeated assessment as well as early consultation with orthopedic, plastic, and vascular surgery teams.
- Supplement neurologic and vascular status with clinical photos of the injured limb.
- Difficult decision between amputation and limb salvage with reconstruction.
  - Often decide after initial operative debridement and examination under anesthesia.
- Good long-term function of both amputation and limb salvage.
- Early amputation is appropriate for complete nonreconstructible vascular injury.
- Consider early amputation if neurologic injury will leave an insensate hand or foot without motors.
- Definitive decision to amputate or reconstruct is made after intraoperative assessment, or within the first few days.
- Adult scoring systems (mangled extremity severity score) do not accurately predict which pediatric limbs are surgically reconstructible.[12]

Vascular Injuries
- Gently realign fractured extremities with diminished or absent pulses.
  - Extension for the lower extremity.
  - Flexion of 30 to 45 degrees for the upper extremity.

- Do not delay orthopedic consultation even if the pulse has returned.
- Some fractures are high risk for occult vascular injury even if distal pulses are normal.
  - High incidence of popliteal artery injury in proximal tibial and distal femoral growth plate injuries.
  - Knee dislocations in adolescents and adults, due to tethering of the artery close to bone distal to the knee.
- Repeated documentation of vascular status is required.
  - Injured arterial intima may extend or thrombose.
  - Complete vessel occlusion may occur hours after injury.

Open Fractures
- Missed diagnoses increase the risk of infectious complications.
- Children's skin is very elastic.
  - Tiny wounds can indicate a location where the bone shaft completely penetrated the skin from within, picked up a plug of earth, and then withdrew completely into the limb.
- Any wound on a fractured limb could potentially communicate with the fracture.
- Signs suggestive of open fracture:
  - Excessive bleeding for the size of the wound.
  - Venous coloration of bleeding.
  - Blood with fat globules.
  - Air in soft tissues (detected clinically or radiographically).

Compartment Syndromes
- Pressure in a fascial compartment exceeds venous pressure.
- Impairs circulation.
- Vicious cycle:
  - Decreased circulation.
  - Ischemic damage to muscle and nerve.
  - Increased swelling and pressure.

Risk Factors
- High-energy trauma.
- Crushing injuries.
- Vascular damage.
- Can occur in the presence of open fractures.[13]
- Double-level injuries.[14]
  - High-energy trauma to the extremity.
    - Ipsilateral femur and tibia fractures (floating knee).
    - Ipsilateral humerus and forearm fractures (floating elbow).
  - Proximal injury swelling produces a tourniquet effect.
  - Impedes venous return.
  - Severe swelling or compartment syndrome results at the distal injury.

Diagnosis
- The diagnosis is clinical.[15]
- Pain out of proportion to underlying injury.
- Pain on passive stretch of muscles.
- Fullness and tenderness of muscle compartment.
- Paresthesias (late).
- Muscle weakness or paralysis (late).
- The absence of pulses (late).

Compartment Pressure Measurement or Monitoring
- Painful, invasive.
- Not a gold standard to rule in or rule out compartment syndrome.
- Useful in unconscious patient at risk of compartment syndrome.
- Rarely indicated in conscious children in the emergency room.

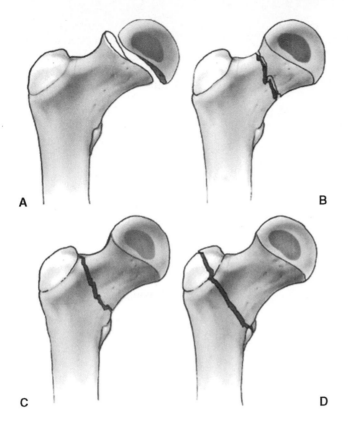

A

B

C

D

FIGURE 12-4 ● Femoral neck fractures are high-energy injuries in children, and carry a high risk of avascular necrosis. This risk approaches 100% with acute transphyseal fractures **(A)** that are displaced or associated with dislocation, is approximately 50% for midcervical fractures **(B)**, 10% to 30% for basicervical fractures **(C)**, and about 10% for intertrochanteric fractures **(D)**. (From Beaty JH, Kasser JR. *Rockwood and Wilkins' fractures in children.* 6th ed. Philadelphia: Lippincott Williams & Wilkins; 2006.)

Treatment
- Decompressive fasciotomy.
- Under general anesthesia, the limb is opened with a generous longitudinal incision(s) and each fascial compartment is opened.
- Type and cross blood if this is anticipated.
- Operative stabilization of associated fractures.

Neck of Femur Fractures
- High-energy injuries in children and young adults.
- Avascular necrosis (AVN) is a much higher risk.
- Due to high-energy mechanism.
- Hip replacement is not an option at this age.
- AVN has long-term consequences.
- Lifelong disability is possible.
- Risk of AVN is[16]:
  - 10% to 30% for basicervical fractures.
  - ~50% for midcervical fractures.
  - Up to 100% for transphyseal fractures, especially if dislocation (Fig. 12-4).

Bilateral Femoral Fractures
- Femoral fracture results in ~20% blood volume loss.
  - Unilateral femur fractures do not result in hemodynamic instability.[17]
  - Suspect pelvic or abdominal injury in hemodynamically unstable children.
- Bilateral femoral fractures can result in ~40% blood volume loss.
  - Can produce hemodynamic instability requiring resuscitation.
- Thomas splint stabilization reduces blood loss.

DEFINITIVE MANAGEMENT
Closed Fractures and Dislocations
- Realignment of the limb.
- Gentle fracture reduction and immobilization.
- Provide analgesia or conscious sedation as required (see Chapter 18 on Pain Management for details).
- Splint fractures even if they require further open or closed reduction.
- Growth plate injuries:
  - Single attempt at gentle reduction.
  - Provide analgesia or conscious sedation.
  - Avoid repeated manipulations, which risk further damage to growth plate.

Open Fractures
- Verify tetanus immune status.
- Administer tetanus toxoid and/or tetanus immune globulin as needed (Table 12-2).
- Pour saline over wound to gently remove gross debris.
- After cleansing, dress with sterile dressing.
- Document motor status of the limb.
- Administer antibiotics according to Gustillo classification of wound (Table 12-1).

Neurologic and Vascular Injuries
- Limb realignment.
- Fracture reduction.
- Splinting.
- Reassessment.
- Early involvement of care team.
  - Orthopedics for stabilization of skeleton.
  - Vascular and/or plastic surgery for vessel repair.
- Vascular imaging as required by surgical team.
  - CT angiogram, conventional angiogram, or on-table angiogram.

CLINICAL PEARLS
DO
- Protect C-spine during airway management, positioning, resuscitation.
- Splint pelvis and long bone fractures to control blood loss and pain.
- Externally compress bleeding open wounds.
- Start IVs in uninjured limbs where possible.
- Perform systematic examination of spine, pelvis, and four extremities.
- Document neurologic and vascular function.
- Realign and splint limbs if neurologic or vascular compromise.
  - Prompt orthopedic referral.
- Document and treat open fractures.
  - Surface irrigation, sterile dressing, splint, and antibiotics/tetanus.

DON'T
- Delay orthopedic referral if neurologic or vascular compromise.
- Attempt repeated forceful manipulations of growth plate injuries.
- Miss open fractures—any small or remote wound on the limb may communicate.
- Miss compartment syndromes—repeated clinical assessment of high-energy or open fractures.
- Repeatedly examine unstable pelvic fracture—it causes bleeding.
- Examine for fracture crepitus—it causes pain.

REFERENCES

1. Swischuk LE, Hernandez JA. Frequently missed fractures in children (value of comparative views). *Emerg Radiol* 2004;11:22–8.
2. Campbell RM Jr., Schrader T. Child abuse. In: Rockwood CA, Wilkins KE, Beaty JH, et al., *Rockwood and Wilkins' fractures in children*. 5th ed. Philadelphia: Lippincott Williams & Wilkins; 2001.
3. Oral R, Blum KL, Johnson C. Fractures in young children: are physicians in the emergency department and orthopedic clinics adequately screening for possible abuse? *Pediatr Emerg Care* 2003;19: 148–153.
4. Salter RB, Harris R. Injuries involving the epiphyseal plate. *J Bone Joint Surg Am* 1963;45A:587.
5. Gustillo RB, Anderson JT. JSBS classics. Prevention of infection in the treatment of one thousand and twenty-five open fractures of long bones. Retrospective and prospective analyses. *J Bone Joint Surg Am* 2002;84A:682.
6. Hope PG, Cole WG. Open fractures of the tibia in children. *J Bone Joint Surg Br* 1992;74:546–553.
7. Chia JP, Holland AJ, Little D, et al. Pelvic fractures and associated injuries in children. *J Trauma* 2004;56:83–88.
8. Demetriades D, Karaiskakis M, Velmahos GC, et al. Pelvic fractures in pediatric and adult trauma patients: are they different injuries? *J Trauma* 2003;54:1146–1151; discussion, 1151.
9. Junkins EP, Furnival RA, Bolte RG. The clinical presentation of pediatric pelvic fractures. *Pediatr Emerg Care* 2001;17:15–18.
10. Macpherson AK, Rothman L, McKeag AM, et al. Mechanism of injury affects 6-month functional outcome in children hospitalized because of severe injuries. *J Trauma* 2003;55:454–458.
11. Widmann RF. Fractures of the pelvis. In: Rockwood CA, Wilkins KE, Beaty JH, et al., eds. *Rockwood and Wilkins' fractures in children*. 5th ed. Philadelphia: Lippincott Williams & Wilkins; 2001.
12. Fagelman MF, Epps HR, Rang M. Mangled extremity severity score in children. *J Pediatr Orthop* 2002;22:182–184.
13. Grottkau BE, Epps HR, Di Scala C. Compartment syndrome in children and adolescents. *J Pediatr Surg* 2005;40:678–682.
14. Blakemore LC, Cooperman DR, Thompson GH, et al. Compartment syndrome in ipsilateral humerus and forearm fractures in children. *Clin Orthop Relat Res* 2000;376:32–38.
15. Cascio BM, Wilckens JH, Ain MC, et al. Documentation of acute compartment syndrome at an academic health-care center. *J Bone Joint Surg Am* 2005;87:346–350.
16. Blasier RD, Hughes LO. Fractures and traumatic dislocations of the hip in children. In: Rockwood CA, Wilkins KE, Beaty JH, et al., eds. *Rockwood and Wilkins' fractures in children*. 5th ed. Philadelphia: Lippincott Williams & Wilkins; 2001.
17. Unal VS, Gulcek M, Unveren Z, et al. Blood loss evaluation in children under the age of 11 with femoral shaft fractures patients with isolated versus multiple injuries. *J Trauma* 2006;60:224–226; discussion, 226.

CHAPTER 13

Thoracic and Lumbar Spine Injuries

Andrew Jea, MD

James M. Drake, BSE, MBBCh,

iMSc, FRCSC, FACS

EPIDEMIOLOGY
- Spinal cord injury (SCI) in children is uncommon.
  - Children account for only 0.65% to 9.47% of all SCI.[1–4]
  - The incidence of spinal cord injury without radiographic abnormality (SCIWORA) is 15% to 66% of all SCI.[3–7]
- Spine fractures in children represent 1% to 2% of all pediatric fractures.[8]
  - The thoracic region (T2-T10) is most commonly injured followed by the lumbar region (L2-L5).[9]
- Trauma to the lower thoracic or lumbar spine in children is rarely associated with spinal cord injury.[8]
- Each year 1,000 new spinal cord injuries are reported in children.[10]
  - Adolescent boys are most affected.[11]
  - Causes of pediatric spine injury include falls, athletic activities, child abuse, and motor vehicle trauma.[11–16]

ANATOMY
- Embryology of the thoracic and lumbar vertebrae.
  - Three main ossification centers:[8]
    - One each for the left and right sides of the neural arch.
    - One for the body.
  - Junction of the arches with the body occurs at the neurocentral synchondrosis.
    - Remains visible radiographically until 3 to 6 years old.
    - Lies just anterior to the pedicle base.
    - Often mistaken for a congenital anomaly or fracture in younger children.[8]
  - Secondary centers of ossification occur in flattened, disc-shaped epiphyses superior and inferior to each vertebral body.
    - Provides longitudinal growth.[17]
    - Ossification of these growth plates at age 7 to 8 years creates the radiographic impression of a groove at the corner of each vertebral body.
    - Ligaments and discs attach to this groove, which is an apophyseal ring.
    - The ring develops its own ossification center by the age of 12 to 15 and fuses with the remainder of the vertebra at skeletal maturity.[18]
- Differences in the pediatric spinal column compared to adults predispose infants and small children to flexion and extension injuries.
  - Pediatric spine has ligamentous laxity, elasticity, and incomplete ossification.[3,19]
  - Small children have proportionally larger heads with underdeveloped neck musculature.[3,8]
  - Small children's facet joints are more horizontally oriented.
    - Results in greater mobility and less stability.[3,20,21]

- Physiologic wedging of the vertebral bodies.
  - Particularly of the upper cervical spine.
  - Facilitates forward movement of the vertebra.
  - Predisposes children to flexion injuries.[3,20,21]
- Hyperextension coupled with the hypermobility:
  - Results in momentary dislocation then spontaneous reduction.
  - Results in spinal cord damage with a normal-appearing vertebral column.[3,22]

EVALUATION
History
- Back pain from a major accident or fall increases suspicion for spine injury.
  - Major accident includes significant vehicular damage, head-on, high-speed collision, rollover, or death at the scene.
- Accidents involving the lack of seatbelts, prolonged extrication, airbag deployment, steering wheel or windshield damage, passenger ejection, or space intrusion can be associated with spine injuries.
- Vehicle accidents involving motorcycles, bicycles, or pedestrians have a high association with spine injuries.
- Transient or persistent symptoms include pain, weakness, numbness, and tingling.

Physical Exam
- A seatbelt mark across the abdomen, or intra-abdominal injury, should increase suspicion for possible thoracic or lumbar fracture.[8]
- Look for tenderness, swelling, ecchymosis, or a palpable defect posteriorly along the spinous processes.[8]
- Lower thoracic and upper lumbar injuries (T11-L1) are associated with increased risk of gastrointestinal injury.
- Lumbar and sacral injuries (L2-sacral) are associated with risks of orthopedic and gastrointestinal injuries.[11]
- Accurately document any loss of sensation or motor function.[8]
- Spinal cord injury above the T6 level can present with **spinal or neurogenic shock** (bradycardia and hypotension).[23]
  - Represents a loss of descending sympathetic tone.
  - Spinal shock must be recognized early.
  - Pure fluid and blood resuscitation may not be effective.
  - A vasopressor may be needed to restore adequate perfusion.

INITIAL MANAGEMENT
Spine Stabilization
- The mainstay of spinal injury management is to immobilize the affected levels.
  - In the field, this means immobilizing the entire spinal axis.[23]
- Use an appropriately sized cervical collar!
  - If proper collar is unavailable, blocks and tape are effective for immobilizing the head on the backboard.[23]
- Children's disproportionate large head places them in *flexion* when positioned on a neutral board.
  - Proper immobilization requires either:
    - A special board with a recess for the occiput, allowing the head to rest in line with the body.
    - Placement of a thin cushion under the torso relative to the head.[23]
- See Chapter 9 on C-spine Injuries for details.

SPINAL IMAGING
Plain Radiographs
- AP and lateral radiographs can detect most osseous injuries in children and give an excellent global view of the spine.[23]

- Flexion/extension x-rays are important to rule out subluxation in any patient with reported transient neurologic symptoms.[20]
- Paraspinous muscles will often "splint" the spine, rendering any subluxation undetectable in the acute setting.
- Obtain follow-up x-rays 5 to 7 days after muscle spasm subsides.[20]

Computed Tomography
- If plain films are negative but clinical suspicion remains high, high-quality CT scans may be obtained to identify an occult, and possibly surgically correctable, vertebral fracture or dislocation.[20]
- CT seems less helpful in pediatric spine's routine evaluation because children are more likely than adults to have ligamentous injury without fracture.

Magnetic Resonance Imaging
- The modality of choice in the pediatric patient with apparent spinal cord injury but negative radiographic studies.
- Sensitive at detecting ligamentous disruptions and instability not seen on plain radiographs.[24]
- Demonstrates extent of actual spinal cord damage, ranging from mild hemorrhage and/or edema to cord transection.[25]
- Findings are prognostic of patient outcome.[25]
- A normal-appearing MRI suggests excellent recovery.
- Findings of major hemorrhage or cord transection are associated with permanent cord injury.
- Can also rule out surgical lesions (those causing persistent cord compression, such as epidural hematoma or traumatic disc herniation).[26-28]

MANAGEMENT
- Assess in hospital using a systematic approach to spine fractures (Fig. 13-1).
- Issue of immediate stability (e.g., whether or not there is a need for rigid immobilization at the time of presentation) based on the specific fracture type (Table 13-1).[29]
  - Definition of stability based on the injured spinal column's remaining ability to bear normal physiologic loads without further neurologic compromise.[29]
  - Majority of thoracic and lumbar spine fractures in children and younger adolescents are minor, stable, and without neurologic deficit.[8]
  - Bed rest and gradual resumption of activities are generally sufficient for managing these injuries.[8]
- Determining need for neurologic decompression (Fig. 13-1).[29]
  - In most instances, emergent decompression is unnecessary for the patient with a complete thoracic spinal cord injury associated with a spinal fracture.[29,30]
  - Spinal cord injury in this setting involves "supra-threshold" forces causing irreversible damage regardless of treatment.[29,30]
- Thoracic spinal cord made up primarily of delicate white matter tracts.
- T4-T8 levels represent the spinal cord's primary vascular watershed zone.
- Emergent decompression justified for:
  - Thoracic spinal cord compression by "sub-threshold" forces causing a rare, incomplete injury (e.g., bone fragment, hematoma, and/or herniated disc).
  - Compression of the conus medullaris at the thoracolumbar junction.
  - Compression of the cauda equina at the lumbar spine.[29]
- Determination of late stability (e.g., knowing the potential for long-term healing if properly immobilized) based on the specific fracture type (Table 13-1).[29]
  - Fractures predominantly osseous have **good** healing potential.
  - Fractures predominantly disco-ligamentous have **poor** healing potential.[29]
- Steroid use in spinal cord injury.
  - Corticosteroids have NOT been conclusively proven to be of value in spinal cord injury.[23,31,32]
  - Only cautious use of corticosteroids in children as they were excluded from the National Acute Spinal Cord Injury Study (NASCIS).[33,34]

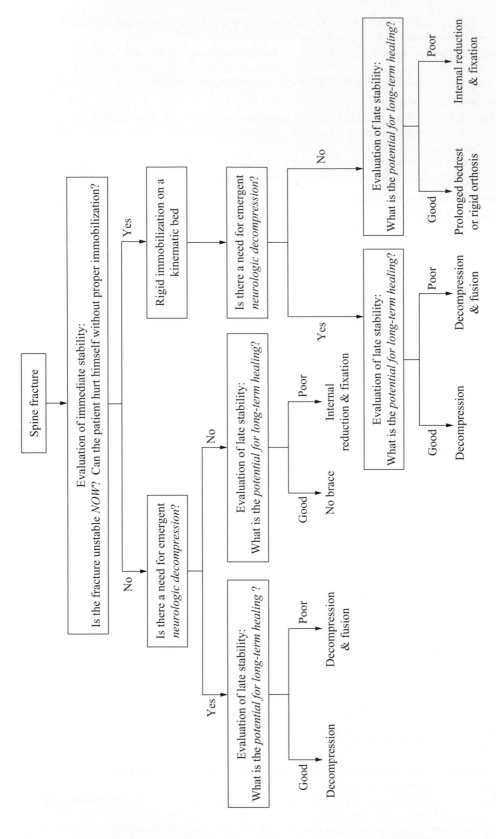

FIGURE 13-1 ● Systematic approach to thoracic and lumbar spine fractures.

TABLE 13-1

Properties of Specific Thoracic and Lumbar Spine Fractures

Fracture Type	Associated Spinal Cord Injury	Stability	
		Immediate	Late
Compression	Uncommon	Good	Good
Burst	Possible	Fair	Good
Fracture-distraction	Possible	Fair	Good
Fracture-rotation	Common	Poor	Poor

SPECIFIC TYPES OF INJURY PATTERNS
Thoracic and Lumbar Spine Fractures
- Classification systems for thoracic and lumbar spine fractures in children have not been proposed.[8]

Compression Fractures[8,35]
- Figure 13-2.
- Mechanism of injury:
  - Axial load with flexion and affect almost exclusively the vertebral body.
- Characteristics:
  - Vertebral body deformation due to compression of the cancellous bone rather than to fragmentation.
  - Posterior column is intact.
  - No spinal canal compromise occurs.
  - Majority of compression fractures in children occur in the thoracic spine.[8]
  - Multiple compression injuries are common.[8]
- Associated spinal cord injury:
  - Neurologic deficit is **very rare** in this stable fracture.[35]
- Conservative management:
  - When the kyphotic wedge of the thoracic or lumbar vertebra is <10 degrees, treatment consists of bed rest and gradually resuming activities as tolerated.[8]
  - When kyphotic deformity is >10 degrees in an immature spine, immobilization in hyperextension is recommended for 2 months, followed by bracing for 1 year or more.[14]
- Surgical indications:
  - Anterior and/or posterior surgical stabilization is recommended for >30 degrees of kyphosis in adolescents near skeletal maturity.[14,36]

Burst Fractures[8,35]
- Figure 13-3.
- Mechanism of injury:
  - Axial compression without flexion, affecting almost exclusively the vertebral body.
- Characteristics:
  - Vertebral body is partially or completely comminuted with centrifugal extrusion of fragments.
  - Fragments of the posterior wall retropulsed into the spinal canal.
- Associated spinal cord injury:
  - Severe compression of vertebral body may cause extrusion of fragments into the spinal canal and thus compress the spinal cord or cauda equina.

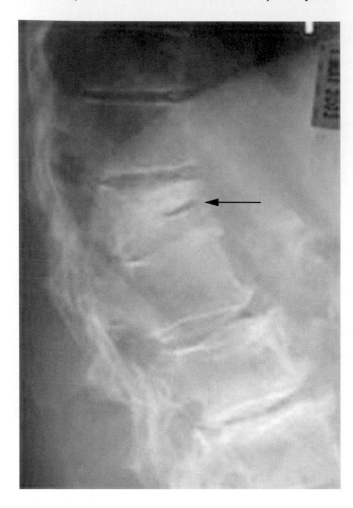

FIGURE 13-2 ● Lateral lumbosacral spine x-ray shows a compression fracture *(arrow)*.

- Conservative management:
  - Can be managed conservatively when there is no neurologic injury.[14,36,37,38]
  - Treatment of this unstable fracture consists of hyperextension casting for 2 to 3 months and bracing for an additional 6 to 12 months.[8]
- Surgical indications:
  - >50% loss of body height.
  - >50% canal compromise from retropulsed bone fragments.
  - >30 degrees of kyphosis.
  - Absolute indications for surgical decompression and/or fusion include neurologic deficits[36,37] or progressive kyphosis.
  - Anterior decompression recommended for multiple nerve root palsies or SCI.

Anterior and Posterior Element Injuries with Distraction[8,35]

- Figure 13-4.
- Mechanism of injury:
  - Flexion-distraction injury associated with use of lapbelt restraints.
  - Lapbelt slides up torso and rests over the abdomen instead of the proximal thighs and hips.[39]
- Characteristics:
  - Main criterion is transverse disruption of one or both spinal columns.
  - Nonspecific findings of posterior tenderness, swelling, and subcutaneous hematoma.

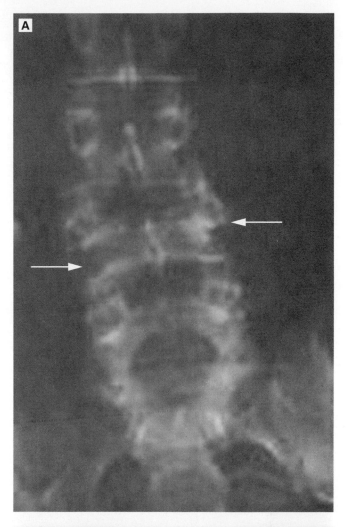

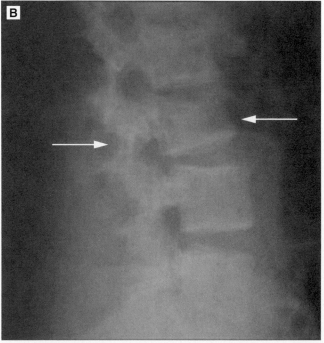

FIGURE 13-3 ● AP (**A**) and lateral (**B**) lumbosacral spine x-rays show an L3 burst fracture *(arrows)*.

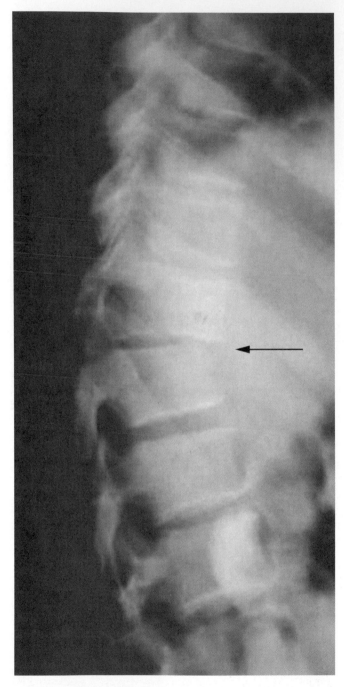

FIGURE 13-4 ● Lateral thoracic spine x-ray shows a lapbelt injury to the spine *(arrow)*.

- Associated spinal cord injury:
  - Neurologic deficits are infrequent and may be due to kyphotic angulation or to fragments retropulsed into the spinal canal.
  - Intra-abdominal injury is common and may obscure diagnosis of spine trauma.[8,35]
- Conservative management:
  - This unstable injury often requires cast immobilization for 8 to 10 weeks when there is minimal displacement and the fracture line goes through bone.[8]

- Surgical indications:
  - Posterior surgical stabilization is indicated in the presence of:
    - Persistent or progressive displacement >17 degrees of kyphosis (FJ Eismont, personal communication, March 24, 2006.)
    - Neurologic deficits.
    - Predominantly discoligamentous injury instead of bony.[40]

Anterior and Posterior Element Injuries with Rotation[8,35]

- Figure 13-5.
- Mechanism of injury:
  - Fall from great heights, a heavy object falling on a bent back, or patient is thrown some distance.[35]
- Characteristics:
  - Most severe and unstable injuries of the thoracic and lumbar spine.
  - Highest rate of neurologic deficit.[35]

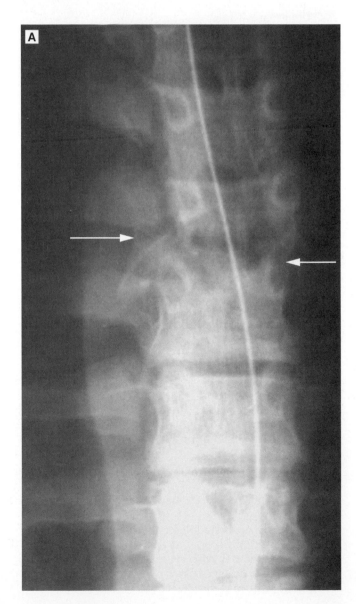

FIGURE 13-5 ● AP **(A)** and lateral **(B)** thoracic spine x-rays show a fracture-dislocation of T5-6 (arrow).

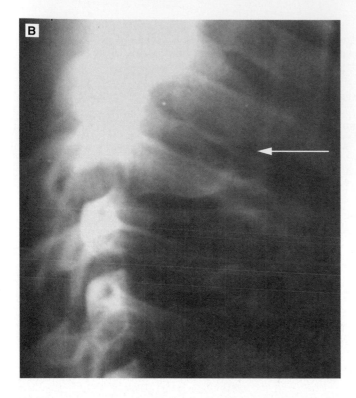

FIGURE 13-5 ● *(Continued)*

- Radiologic signs of rotation and axial torque include:
  - Rotational displacement.
  - Potential for translational displacement in all directions of the horizontal plane.
  - Disruption of all longitudinal ligaments and discs.
  - Fractures of articular processes, usually unilateral.
  - Fracture of transverse processes.
  - Rib dislocations and/or fractures close to the spine.
  - Lateral avulsion fracture of the end plate.
  - Irregular fractures of the neural arch.
  - Asymmetrical fractures of the vertebral body.[35]
- Associated spinal cord injury:
  - Neural injury is caused by fragments dislocated into the spinal canal and/or by encroachment of the spinal canal resulting from translational displacement.[35]
- Surgical indication:
  - Treatment should be surgical through a posterior approach.[35,41]
  - Due to high degree of instability and poor healing potential of mainly discoligamentous rotational injuries.

Limbus Fracture (Apophyseal Fracture)[8]
- Mechanism of injury:
  - Lifting a heavy object; may also occur from falls or twisting injuries.[8]
- Characteristics:
  - Typically seen in adolescents or young adults and presents clinically like a herniated disc.[8]
  - The patient may describe a "pop" at the time of injury, followed by radiculopathy.[8]
- Conservative management:
  - Nonoperative management rarely successful.[36,42]

- Surgical indication:
  - Surgical excision of the limbus fragment.[8]
  - Use MRI and/or CT to determine lesion's exact location and configuration.

Thoracic and Lumbar Spinal Cord Injuries

- SCIWORA coined by Pang and Wilberger in 1982[20] (Fig. 13-6).
- Mechanisms of injury—four suspected mechanisms of SCIWORA:
  - Longitudinal distraction.
  - Hyperflexion.
  - Hyperextension.
  - Ischemic spinal cord damage.[3]
- Suspected mechanisms of thoracic SCIWORA:
  - Ribcage makes thoracic spine resistant to flexion and extension forces.[3,25,43]
  - Proposed mechanism is distraction, which can occur in two situations:[3,43]
    - Crush injury if patient is prone with the spine's "ventral bowing" (hyperextension) into the thoracic and abdominal cavities.
    - Restrained in a motor vehicle using only a lapbelt. Injury results from longitudinal distraction on the thoracic spinal cord.
- Characteristics:
  - Describes phenomenon of closed spinal trauma with significant neurologic injury but without vertebral fracture or subluxation.[44]

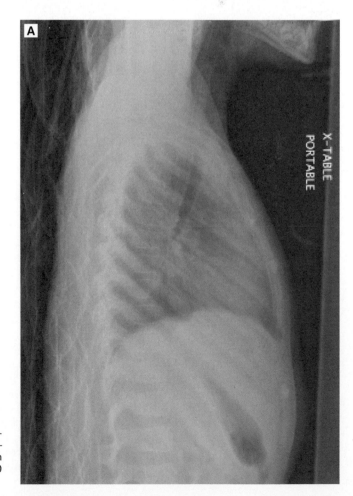

FIGURE 13-6 ● Example of SCIWORA. 6-year-old girl with T10 complete paraplegia after a motor vehicle accident. Neurologic exam unexplained by the admission normal-appearing plain x-ray of the thoracic spine **(A)**. Further workup with MRI shows cord signal change (*white arrow*) at the T10 level on the sagittal T2-weighted sequence **(B)**, indicating a spinal cord injury without evidence of abnormality on the plain radiograph at the T10 level.

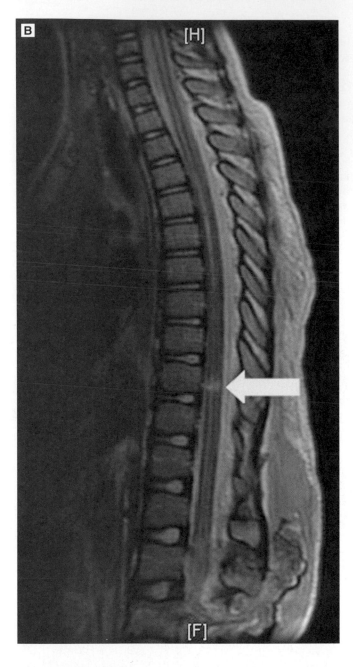

FIGURE 13-6 ● *(Continued)*

- Infantile bony spinal column elastic stretching up to 5 cm.
- The spinal cord is not so pliable, rupturing with only 5 or 6 mm of traction.[20,45]
- Spinal cord is anchored by cauda equina inferiorly and superiorly by brachial plexus.
- Children under 8 years old are similarly susceptible to SCIWORA because of their spinal column's elasticity.
- Over 8 years old, the spine progresses to the stiffer and stronger adult spine, reducing the probability of hypermobility leading to spinal cord injury.[7,20,46]
  Spinal cord syndromes associated with SCIWORA (Fig. 13-7)[44]:
- *Central cord syndrome:* Lesion occurring in central part of the upper cervical spinal cord, producing upper limb weakness (particularly hands) "out-of-proportion" compared to lower limbs (Fig. 13-7A).

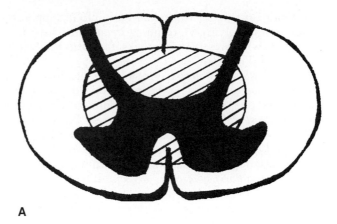

A

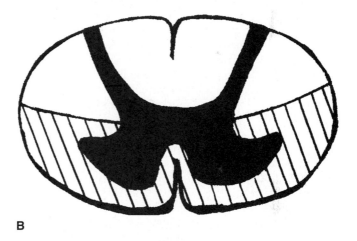

B

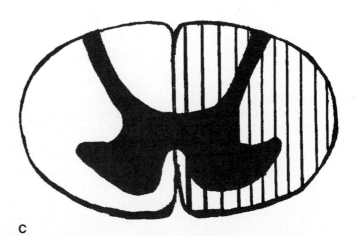

C

FIGURE 13-7 ● Site of lesion (*shaded area*) within the spinal cord for (**A**) central cord syndrome, (**B**) anterior cord syndrome, and (**C**) Brown-Séquard syndrome.

- *Anterior spinal cord syndrome:* Main blood supply to the spinal cord is interrupted (anterior spinal artery), resulting in complete loss of motor function, pain, and temperature with preservation of vibratory sensation, proprioception, and light touch sensation (Fig. 13-7B).
- *Brown–Séquard syndrome:* Physiologic "hemisection" of the spinal cord with motor and position sense loss on the ipsilateral side, and pain and temperature sensation loss beginning one or two levels below injury on the contralateral side (Fig. 13-7C).
- *Complete spinal cord injury:* No function below the level of the lesion, including motor, sensation, reflexes, and sphincter (bowel/bladder function).
- *Incomplete, or partial, spinal cord injury:* Any cord injury short of complete that does not closely reproduce classic spinal cord injury syndromes.
- *Conus medullaris syndrome:* Associated with a thoracolumbar junction spine fracture, early loss of sexual and sphincter function, and symmetric "saddle" loss of motor and/or sensory function in the lower extremities.
  - May be a complex constellation of upper and lower motor neuron findings.
- *Cauda equina syndrome:* Associated with a lumbar spine fracture, asymmetric loss of motor and/or sensory function in the lower extremities, and late sexual and sphincter dysfunction.

Special Considerations in Management of Sciwora

- Treatment in SCIWORA has minimal effect on the primary injury but has extreme importance in preventing reinjury, which can lead to more severe neurologic injury.[3,6,47]
- Up to half of patients with SCIWORA experience a delayed neurologic deterioration believed to be caused by repeated mechanical trauma to the cord because of undiagnosed spinal instability or ongoing ischemia.[20]
- Question patients and their parents for symptoms such as transient weakness, paresthesias, numbness, or "shock-like" sensations in the extremities after any cranial-spinal axis trauma.[44]
- If suspicious, admit the child for observation and/or immobilization.
- Patients with minor symptoms (like transient paresthesias without motor deficit) and who are neurologically intact at presentation with negative flexion/extension films, should refrain from physical activity for several weeks with clinical follow-up.[44]
  - Patients with persistent deficits, convincing histories of myelopathic symptoms (often transient) after trauma, or documented ligamentous instability on dynamic films, must be admitted for observation and immobilization.[3]
- Patients with thoracic injuries should be on strict bed rest until a properly fitted external orthosis can be made.
- Obtain upright x-rays in the orthosis to ensure that there is no progressive kyphosis or subluxation, which would indicate internal fixation.
  - Otherwise, a rigid external orthosis should be worn for a minimum of 3 months.[3,43,47]
- Take flexion and extension x-rays after 3 months of bracing. Any late development of instability requires surgical stabilization.[8]
- Admit and observe patients with significant deficits (like temporary paralysis), even if fully resolved at presentation.
  - At high risk for delayed deterioration.[44]
  - MRI of the spine is indicated for these patients.[3,20]
    - Infants and younger children with severe, persistent neurologic deficits have a grim prognosis and rarely recover function.[20,26,28,48,49]
  - These patients are subject to spinal shock, which exacerbates any cord injury through poor perfusion of an already damaged and sensitive spinal cord.

CLINICAL PEARLS

DO

- Consider the large head of a child during immobilization on a neutral backboard.
  - Avoid placing the neck into flexion.
  - Keep the neck in line with the rest of the spinal axis.
- Approach spine fractures systematically, taking into account immediate stability, the need for neurologic decompression, and late stability.
- Consider SCIWORA in the pediatric population.
- Consider spinal shock in cases of hypotension unresponsive to aggressive fluid and blood resuscitation.
  - Treat spinal or neurogenic shock with vasopressors.
  - Neurogenic shock seen with spinal cord injury above the T6 level.
- Majority of thoracic and lumbar spine fractures in children and young adolescents are minor, stable, and without neurologic deficit.

DON'T

- Compromise the immediate stability of the spine. Use proper cervical and spinal immobilization.
- Use steroids to treat spinal cord injury as their use in children is NOT currently supported by literature. Please consult your local referral center for advice.
- Rush for emergent decompression and fusion of complete thoracic spinal cord injuries after a high-velocity fracture.
  - Not usually indicated.
  - It is more imperative to stabilize the patient systemically first.

REFERENCES

1. Babock JL. Spinal injuries in children. *Pediatr Clin North Am* 1975;22:487–500.
2. Kewalramani LS, Kraus JF, Sterling HM. Acute spinal cord lesions in a pediatric population: epidemiological and clinical features. *Paraplegia* 1980;18:206–219.
3. Pang D, Pollack IF. Spinal cord injury without radiographic abnormality in children: the SCIWORA syndrome. *J Trauma* 1989;29:654–664.
4. Ruge JR, Sinson GP, McLone DG. Pediatric spinal injury: the very young. *J Neurosurg* 1988;68:25–30.
5. Dickman CA, Rekate HL, Sonntag VK, et al. Pediatric spinal trauma: vertebral column and spinal cord injuries in children. *Pediatr Neurosci* 1989;15:237–256.
6. Dickman CA, Zabramski JM, Hadley MN. Pediatric spinal cord injury without radiographic abnormalities: report of 26 cases and review of the literature. *J Spinal Disord* 1991;4:296–305.
7. Hadley MN, Zabramski JM, Browner CM, et al. Pediatric spinal trauma. Review of 122 cases of spinal cord and vertebral column injuries. *J Neurosurg* 1988;68:18–24.
8. Vialle LR, Vialle E. Pediatric spine injuries. *Injury* 2005;36(suppl):B104–B112.
9. Reddy SP, Junewick JJ, Backstrom JW. Distribution of spinal fractures in children: does age, mechanism of injury, or gender play a significant role? *Pediatr Radiol* 2003;33:776–781.
10. Hu R, Mustard CA, Burns C. Epidemiology of incident spinal fracture in a complete population. *Spine* 1996;21:492–499.
11. Cirak B, Ziegfeld S, Knight VM, et al. Spinal injuries in children. *J Pediatr Surg* 2004;39:607–612.
12. Finch GD, Barnes MJ. Major cervical spine injuries in children and adolescents. *J Pediatr Orthop* 1998;18:811–814.
13. McPhee IB. Spinal fractures and dislocations in children and adolescents. *Spine* 1981;6:533–537.
14. Pouliquen JC, Kassis B, Glorion C, et al. Vertebral growth after thoracic or lumbar fracture of the spine in children. *J Pediatr Orthop* 1997;17:115–120.
15. Schwartz GR, Wright SW, Fein JA, et al. Pediatric cervical spine injury sustained in falls from low heights. *Ann Emerg Med* 1997;30:249–252.
16. Turgut M, Akpinar G, Akalan N, et al. Spinal injuries in the pediatric age group: a review of 82 cases of spinal cord and vertebral column injuries. *Eur Spine J* 1996;5:148–152.
17. Bick EM, Copel JW. Longitudinal growth of the human vertebra. *J Bone Joint Surg Am* 1950;32:803–814.
18. Bick EM, Copel JW. The ring apophysis of the human vertebra; contribution to human osteogeny. *J Bone Joint Surg Am* 1951;33:783–787.
19. Roche C, Carty H. Spinal trauma in children. *Pediatr Radiol* 2001;31:677–700.
20. Pang D, Wilberger JE. Spinal cord injury without radiographic abnormalities in children. *J Neurosurg* 1982;57:114–129.
21. Swischuk LE, Swischuk PN, John SD. Wedging of C-3 in infants and children: usually a normal finding and not a fracture. *Radiology* 1993;188:523–526.
22. Marar BC. Hyperextension injuries of the cervical spine: the pathogenesis of damage to the spinal cord. *J Bone Joint Surg Am* 1974:56:1655–1662.

23. Proctor MR. Spinal cord injury. *Crit Care Med* 2002;30:S489–S499.
24. Keiper M, Zimmerman R, Bilaniuk L. MRI in the assessment of the supportive soft tissues of the cervical spine in acute trauma in children. *Neuroradiology* 1998;40:359–363.
25. Grabb PA, Pang D. Magnetic resonance imaging in the evaluation of spinal cord injury without radiographic abnormality in children. *Neurosurgery* 1994;35:406–414.
26. Ahmann PA, Smith SA, Schwartz JF, et al. Spinal cord infarction due to minor trauma in children. *Neurology* 1975;25:301–307.
27. Davis PC, Reisner A, Hudgins PA, et al. Spinal injuries in children: role of MRI. *AJNR Am J Neuroradiol* 1993;14:607–617.
28. Walsh JW, Stevens DB, Young AB. Traumatic paraplegia in children without contiguous spinal fracture or dislocation. *Neurosurgery* 1993;12:439–445.
29. Ogilvy CS, Heros RC. Spinal cord compression. In: Ropper AH, Kennedy SK, Zervas NT, eds. *Neurological and neurosurgical intensive care.* Baltimore: University Park Press; 1983:309–322.
30. Geisler FH, Coleman WP, Grieco G, et al. Measurement and recovery patterns in a multicenter study of acute spinal cord injury. *Spine* 2001;26:S68–S86.
31. Hurlbert RJ. The role of steroids in acute spinal cord injury: an evidence-based analysis. *Spine* 2001;26:S39–S46.
32. Nesathurai S. The role of methylprednisolone in acute spinal cord injuries. *J Trauma* 2001;51:421–423.
33. Bracken MB, Collins WF, Freeman DF, et al. Efficacy of methylprednisolone in acute spinal cord injury. *JAMA* 1984;251:45–52.
34. Bracken MB, Shephard MJ, Collins WF, et al. A randomized, controlled trial of methylprednisolone or nalaxone in the treatment of acute spinal cord injury: results of the second national acute spinal cord injury study. *N Engl J Med* 1990;322:1405–1411.
35. Magerl F, Aebi M, Gertzbein SD, et al. A comprehensive classification of thoracic and lumbar injuries. *Eur Spine J* 1994;3:184–201.
36. Crawford AH. Operative treatment of spine fractures in children. *Orthop Clin North Am* 1990;21:325–339.
37. Andreychik DA, Alandar DH, Senica KM, et al. Burst fractures of the second through fifth lumbar vertebrae. Clinical and radiographic results. *J Bone Joint Surg Am* 1996;78:1156–1166.
38. Cantor JB, Lebwohl NH, Garvey T, et al. Nonoperative management of stable thoracolumbar burst fractures with early ambulation and bracing. *Spine* 1993;18:971–976.
39. Voss L, Cole PA, D'Amato C. Pediatric chance fractures from lapbelts: unique case report of three in one accident. *J Orthop Trauma* 1996;10:421–428.
40. Gumley G, Taylor TK, Ryan MD. Distraction fractures of the lumbar spine. *J Bone Joint Surg Br* 1982;64:520–525.
41. McCormack T, Karaikovic E, Gaines RW. The load sharing classification of spine fractures. *Spine* 1994;19:1741–1744.
42. Epstein NE, Epstein JA. Limbus lumbar vertebral fractures in 27 adolescents and adults. *Spine* 1991;16:962–966.
43. Pollack IF, Pang D. Spinal cord injury without radiographic abnormality. In: Pang D, ed. *Disorders of the pediatric spine.* New York: Raven; 1995:509–516.
44. Kriss VM, Kriss TC. SCIWORA (spinal cord injury without radiographic abnormality) in infants and children. *Clin Pediatr (Phila)* 1996;35:119–124.
45. Scher AT. Trauma of the spinal cord in children. *S Afr Med J* 1976;50:2023–2024.
46. Hamilton MG, Myles ST. Pediatric spinal injury: review of 174 hospital admissions. *J Neurosurg* 1992;77:700–704.
47. Pollack IF, Pang D, Schlabassi R. Recurrent spinal cord injury without radiographic abnormalities in children. *J Neurosurg* 1988;69:177–182.
48. Chesire DJE. The pediatric syndrome of traumatic myelopathy without demonstrable vertebral injury. *Paraplegia* 1978;15:74–85.
49. Glasauer FE, Cares HL. Traumatic paraplegia in infancy. *JAMA* 1972;219:38–41.

CHAPTER 14

Pediatric Thermal Injury

Laura Snell, MD

Howard Clarke, MD, PhD, FRCS, FAAP, FACS

EPIDEMIOLOGY
- 50% of all burns are in the pediatric population.
- 70% of pediatric burns are caused by hot liquid.[1]
  - Flame burns make up the majority of the remaining 30%.
- Younger children are at higher risk of burn injury.
- Up to 20% of burn injuries in younger children are the result of abuse or neglect.[2]

PATHOPHYSIOLOGY
- Many systemic derangements caused by burn injury contribute to fluid shifts.
  - Significant fluid shifts result in burn wound edema and systemic hypovolemia.
- Loss of cutaneous barrier function.
  - Insensible losses.
- Increased capillary permeability.
  - Local in all burn wounds, systemic if >25% TBSA (total body surface area).
  - Hypoproteinemia.
  - Increased fluid shift from vessels to interstitial tissues.
- Release of arachidonic acid cascade metabolites including prostaglandins, histamine, serotonin.
- Hormonal derangements (increase in ADH and aldosterone).

BURN CLASSIFICATION
- Early assessment and documentation of burn depth, extent, and involvement of hands/face/perineum is very important for treatment planning and must be done.

Depth
- First degree/superficial:
  - Red, dry, painful.
  - Will heal after several days, no scar.
- Second degree/partial thickness:
  - Red, wet, very painful.
  - May be superficial or deep partial thickness.
  - Will likely heal after days to weeks of adequate wound care including debridement, daily wound check and dressing changes.
  - May require skin grafting and may scar.
- Third degree/full thickness:
  - Leathery, dry, insensate, waxy.
  - Will not heal without excision and grafting.
- Fourth degree:
  - Involves underlying subcutaneous tissue, tendon, bone.

Total Burn Surface Area (TBSA) (Fig. 14-1)
- Lund—Browder chart.
  - Age-specific.
- Rule of nines (Fig. 14-1).
  - Assuming adult body proportions—appropriate for use in teenagers.
  - Larger head and neck in proportion for younger children and infants.
- Exclude first-degree burns when calculating TBSA.

PEDIATRIC BURNS: INITIAL MANAGEMENT
Primary Survey
Airway Management
- Airway is first priority during primary survey.
- Must be secured prior to transport.
- Suspect inhalation injury if:
  - The fire occurred in an enclosed space.
  - Patient has:
    - Carbonaceous sputum.
    - Singed nasal hairs or eyebrows.
    - Hoarseness or stridor.
    - Elevated carboxyhemoglobin level (>10%).
- Confirm airway injury with bronchoscopy at the bedside.
- Hot liquid aspiration can also cause airway compromise.[3]
- Indications for intubation:
  - Inhalation injury
    - Stridor.
    - Respiratory distress.
    - $PaO_2 < 60$ mmHg, $PaCO_2 > 55$ mmHg.
  - Need for transport to another facility.
  - Significant facial ± neck burns.
  - Anticipated aggressive fluid resuscitation.
- Important to secure the endotracheal tube (ETT) at the time of intubation.
  - Do not cut the ETT shorter as facial edema will likely progress.

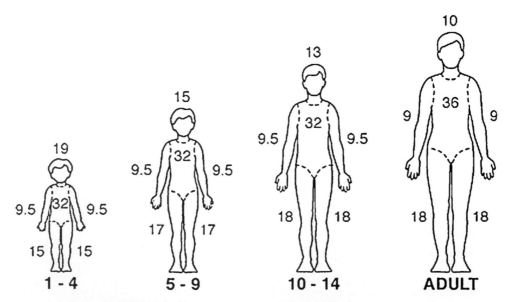

FIGURE 14-1 ● Total body surface area (TBSA) estimation.

- Ensure the ETT is secured properly.
- Consider use of reinforced ETT.
- 24-gauge wire around the molars and then around the tube.
- Do not use suture material (not strong enough).
- See Chapter 3 on Airway Management for details.

Fluid Resuscitation
- Important to establish early secure venous access.
  - Can be difficult in the hypovolemic patient.
  - May require intraosseous access to begin resuscitation.
  - See the "Definitive Management" section later in this chapter for details.
- Aggressive fluid resuscitation with normal saline required for burns >15%.
- Burns <15% are generally not associated with extensive capillary leak.
  - Encourage PO fluid intake.
  - Closely monitor urine output. Goal = 1-2 mL/kg/hr.
- Parkland resuscitation formula (Ringer lactate): **4 mL/kg/%TBSA.**
  - Note: Time zero for fluid resuscitation = time of burn injury.
  - An estimation of fluid requirements for the initial 24 hours following a significant burn injury ABOVE normal maintenance requirements.
  - Give first half of calculated volume over 8 hours from time of injury.
  - Give the remaining half of calculated volume over the following 16 hours.
  - Remember to consider other ongoing losses as well (e.g., vomiting).
  - Monitor urine output closely and adjust rate of fluid infusion as needed for target urine output of 1-2 mL/kg/hr.

EVALUATION
History
- Details of the events surrounding the injury.
  - Where did it occur? When did it occur? How did it occur?
  - Was anyone else injured?
  - What was the fluid involved—grease versus water/steam?
- Symptoms:
  - Pain related to burns.
  - Chest pain, shortness of breath, coughing.
  - Vomiting or abdominal pain.
  - Dizziness or lightheadedness, syncope, headache, visual changes.
  - Extremity pain, numbness, tingling.
- Past medical history:
  - Underlying cardiac, respiratory, or neurological disease.
  - Tetanus status.
  - NPO status.

Physical Examination/Burn-Specific Secondary Survey
- Neurologic exam:
  - Rule out intracranial trauma.
  - Carbon monoxide poisoning.
    - Administer 100% O_2 until COHB <10%.
    - See Chapter 15 on Smoke Inhalation for further details.
  - Assess for and manage pain/anxiety.
    - See Chapter 18 on Pain Management for further details.
- Ophthalmologic and otolaryngologic exam.
  - Cornea:
    - Fluorescein exam to rule out corneal injury.
  - External ear:
    - Assess for burns and exposed cartilage.

- Chest:
  - Inhalation injury.
    - See Chapter 15 on Smoke Inhalation for further details.
  - Decreased compliance.
    - Escharotomy (Fig. 14-2).
      - Should be considered if burn is circumferential around the chest, airway pressures increased, lung compliance decreased due to chest wall noncompliance.
      - Incision made through thick, leathery eschar of third-degree burns to increase compliance.
- Cardiac:
  - If mechanism unknown or suspected electrical injury, arrhythmias may develop.
    - See Chapter 16 on Electrical Injury for further details.
- Abdomen:
  - Exclude associated injuries.
  - Abdominal compartment syndrome can occur.
    - Easiest method of measuring is transducing through a Foley catheter.
    - Rarely, children require drainage of peritoneal fluid to decompress increased abdominal pressure.[4]
- GU:
  - Reduce the foreskin over the glans.
- Musculoskeletal:
  - Serial examinations of the extremities including:
    - Pain with voluntary motion.
    - Pain with passive motion.
    - Pulses.
    - Capillary refill.
    - Temperature.
    - Pliability.
  - Consider escharotomy when physical exam of burned extremity is suggestive of compartment syndrome:
    - Pain out of keeping with injury, pain when muscle is stretched, pallor, pulselessness, paresthesias, muscle tightness/fullness.
    - Can do escharotomies with electrocautery, most often in the OR in children due to unpredictable amount of blood loss.
    - See Figure 14-2 for escharotomy sites.
- Tetanus prophylaxis.
- No role for prophylactic systemic antibiotics.

Lab Testing
- CBC, electrolytes, and renal function for all burns requiring admission.
- Carboxyhemoglobin level, blood gases if inhalation injury is suspected.
- Monitor for hypoalbuminemia in severe burns.

Imaging
- Chest x-ray for all patients requiring fluid resuscitation as a baseline, or if other injuries including inhalation injury suspected.
- Any other imaging as per ATLS protocol: See Chapter 2 on Primary and Secondary Survey for details.

DEFINITIVE MANAGEMENT
Unique Aspects of Pediatric Burn Care
- Survival rates have improved as resuscitation efforts have become more aggressive and standardized.
  - In children with TBSA >60%, a survival rate of 14% is estimated.[5]
- Electrolytes must be closely monitored; watch for the development of hypoglycemia.

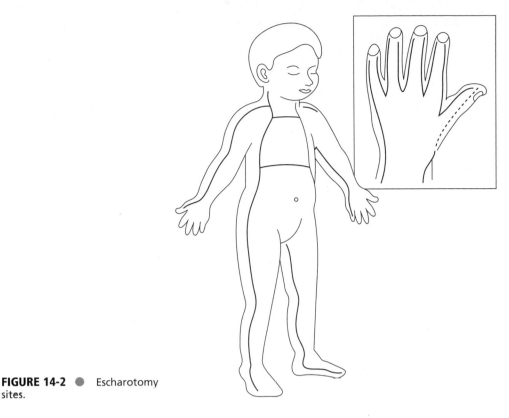

FIGURE 14-2 ● Escharotomy sites.

- Tight control of fluid resuscitation.
  - Tendency toward over-resuscitation.
  - Keep in mind age-appropriate fluid goals, include all IV meds in calculations.
  - Furosemide (Lasix) is counterproductive.
- Reduction of hepatic albumin synthesis.
  - Combined with a loss of albumin through open wounds, leads to predictable hypoalbuminemia.
  - Use of albumin during resuscitative phase (initial 48 hours) is not indicated and may be harmful.[7]
- Monitor for predictable hypermetabolic response postburn:
  - Fever.
  - Increased metabolic rate.
  - Increased minute ventilation.
  - Increased cardiac output.
  - Decreased afterload.
  - Increased gluconeogenesis.
  - Increased skeletal and visceral muscle catabolism.
- Enteral nutritional support.
  - Should begin during resuscitation and reduces the risk of systemic sepsis if begun within 6 hours of the injury.
- Global immunosuppression postburn.
  - At risk for sepsis, pneumonia but NO role for prophylactic systemic antibiotics.

Parental Issues
- Abuse.
  - See Chapter 19 on Nonaccidental Injury for further details.

- Obtain full history, including temperature of liquid if relevant, length of contact, caregivers involved, documentation of conflicting reports from involved caregivers, delay in seeking treatment, prior injuries.
- At-risk children:
  - <3 years old.
  - Single-parent homes.
  - Impoverished.
  - Scald or contact burn.
- Red flags:
  - "Dipping" burn.
  - "Punched-out" burn (cigarettes).
  - Repeated history of trauma.
  - Reports that the burn is caused by other siblings or the child him/herself.
  - Child accompanied by someone other than a parent.[6]

Dressings
- Goal of initial dressing is to:
  - Control pain.
  - Decrease vapor loss.
  - Prevent dessication.
  - Slow bacterial growth.
- Initial dressing:
  - Superficial partial thickness.
    - Polysporin + Bactigras + gauze.
    - Daily wound check and dressing change.
  - Deep partial thickness/full thickness:
    - Flamazine (silver sulfadiazine) + gauze.
    - If a consult to plastic surgery is pending, initially apply Polysporin + Bactigras as flamazine can obscure initial burn evaluation.
    - Daily cleansing, wound check, dressing change (Table 14-1).

Criteria for Referring a Patient to a Specialized Burn Center
- Inhalation injury.
- Burn size >10% TBSA in patients <10 years.
- Burn size >20% in any patient.
- Full-thickness burns >5% TBSA.
- Burn involving face, hands, feet, perineum, genitalia.
- Associated trauma.
- Significant comorbidities.
- Special social circumstances (e.g., nonaccidental injury suspected).
- Chemical or electrical injuries.

TABLE 14-1

Common Burn Dressings

Agent	Application	Contraindications	Important Side Effects
Silver sulfadiazine	Deep partial-thickness/full-thickness burns	Sulfa allergy	Rare reports of neutropenia, leukopenia
Polysporin	Superficial partial-thickness/healing burns	Grossly infected wounds	Can cause dermatitis after several days

- Other pediatric issues to consider:
  - Pain control.
  - Nutritional support.
  - Wound care—no adequate available options as outpatient.
  - Social situation—concern regarding the family's ability to cope.

Transport—What Must Be Done Prior to Transport
- Primary survey:
  - **Must** ensure airway safety.
  - If any concerns, secure the airway.
  - Ensure appropriate venous access.
- Initiation of fluid resuscitation (according to Parkland formula and urine output).
- Ensure adequate analgesia (see Chapter 18 on Pain Management for details).
- Secondary survey: Assess for other injuries.
- Place NG tube and Foley catheter when appropriate.
- Dressing for transport: Dry dressing rather than wet (hypothermia a risk during transport).
- Tetanus prophylaxis—either give prior to transport, or ensure given on arrival if indicated.
- Appropriate and complete paperwork, including assessment of burn wounds (depth, extent).
  - Diagrams are helpful.
- See Chapter 22 on Transport of the Pediatric Trauma Patient for further details.

SPECIFIC INJURIES
- Scald burns:
  - The majority of patients do not require surgery if aggressive wound care is done (daily wound cleansing and dressing changes).
  - Ensure adequate analgesia.
- Facial burns:
  - Rule out corneal injury.
  - Lubrication important as eyelids swell.
  - Securing the ETT is very important with wire (can't use tape).
- Scalp burns:
  - MUST shave hair in the burned area to properly assess burn and keep wound clean.
- Commisure burns:
  - Late bleeding.
  - Parents must be warned about potential for massive bleeding at 5 to 10 days as eschar separates and exposes labial artery.
  - See Chapter 16 on Electrical Injury for further details.
- Hand burns:
  - Occasionally require surgery but require close follow-up for wound healing, contractures, and physiotherapy.

CHEMICAL BURNS
- Three main groups:
  - Acid burns.
  - Alkali burns.
  - Chemical injection injuries (extravasation injuries).
- Acids cause coagulation necrosis.
- Alkalis cause saponification, liquefactive necrosis.
  - Penetrate deeper than acids, often cause more tissue destruction.
- Irrigate wounds with clean water for at least 30 minutes, much longer (hours) for alkali burns.

- Elemental sodium, potassium, and lithium ignite when exposed to water—extinguish these burns with a fire extinguisher.
- Irrigation is also contraindicated for phenol burns as dilution allows phenol to penetrate better.
  - Use polyethylene glycol wipes.
- Irrigate globe with isotonic crystalloid solution if available.
  - Morgan lens may be helpful.
  - Ensure adequate topical anesthesia (e.g., Tetracaine).
- Inspect nails, hair, web spaces for residual chemical.
- Tar and grease removal—use Vaseline or Polysporin ointment.
- Exposures to concentrates or anhydrous hydrofluoric acid (industrial cleaning, tile etching) may cause a life-threatening hypocalcemia.
  - Sub-eschar injections of 10% calcium gluconate solution should be given in cases of hypocalcemia.

EXTRAVASATION INJURIES
- See Table 14-2 for agents that cause extravasation injuries.
- Manage by removing the IV line, elevate the involved extremity, use an antidote if available, splinting of involved extremity.
- Antidotes should be used only after consultation with a specialist:
  - Hyaluronidase—for extravasations of 10% dextrose, calcium, potassium, radiocontrast media, TPN.
  - Phentolamine—for vasopressors.
  - Topical dimethyl sulfoxide (DMSO)—for doxorubicin.
  - Contact the local plastic surgery center or toxicologist for further guidance.
- Role of surgery is minimal in extravasation injuries (Table 14-2).

COLD INJURY
- Tissue freezing (frostbite), non-tissue freezing (trenchfoot), hypothermia.
- Frostbite: Formation of intracellular ice crystals and microvascular occlusion.
- Trenchfoot: Skin chronically exposed to high humidity, low temperatures without tissue freezing.
  - Numbness, tingling, pain, itching, erythema, edema.
- Very young children at risk for frostbite.
- Treatment of frostbite:
  - Rewarming of involved area.
  - Adequate analgesia.
  - **Do not** massage area—crystals further damage tissues.
  - Once rewarmed, debride clear blisters, leave hemorrhagic blisters intact, elevate affected areas, give ASA, tetanus prophylaxis, topical aloe vera, wait for the area to demarcate before surgical intervention may be warranted (weeks).

TABLE 14-2

Common Agents Causing Extravasation Injuries

Mechanism of Action	Agents
Osmotically active agents	Hypertonic solutions, calcium gluconate, potassium, calcium chloride, TPN
Ischemia-inducing agents	Catecholamines, vasopressin
Agents with direct cellular toxicity	Antineoplastic agents, sodium bicarbonate, sodium thiopental, digoxin, tetracycline

CLINICAL PEARLS

DO
- Ensure airway safety prior to transport.
- Provide tetanus prophylaxis if immunizations are not up to date.
- Rule out corneal injury for facial burns.

DON'T
- Cut endotracheal tube in burn patient as facial edema will likely progress.
- Give systemic antibiotics for burn injuries unless otherwise clinically indicated.
- Give furosemide during resuscitation phase of burn care unless otherwise clinically indicated.

REFERENCES

1. Rossignol AM, Boyle CM, Locke JA, et al. Hospitalized burn injuries in Massachusetts: an assessment of incidence and product development. *Am J Public Health* 1986;76;1341–1343.
2. Sheridan RL, Ryan CM, Petras LM, et al. Burns in children younger than two years of age: an experience with 200 consecutive admissions. *Pediatrics* 1997;100;721–723.
3. Sheridan RL. Recognition and management of hot liquid aspiration in children. *Ann Emerg Med* 1996;27;89–91.
4. Greenhalgh DG, Warden GD. The importance of intra-abdominal pressure measurements in burned children. *J Trauma* 1994;36;685–690.
5. Sheridan RL, Remensnyder JP, Schnitzer JJ, et al. Current expectations for survival in pediatric burns. *Arch Pediatr Adolesc Med* 2000;154:245–249.
6. Passaretti D, Billmire D. Clinical experience: management of pediatric burns. *J Craniofac Surg* 2003;14 14(5):713–8.
7. Cochrane Review. Human Albumin Administration in Critically Ill Patients: Systematic review of randomized controlled trials. Cochrane Injuries Group Albumin Reviewers. *BMJ.* 1998;317(7153):235–40.

CHAPTER 15

Smoke Inhalation

Sanjay V. Mehta, MD, MEd, FRCPC, FAAP, FACEP

EPIDEMIOLOGY

- Most life-threatening burns are from house fires, followed by ignition of non-flame-retardant clothes.
- Of fire-related deaths in children, 82% die at the scene of the fire, 7% die at local hospitals, and 11% die at burn centers.[1]
- House fires victims have a higher case fatality rate compared to burns from other causes, presumably from the added trauma of an inhalation injury.
- Pulmonary failure is one of the leading causes of death in the burn patient, with a 3.6-fold increase in the death rate as the result of concomitant burn and inhalation injury.
  - Children under 3 years are at a higher risk both with and without inhalation injury.

PATHOPHYSIOLOGY

- The airway is most commonly affected by smoke, superheated air, and/or steam.
  - Frequently occurs in the absence of significant burns.
- Inhaling hot gases burns the upper airway, leading to progressive edema and airway obstruction.
  - Heat, asphyxiants, particulate matter, and irritants damage the airway.
  - Lower airway injury is from exposure to toxic combustion products.
- Numerous chemicals are produced in house fires: Hydrochloric acid, chlorine gas, carbon monoxide (CO), acrolein, aldehydes, benzene, phosgene, and cyanide.
  - Can cause chemical asphyxia, local anesthesia, and mucosal and cellular damage.
  - Pulmonary irritation can lead to:
    - Bronchospasm.
    - Increased secretions.
    - Debris.
    - Atelectasis.
    - Acute respiratory distress syndrome.
- Respiratory failure can result from:
  - Loss of airway patency.
  - Bronchospasm.
  - Pulmonary edema.
  - Diminished ciliary activity.
  - Intrapulmonary shunting from small airway occlusion (i.e., bronchiolar obstruction).
  - Diminished lung compliance.
  - Pneumonia.

CLASSIFICATION

- See Chapter 14 on Thermal Injury for details.
- Burns are differentiated based on the depth and layer involved:
  - Superficial (first degree)—epidermis.
  - Partial thickness.

- Superficial (second degree)—dermis.
- Deep (third degree)—subcutaneous tissue.
- Full thickness (fourth degree)—fascia, muscle, or bone.

INITIAL MANAGEMENT

- Maintain ABCs.
- Provide 100% oxygen.
- When to consider smoke inhalational injury[2,3]:
  - Altered mental status.
  - Chest pain.
  - Dyspnea.
  - Respiratory compromise.
  - Need for cardiopulmonary resuscitation on-scene.
  - Burn in a closed space.
  - Potential CO poisoning.
- Intubation should be considered if (Table 15-1):
  - Upper airway patency is threatened.
  - Gas exchange or lung compliance is altered.
  - Mental status is altered.
- Early intubation prevents the later, difficult intubation of a child with severe pharyngeal and subglottic swelling.
  - Ensure bag-valve mask ventilation is possible before attempting laryngoscopy.
  - If rapid-sequence intubation is required, consider:
    - Backup with ENT and anesthesia.
    - Having alternative, difficult airway equipment ready (e.g., difficult airway cart with fiberoptic laryngoscope, gum bougie, and surgical airway equipment).
    - Ketamine for sedation if any evidence of bronchospasm.
    - Using a narrower, reinforced tube.
    - See Chapter 3 on Airway Management for details.
  - If successful intubation, do not cut the endotracheal tube.
    - Oropharyngeal edema will progressively increase and require a longer tube over the next 1 to 3 days.
- If unable to oxygenate or ventilate, needle cricothyroidotomy is needed.
  - See Chapter 21 on Procedures for details.
- Consider at least two large-bore intravenous cannulae to provide fluid resuscitation, as in all trauma patients.

EVALUATION
History
- Associated trauma.
- Impaired mentation.

TABLE 15-1

Potential Indications for Early Intubation[1–4]

Face, mouth, or neck burns or swelling
Singed nasal hair
Soot in mouth
Carbonaceous sputum
Early onset of hoarse voice or stridor
Wheezing
Progressive respiratory insufficiency
Inability to protect airway due to coma or secretions
Carboxyhemoglobin levels >50%

- Confinement in a closed, burning environment with gas, fumes, or steam exposure.
- Nature of materials at scene, and agents involved (grease, oil, plastic substances, fumes, chemical exposure, etc.).

Physical Exam

- CO poisoning may have minimal or multiorgan signs:
  - Chest pain, palpitations, dysrhythmias.
  - Pulmonary edema.
  - Signs of disseminated intravascular coagulation.
  - Skin may be blistered.
  - Cherry-like appearance (due to darker, red color of carboxyhemoglobin) is a late sign.
  - Subtle neurologic findings may be noted.
  - Be wary of the SaO_2, which can be falsely normal in CO poisoning.
- Signs of CN poisoning on exam:[3,4]
  - Low vapor exposure:
    - Tachypnea.
    - Akisthesia.
    - Presyncope.
    - Weakness.
    - Headache.
    - Nausea and vomiting.
  - High vapor exposure:
    - Loss of consciousness.
    - Seizures.
    - Apnea.
- Direct laryngoscopy with thermal injury or signs of upper airway obstruction (Table 15-2).
  - Elective intubation with significant supraglottic or glottic edema.

Laboratory Investigations to Consider

- Complete blood count.
- Type, screen, and crossmatch for blood.
- Blood gas.
  - Be wary of PaO_2 on arterial samples as this only measures dissolved oxygen, and can be falsely normal with CO poisoning.
  - Request CO levels with co-oximetry.
  - pH is most useful data, and values venous may be as helpful as an arterial or capillary one.
- Lactate level.
  - Levels >10 mmol/L (responsible for a large anion gap metabolic acidosis) correlate with cyanide poisoning.
- Carboxyhemoglobin level.
- Serum creatinine kinase and urinalysis.
  - Watch for rhabdomyolysis and/or acute tubular necrosis.

TABLE 15-2

Signs of Thermal Injury to Consider Early Intubation[1–4]

Singed nasal hairs and eyebrows
Carbonaceous deposits in the oropharynx, sputum, or on face
Oropharyngeal edema
Voice change, hoarseness, persistent coughing, or stridor
Pulmonary aspiration
Facial, neck, or upper torso burns
Airway burns can still occur in the absence of these signs

IMAGING

- Chest x-rays:
  - Normal chest x-ray does not exclude significant pulmonary injuries.
  - Early findings on x-ray suggest more severe injury.
  - Diffuse interstitial infiltrates are consistent with smoke inhalation.
  - Focal infiltrates in the first 24 hours indicate atelectasis.
  - Bronchopneumonia usually presents after 72 hours.
  - Pulmonary edema typically appears 6 to 72 hours after exposure, especially with aggressive fluid resuscitation.
  - Pneumothorax is more likely from barotrauma following intubation and positive pressure ventilation.
  - Overall, chest x-rays are insensitive in determining lung injury and rarely dictate emergency management.
- Consider C-spine x-rays or head CT if head and neck trauma are a concern.
- If evidence of seizure, obtain an urgent CT of the head to rule out intracranial bleed or changes in parenchyma.

SPECIFIC INJURIES

- CO poisoning:
  - Mimics numerous other illnesses.
  - Is colorless, tasteless, and odorless at room temperature.
  - CO binds hemoglobin with ~230 times the affinity of oxygen.
  - Carboxyhemoglobin left-shifts the oxyhemoglobin dissociation curve.
  - CO also binds cytochrome oxidase and blocks electron transport, facilitating free radicals and disrupting mitochondria.
  - Carboxyhemoglobin has a half-life of 5 hours in room air, 80 minutes on 100% oxygen, and 20 minutes in hyperbaric oxygen (usually at 2.5 to 3 atmospheres).
  - Dissociative shock is produced, with tissue hypoxia and metabolic acidosis.
  - Causes direct neurotoxicity and lipid peroxidation of cell membranes, with characteristic lesions in the globus pallidus, putamen, caudate, ventricles, and cortex associated with motor and learning dysfunction (Table 15-3).[5]
- Hyperbaric oxygen early for CO poisoning (Table 15-4).
  - Early consultation with hyperbaric chamber physician and toxicologist recommended.
  - Multiple therapeutic actions:
    - Rapidly reduces carboxyhemoglobin levels.
    - Inhibits lipid peroxidation.
    - Directly oxygenates tissues by raising PaO_2 levels.
    - Reduces cerebral edema.
    - May reverse cyanide poisoning.
    - Reduces delayed neuropsychological sequelae of CO poisoning.
  - Younger patients may not be able to self-modulate eustachian tube pressures.
    - May suffer tympanic membrane barotrauma in the hyperbaric oxygen chamber.
    - May need otolaryngology consultation to provide emergent myringotomy.
  - Parent may need to accompany child in the chamber.
  - Consider the numerous barriers to, and risks of, hyperbaric chamber use.
  - Barriers include:
    - Expense.
    - Logistics (availability, distance, timing).
    - Patient instability.
    - Need for increased staffing.
    - Limited evidence for duration, number of treatments, and use in pediatrics.
  - Risks include:
    - Patient intolerance of solitary-patient or multiple-patient chambers.
    - Oxygen toxicity (may rarely cause seizures).[5]
    - Air emboli, pneumothoraces, and perforated tympanic membranes.[5]
    - Risk of fire within chamber.[5]

TABLE 15-3

Symptoms of Carbon Monoxide Poisoning

Symptoms of CO Poisoning[3]	CO Levels[3]
Headache	Mild elevation (5–20%)
Dyspnea	
Visual changes	
Confusion	
Malaise or fatigue	
Drowsiness	
Faintness	
Nausea and/or vomiting	
Tachycardia	
Dulled sensation	
Decreased awareness of danger	Moderate elevation (20–40%)
Weakness	
Incoordination	
Loss of recent memory	
Cardiovascular collapse	
Neurological collapse	Severe elevation (40–60%)
Coma	
Convulsions	
Death	Extreme elevation (>60%)

- Long-term neuropsychiatric effects of CO poisoning include:
  - Parkinsonism and/or akinetic mutism.
  - Hearing and/or memory impairment.
  - Speech and/or gait disturbances.
  - Hemiplegia.
  - Epilepsy.
  - Dementia, hysteria, and/or personality changes.
  - Cortical blindness.
  - Peripheral neuropathy.

TABLE 15-4

Indications for Hyperbaric Oxygen[1,2,4]

Carboxyhemoglobin levels >20%
Neurologic symptoms
- Confusion
- Visual disturbances
- Ataxia
- Syncope
- Seizures
- Focal findings
- Coma

Cardiac symptoms
- Myocardial ischemia
- Dysrhythmias

Pregnancy
- Fetal hemoglobin has higher affinity for CO than maternal hemoglobin

- Cyanide poisoning
  - Consider cyanide poisoning in all patients with smoke inhalation.
  - Cyanide binds to cytochrome A3, inhibiting mitochondrial electron transport and aerobic metabolism.
  - Most patients will have immediate (usually within 8 minutes) and life-incompatible effects, or delayed and minimal effects.
  - Symptoms of CN poisoning[3,4]:
    - Low vapor exposure:
      - Dyspnea.
      - Inner sense of restlessness.
      - Faintness.
      - Weakness.
      - Headache.
      - Nausea and vomiting.
    - High vapor exposure:
      - Coma.
      - Seizures.
      - Respiratory failure or arrest.
  - Treatment:
    - First, crush amyl nitrite (to form ~5% methemoglobin and decrease cyanide effects) pearls onto gauze within bag-valve mask apparatus while the other two components are being made up.
    - Second, give sodium nitrite (to form ~ 20–30% methemoglobin, and further decrease cyanide effects) 0.33 mL/kg of 3% solution intravascularly (usually 300 mg, or 10 mL, in adults) over 5 minutes, watching for orthostatic hypotension.
    - Finally, give sodium thiosulfate (to metabolize cyanide into thiocyanate for rhodanese detoxification and renal excretion) 1.65 mL/kg of 25% solution intravascularly (usually 12.5 g, or 50 mL, in adults) over 10 minutes.
    - Hydroxocobalamin (to directly extract and bind cyanide into vitamin B_{12}) is not currently approved for this use in Canada.

PREVENTION

- Older buildings, crowded living conditions, open heaters, and flammable clothing increase the chance of fire-related deaths.[6]
- 50% of fire-related deaths can be avoided with smoke detectors.
- 90% of childhood fire-related deaths occur in homes without properly functioning smoke detectors.
- Most children in house fires die from smoke inhalation rather than burns.

CLINICAL PEARLS

DO
- Consider inhalation injury in *any* exposure to fire or severe burns.
- Intubate potential inhalational injury patients early.
- Always consider carbon monoxide poisoning in all fire-related injuries.
- Have difficult airway equipment and personnel available.

DON'T
- Rely on pulse oximetry and arterial blood gas PaO_2 levels.
- Cut the endotracheal tube too short postintubation.

REFERENCES
1. Selbst S, Cronan K, eds. *Pediatric emergency medicine secrets*. Philadelphia: Hanley & Belfus; 2001.
2. Baldwin GA, ed. *Handbook of pediatric emergencies*. 2nd ed. Boston: Little, Brown; 1994.
3. Fleisher GR, Ludwig S, eds. *Textbook of pediatric emergency medicine*. 4th ed. Philadelphia: Lippincott, Williams & Wilkins; 2000.
4. Gausche-Hill M, Fuchs S, Yamamoto L, eds. *APLS: the pediatric emergency medicine resource*. 4th ed. Sudbury, MA: Jones & Bartlett; 2004.
5. Chou KJ, Fisher JL, Silver EJ, Characteristics and outcome of children with carbon monoxide poisoning with and without smoke exposure referred for hyperbaric oxygen therapy. *Pediatr Emerg Care*. 2000;16:151–155.
6. Barrow RE, Spies M, Barrow LN, et al. Influence of demographics and inhalation injury on burn mortality in children. *Burns* 2004;30:72–77.

CHAPTER 16

Electrical Injury

Amina Lalani, MD, FRCPC

EPIDEMIOLOGY[1,2]
- Electrical injuries cause over 500 deaths per year in the United States.
- Electrical burns account for 2% to 3% of burns assessed in the pediatric emergency department.
- Most electrical burns in children occur at home due to:
  - Electrical appliances.
  - Extension cords.
  - Electrical wall outlets.
- Deaths are more common in school-aged children.
  - More likely due to high-voltage and lightning strikes.
- Minor injuries and emergency department visits are more common in younger children.
  - Tend to be low-voltage injuries.

DEFINITIONS AND CLASSIFICATION[2]
- Definitions:
  - Electricity is the flow of electrons through a conductor.
  - Electric current is the flow of electrons away from an object through a conductor.
  - Voltage = force causing electrons to flow.
  - Resistance = impedance to flow through the conductor.
- Electrical injury occurs when contact is made with an electric current that can cause internal and external injuries.
- Two types of electric current.
  - Alternating current (AC):
    - Most common in home outlets, and more efficient than DC.
    - More dangerous than DC, as it causes tetanic muscle contractions that prolong contact with source.
  - Direct current (DC):
    - Used in batteries, defibrillators, and pacemakers.
- Electrical injuries can be classified as low voltage, high voltage, or lightning injuries.
  - Low voltage: <600 V
  - High voltage: >1,000 V.
  - Lightning injury: $>30 \times 10^6$ V.
- Contact with electrical current causes injury through muscle contraction, thermal burns, blunt trauma, and depolarization of inducible tissue.
  - Direct injury is due to the effect of current on tissues or conversion to thermal energy.
  - Indirect injury is due to severe muscle contractions and secondary injury to other systems (e.g., myocardium and tympanic membranes).

FACTORS AFFECTING SEVERITY OF ELECTRICAL INJURY[4]
Intensity of Current
- Current is proportional to voltage and inversely proportional to tissue resistance.
- Ohm's law: Voltage = Intensity of current × Resistance.
- The effects of current vary depending on the amount (Table 16-1).

TABLE 16-1

Effects of Varying Current Intensity

Current (mA)	Effect
1	Tingling sensation
3–5	"Let-go" current for a child
10–20	Tetanic muscle contractions
20–50	Paralysis of respiratory muscles
50–100	Ventricular fibrillation

Duration of Contact
- Prolonged contact results in more injury due to thermal injury and burn.

Resistance of Tissues
- Increased resistance decreases current flow forward, and therefore results in increased heat production.
- Least resistance: Nerves, blood vessels, mucous membranes, wet skin.
- Highest resistance: Fat, bones, tendons.

Pathway of Current
- Affects type and severity of injury.
- Most dangerous: Vertical pathway along axis of body, as it involves all vital organs.
- Hand-to-hand flow may involve heart, respiratory muscles, spinal cord.

Type of Current
- Different injury patterns are seen with low versus high voltage.
  - Low voltage (<600 V): Mainly AC, therefore prolonged contact; causes tetanic contractions of respiratory muscles, ventricular fibrillation.
  - High voltage (>1,000 V): DC or AC; causes single muscle contraction that throws victim away from source; causes ventricular fibrillation, indirect trauma.

ASSESSMENT AND EVALUATION
At Scene
- Risk to rescuer: Should not attempt to access patient until current has been cut off or victim has been removed from the source with insulated equipment.

Triage
- Rapidly assess and treat lightning victims who are pulseless (Fig. 16-1).
- Prognosis more favorable with rapid onset of resuscitation.

History
- AMPLE history: Allergies, Medications, Past health including history of cardiac disease, Last meal, Events.
- Type of exposure: Low versus high voltage.
- Duration of contact if witnessed.
- Events post-exposure: Patient thrown? Fall from height?
- Loss of consciousness?

Physical Examination
- Follow ATLS principles of primary and secondary survey with stabilization.
- See Chapter 2 on Primary and Secondary Survey for details.

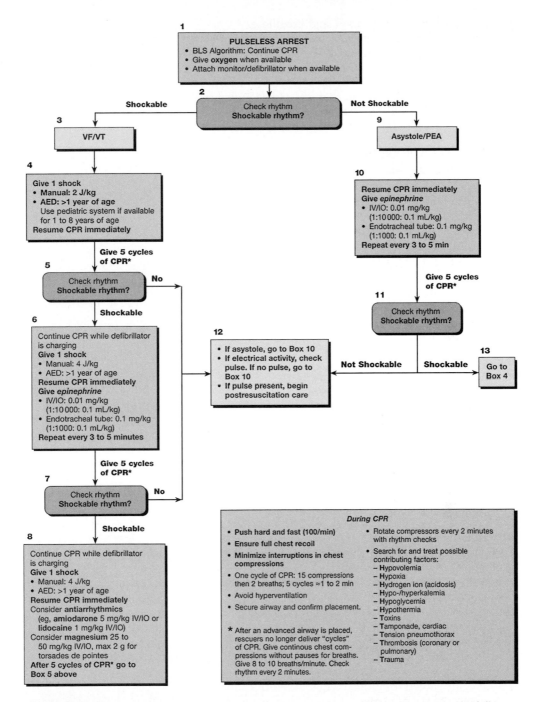

FIGURE 16-1 ● PALS algorithm: pulseless arrest. (From American Heart Association Guidelines for Cardiopulmonary Resuscitation and Emergency Cardiovascular Care. Part 12: Pediatric Advanced Life Support. *Circulation* 2005;112:IV-167–IV-187, with permission.)

- Assess for airway compromise and breathing.
  - Consider early intubation if there is evidence of facial burns.
- Assess cardiovascular status.
  - Ensure cardiac monitoring to rule out arrhythmia.
  - Follow PALS guidelines for management of arrhythmias and asystole.
- Assess for fractures or blunt thoracic or abdominal trauma.
- Assess for entry and exit wounds.
  - Can be deceptively small, but the patient may have profound internal injury.

SYSTEM-SPECIFIC INJURIES[2,3]
Cardiovascular System
- Electrical injury may cause:
  - Direct injury and necrosis to myocardium.
  - Cardiac arrhythmias.
  - Vascular injury with compartment syndrome in the extremities.
- Myocardial injury depends on voltage intensity and type of current.
  - Worse with high voltage and alternating current.
  - High voltages tend to cause asystole.
  - Low voltages may cause ventricular fibrillation, heart block, bundle branch block, ST-T changes, supraventricular tachycardia, atrial fibrillation.
  - AC tends to produce ventricular fibrillation while DC may produce asystole or ventricular fibrillation.

Cutaneous Injuries
- May be mild with local erythema, up to severe full-thickness burns.
- Cutaneous injuries may be deceptively minimal.
  - Electrical current may affect deeper tissues before significant skin damage occurs.
  - May cause necrosis and coagulation of deep muscles while sparing the skin.
  - Need to maintain high index of suspicion for internal injury without skin burns in low-voltage injuries.
- Feathering pattern (Lichtenberg figure) is pathognomonic for lightning injury.
- Identification of entry and exit wounds may be difficult.
  - Only small wounds may be present despite extensive internal damage.
  - Size of entry and exit wounds does not predict amount of internal damage.

Orofacial Burns[4]
- Young children often bite on electrical cords and may develop full-thickness burns of the lips and oral commissure.
  - Salivary electrolytes allow conduction of current through tissues in the mouth and surrounding areas.
- Vascular injury to the labial artery may not be immediately apparent due to thrombosis, vasospasm, or overlying tissue.
  - Delayed bleeding may be seen within 5 days after eschar falls off.
  - If meets discharge criteria (see below), ensure plastic surgery clinic follow-up in 2 to 3 days.
  - Parents should be notified when to return to the ED.
- Common to see drooling.
- If severe, may require oral airway before development of edema.
- Criteria for discharge after oral electrical burns:
  - No history of loss of consciousness.
  - No other injuries that require admission to hospital.
  - Normal ECG.
  - The child is able to tolerate fluids in the ED.
  - Parents are reliable for follow-up and when to return to the ED.
  - Follow-up with plastic surgery within 2 to 3 days.

Nervous System
- Often injuries are due to trauma from a fall or cardiorespiratory compromise with anoxia.
- Electrical injury to the brain may cause damage to the respiratory control center and respiratory arrest, seizures, altered level of consciousness, cranial nerve deficits, and visual or auditory disturbances.
- Injury to the spinal cord with hemiplegia or quadriplegia may occur with hand-to-hand flow.

Respiratory System
- Injury may be secondary to:
  - Direct injury to the respiratory control center.
  - Suffocation due to tetanic contractions of respiratory muscles (especially the diaphragm).
  - Anoxia.

Renal System
- Sensitive to ischemia.
- Renal failure may occur from renal tubular damage due to myoglobinuria and release of creatinine phosphokinase.

Musculoskeletal System
- Fractures may occur from falls or tetanic contractions.
- Vertebral compression fractures may cause spinal cord injury.
- Posterior shoulder dislocations.

Eyes
- Fixed pupils may occur transiently after lightning injury.
- Cataracts, retinal detachment, and optic nerve degeneration may occur as late complications.

Ears
- Rupture of tympanic membranes and temporary sensorineural hearing loss.
- Risk of tinnitus, permanent hearing loss.

INITIAL MANAGEMENT
- ABCs with spinal precautions.
- See Chapter 2 on Primary and Secondary Survey for details.
- Oxygen.
- Cardiorespiratory monitoring.
  - Treat arrhythmias.
- IV lines and fluid resuscitation.
  - May have high fluid requirements due to third-spacing of fluids.
- Obtain CBC, electrolytes, renal function, blood gas, CPK, cardiac enzymes, type and cross-match.
- Urinalysis including myoglobin.
- Electrocardiogram.
- CT head as indicated if abnormal neurologic exam, history of loss of consciousness or confusion.
- Radiographs for musculoskeletal injury.
- Consult ICU as needed.

DEFINITIVE MANAGEMENT
- Specific management for electrical injury:
  - Oral cavity for evidence of burns or respiratory compromise.
  - Evaluate for blunt thoracic and abdominal trauma.
  - Evaluate for spinal cord injury.
  - Close monitoring of renal, liver, and pancreatic function.

- Evaluate for rhabdomyolysis and myoglobinuria in high-voltage injury.
- Monitor limbs for compartment syndrome.
- Ophthalmology and otoscopic evaluation.
- Nutritional support.
- Prevention of stress ulcers.
- Tetanus toxoid.
- CT head if:
  - Deterioration in neurologic status or fails to improve.
  - Signs of increased intracranial pressure.

CRITERIA FOR DISCHARGE[2]

- Low-voltage injury or lightning injury with:
  - No cardiac arrest.
  - No loss of consciousness.
  - No burns.
  - Normal neurologic exam.
  - Normal electrocardiogram in emergency department.
- Criteria for 24-hour cardiac monitoring:
  - High-voltage injury.
  - Loss of consciousness.
  - Abnormal electrocardiogram in emergency department.
  - Past history of cardiac disease.

LIGHTNING (ARC) INJURIES[4]

- High-voltage injury but brief massive exposure to DC (100 million V).
- Path of current tends to be more direct to ground than low-voltage currents.
- Type of strike includes:
  - Direct strike (most common form).
  - Side flash (from a nearby object).
  - Contact strike (strikes object the individual is touching).
  - Ground current (transferred from the strike site to where the person is standing).
- Specific injures include:
  - Cardiovascular
    - Dysrhythmias and asystole.
    - Edema, ischemia, and necrosis of tissues and blood vessels.
  - Pulmonary
    - Respiratory failure or arrest.
  - Ophthalmic
    - May present with fixed and dilated pupils due to autonomic disturbance.
    - Common: Ocular damage including corneal lesions, hyphema, vitreous hemorrhage, uveitis, iridocyclitis.
    - Late complications include cataracts and optic atrophy.
  - Cutaneous
    - Usually only superficial burns due to very brief exposure (1–3 ms).
    - Arcing current may ignite clothing and produce thermal burns.
  - Other
    - Rare to develop renal failure or require fasciotomies.
    - Require admission and monitoring for complications.
    - Follow CNS status for cerebral edema, which may develop after days.
    - Require maintenance fluids as rare to see extensive muscle damage.

CLINICAL PEARLS

DO
1. Recognize the factors that contribute to electrical injury, including intensity of current, duration of contact, tissue resistance, and pathway of current.
2. Obtain an ECG and assess for myocardial damage if pathway may have involved the heart.
3. Monitor the CNS status closely in victims of lightning and high-voltage injuries and obtain a CT head if necessary.

DON'T
1. Assume that the size of the entry and exit wounds predicts the extent of internal damage.
2. Assume that tissue that appears viable immediately postinjury will remain intact, as high risk of damage to muscle and blood vessels with high-voltage injury.
3. Forget to arrange follow-up for the child with orofacial burns due to risk of bleeding within 1 to 2 weeks of injury.

REFERENCES

1. Nguyen BH, MacKay M, et al. Epidemiology of electrical and lightning related deaths and injuries among Canadian children and youth. *Inj Prev* 2004;10:122–124.
2. Koumbourlis AC. Electrical injuries. *Crit Care Med* 2002;30:S424–S430.
3. Cherington M. Neurologic manifestations of lightning strikes. *Neurology* 2003;60:182–185.
4. Baum CR. Environmental emergencies. In: Fleisher G, Ludwig S, eds. *Textbook of pediatric emergency medicine*. 4th ed. Philadelphia: Lippincott Williams & Wilkins; 2000:959–963.
5. 2005 American Heart Association guidelines for cardiopulmonary resuscitation and emergency cardiovascular care. Part 12: pediatric advanced life support. *Circulation* 2005;112:IV-167–IV-187.

CHAPTER 17

Drowning and Submersion Injuries

Adam Cheng, MD, FRCPC (Ped EM), FAAP

DEFINITIONS
- Drowning: respiratory impairment from submersion or immersion in a liquid.[1]
- Survival is not considered in the definition. The victim may survive or die.

EPIDEMIOLOGY
- 500,000 drowning deaths occur worldwide annually.[2]
- Annual incidence of drowning in the United States is 15,000 to 70,000.
- >50% of drowning victims are children under 5 years of age.[3]
- Fatality rates are highest in children under 5 years of age.
- Males more commonly affected than females.
- Leading cause of cardiac arrest in children.
- Leading cause of accidental death in children from industrialized countries.
- Site of drowning, as reviewed by Brenner and associates in 2001:[4]
  - <1 year: 55% in bathtubs.
  - 1 to 4 years: 56% in artificial pools.
  - Older children: 63% in natural collections of freshwater.

PATHOPHYSIOLOGY (FIG. 17-1)
- Exact pathophysiologic mechanism of drowning remains unclear.
- Final common pathophysiologic consequence is hypoxemia.
- Hypoxemia results from three main causes:[5]
  - Apnea and breath holding.
  - Laryngospasm.
  - Pulmonary aspiration and lung injury.
- Surfactant disruption.
- Alveolar collapse and atelectasis.
- Pulmonary edema.
- Intrapulmonary shunting.
- Ventilation—perfusion mismatch.
- Cardiac arrest can ultimately occur from:
  - Prolonged hypoxia.
  - Intense peripheral vasoconstriction.
  - Hypothermia.
  - Extravascular fluid shifts, and intravascular fluid loss.
  - Bradycardia.
  - Ventricular fibrillation or other arrhythmias.
- Water tonicity (freshwater vs. seawater) does not influence change in serum sodium, hemoglobin, or intravascular volume status.[6]

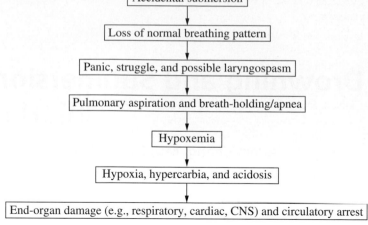

FIGURE 17-1 ●   Pathophysiologic mechanism of drowning.

- Hypothermia often occurs in drowning, particularly with prolonged submersion.
  - Below 32°C, heart rate and blood pressure fall and oxygen consumption and metabolic rate decrease.
  - Severe hypothermia creates risk of bradycardia, ventricular fibrillation, or asystole.
  - Can lead to coagulopathy and platelet dysfunction.
  - Protective effect on brain function possible if hypothermia occurs quickly.

RISK FACTORS FOR DROWNING
- Young age, particularly less than 5 years.
- Child maltreatment and neglect.
- Alcohol intoxication: 40% to 50% of drowning is associated with alcohol use.
- Drug abuse.
- Seizure disorder: 4 to 5-fold increased risk for submersion.
- Cardiac disorder: Prior history of arrhythmias (e.g., long QT syndrome).
- Risk-taking behavior.
- Residential swimming pool: Location of most drownings in 1 to 4 year age group.
- Proximity to rivers, lakes, canals, beaches: Mostly for adolescent age group.

INITIAL MANAGEMENT: PRE-HOSPITAL CARE
At the Scene
- Remove from water immediately.
- Initiate CPR immediately (bystander resuscitation is critical).
- Heimlich maneuver NOT indicated.
- Obtain details: Submersion time, symptoms, vomiting.

During Transport
- Initiate PALS protocols and cardiorespiratory monitoring.
- Airway management.
- Protect C-spine: Jaw thrust if needed.
- Administer 100% oxygen.
- Give IV fluids: Normal saline or Ringer's lactate.
- Remove wet clothing.
- Initiate rewarming: Wrap in blankets.

INITIAL MANAGEMENT: EMERGENCY CARE[5-7]
Airway and Breathing
- Rapid-sequence intubation (RSI) if indicated:
  - Apnea, severe respiratory distress, poor oxygenation, $PaCO_2$ retention, altered mental status, inability to protect airway.
  - See Chapter 3 on Airway Management for RSI technique and medications.
- Consider C-spine stabilization for suspicious cases.[8]
  - 0.5% of submersion victims have C-spine injuries.
  - C-spine immobilization is recommended for:
    - High-impact submersions from diving or motorized vehicle crash.
    - Clinical signs of serious injury.
- Administer 100% oxygen to optimize saturation.
- CPAP/PEEP: Improves oxygenation and corrects ventilation perfusion mismatch.
  - May require PEEP 5 to 15 cm H_2O or greater.
  - Monitor blood pressure as PEEP is increased.
- Maintain normocapnia.

Circulation
- Cardiorespiratory monitoring.
- Rapid IV access: Consider intraosseous access if IV access is unobtainable.
- Aggressive fluid resuscitation may be required for hypotension.
- Give warmed normal saline or Ringer's lactate for fluid resuscitation (20 mL/kg increments).
- Inotropes or vasopressors may be required to help restore adequate perfusion.
- Check bedside glucose.
- Glucose-containing solutions: May use, but monitor bedside glucose carefully as hyperglycemia is associated with poor neurologic outcome.

Disability and Exposure
- Rapid and accurate neurologic assessment: Glasgow Coma Scale and pupils.
- Frequent reassessment of neurologic status.
- Complete exposure and assessment for associated injuries and underlying comorbidity, such as child abuse and drug abuse.
- Measure temperature and consider hypothermia (see "Definitive Management" section later in this chapter).

EVALUATION
History
- Assign an assistant to gather history as resuscitation proceeds.
- Use all available sources of information (police, paramedics, lifeguards, parents, friends, bystanders).
- Details surrounding the submersion.
- Mechanism of injury.
  - Diving? Motorboat?
  - Any trauma witnessed?
  - Quiet submersion? Slipped beneath the water?
- Time elapsed from time of submersion.
- Time spent at the scene.
- Interventions carried out at the scene, and en-route to hospital.
- Patient response to interventions.
- Last meal.
- Past medical history and medications.

Physical Exam
- Primary and secondary survey.
- Assess for signs of end-organ dysfunction (Table 17-1).

TABLE 17-1

End-Organ Effects of Drowning

Central Nervous System	• Hypoxemic encephalopathy and cord injury from hypoxemia • Cerebral edema and increased intracranial pressure
Respiratory	• Decreased pulmonary compliance and increased airway resistance • Noncardiogenic pulmonary edema and potential aspiration
Cardiac	• Myocardial dysfunction from ischemic injury • Dysrhythmias: Bradycardia, atrial/ventricular fibrillation, asystole • Hypovolemia and hypotension
Metabolic	• Combined metabolic and respiratory acidosis in 50% of drowning victims • Hypo/hypernatremia or hypokalemia in some drowning (rarely hyperkalemia due to hemolysis) victims
Renal	• Renal failure and acute tubular necrosis • Hemoglobinuria due to hemolysis or shock-related DIC

Lab Investigations
- Complete blood count (CBC).
- Blood gas, electrolytes, glucose, renal function, calcium, magnesium.
- Coagulation studies.
- Blood type and cross-match as needed.
- Toxicology and alcohol screen.
- 12-lead ECG.
- Urinalysis.

Imaging
- Chest x-ray: May show aspiration, pulmonary edema, atelectasis, pneumothorax, or may be normal (22%).[6]
  - Findings can be delayed.
- C-spine imaging as indicated.
- Patients with known or suspected blunt trauma will require a CXR, C-spine, and pelvic x-rays for trauma assessment.
- Neuroimaging if signs of cerebral injury or increased intracranial pressure.

DEFINITIVE MANAGEMENT
Hypothermia
- Goal is to safely rewarm while maintaining cardiovascular stability.
- Rewarm aggressively to achieve core temperatures of 33% to 36°C.
- Use passive external rewarming if temp >32°C (Table 17-2).
- Use active external and internal rewarming if temp <32°C (Table 17-2).
- A patient who becomes rapidly hypothermic **prior to** becoming hypoxic should not be considered dead until unresponsive to CPR and core temperature is >32°C.
  - Epinephrine and other resuscitation drugs are not efficacious at temperatures <32°C.
- Avoid hyperthermia.

Adjunctive Therapy
- Pulmonary physiotherapy.
- Fluid therapy: Fluid restriction may be required to help maintain normovolemia after initial resuscitation.
- Diuretic therapy: Furosemide 0.5 to 1 mg/kg may improve gas exchange. Forced diuresis required if hemoglobinuria exists.

TABLE 17-2

Rewarming Techniques

Passive Rewarming	• Remove wet clothing • Warm blankets
Active Rewarming: External	• Hot packs • Heat lamps • Warm air blanket
Active Rewarming: Internal	• Warm humidified oxygen • Warm IV fluids • Warm saline lavage of various body cavities: gastric, bladder, chest, abdomen, rectal • Warm peritoneal dialysis • Cardiopulmonary bypass

Controversial Therapies

- Steroids: Not indicated.
- Antibiotics are not indicated for prophylaxis unless:[6]
  - Submerged in contaminated water, such as lake or sewage.
  - Therapy for pneumonia should be guided by clinical and radiographic signs such as evolving infiltrates, leukocytosis, persistent fever, purulent secretions.
- Bronchial lavage with saline is indicated when sand aspiration impairs adequate ventilation (radioopaque particles seen on chest radiograph).
- Bicarbonate: Consider use for correcting severe metabolic acidosis (pH < 7.1) that is unresponsive to fluid therapy.

DISPOSITION

Discharge Criteria[9]

- Asymptomatic and normal level of consciousness.
- Normal physical examination.
- Normal oxygenation by oxygen saturation and/or ABG.
- 4 to 6 hours of observation completed.
- Normal chest radiograph.
- Guaranteed medical follow-up.

Admission Criteria

- Abnormal level of consciousness (Glasgow Coma Scale ≤13).
- Respiratory distress, shortness of breath, cough, chest pain, etc.
- Abnormality on physical examination.
- Abnormal oxygenation or requiring respiratory support.
- Abnormal chest radiograph.
- Tachycardia or dysrhythmia.

OUTCOME

- Death in 25% of drowning victims brought to the emergency department.[10–12]
- 10 to 33% of drowning victims have permanent neurologic sequelae.

Poor Prognostic Factors

- Prolonged submersion >25 minutes.
- Delay in CPR initiation.
- Resuscitation >25 minutes.
- Severe metabolic acidosis, with pH < 7.1.
- Pulseless, cardiac arrest on arrival to emergency department.

- Elevated blood glucose level on arrival.
- Dilated and fixed pupils on arrival to emergency department.
- Abnormal initial CT scan of brain.
- Initial Glasgow Coma Scale score <5.

CLINICAL PEARLS

DO
- Initiate bystander CPR at the scene of the submersion.
- Consider C-spine immobilization for high-impact submersions from diving or motorized vehicle crash, or if there are clinical signs of serious injury.
- Provide aggressive cardiorespiratory support.
- Consider hypothermia and initiate rewarming techniques when indicated.

DON'T
- Perform the Heimlich maneuver as part of initial resuscitation.
- Neglect the airway. Oxygenation is of paramount importance in the resuscitation of drowning victims.
- Forget to monitor glucose levels. Hyperglycemia is associated with poor neurologic outcome.

REFERENCES

1. Van Dorp JCM, Knape JTA, Bierens JJLM. *Recommendations*. World congress on drowning, June 26–28, 2002, Amsterdam. http://www.drowning.nl/. 2003.
2. Peden MM, McGee K. The epidemiology of drowning worldwide. *Inj Control Saf Promot* 2003; 10:195–199.
3. Quan L, Cummings P. Characteristics of drowning by different age groups. *Inj Prev* 2003;9:163–168.
4. Brenner RA, Trumble AC, Smith GS, et al. Where children drown, United States. *Pediatrics* 2001;108:85–89.
5. Zuckerbraun NS, Saladino RA. Pediatric drowning: current management strategies and immediate care. *Clin Pediatr Emerg Med* 2005;6:49–56.
6. Salomez F, Vincent JL. Drowning: a review of epidemiology, pathophysiology, treatment and prevention. *Resuscitation* 2004;63:261–268.
7. Ibsen LM, Koch T. Submersion and asphyxial injury. *Crit Care Med* 2002;30:S402–S408.
8. Watson RS, Cummings P, Quan L, et al. Cervical spinal injuries among submersion victims. *J Trauma* 2001;51:658–662.
9. Causey AL, Tilelli JA, Swanson ME. Predicting discharge in uncomplicated near-drowning. *Am J Emerg Med* 2000;18:9–11.
10. Zuckerman GB, Conway EE. Drowning and near drowning: a pediatric epidemic. *Pediatr Ann* 2000; 29:360–382.
11. Weinstein MD, Krieger BP. Near-drowning: epidemiology, pathophysiology, and initial treatment. *J Emerg Med* 1996;14:461–467.
12. Modell JH. Drowning. *N Engl J Med* 1993;328:253–256.
13. Baum CR. Drowning and near drowning. In: Fleisher GR, Ludwig S, eds. *Textbook of pediatric emergency medicine*. 4th ed. Philadelphia: Lippincott Williams & Wilkins; 2000.

CHAPTER 18

Pain Management and Sedation

Rahim Valani, MD, CCFP-EM, FRCPC, PG Dip Med Ed

ANATOMY OF PAIN[1]

- Pain is a neuro–biochemical phenomenon.
- Nociceptors from the periphery transduce stimuli into neural impulses that are propagated to cell bodies and up the spinal cord.
  - Neuron cell bodies are in the spinal cord's dorsal root ganglion (DRG).
- Each spinal cord level has its own DRG, while the face has the trigeminal ganglion.
- Two main types of receptors, the slow C-fibers and the fast Aδ fibers (Table 18-1).
- Impulse-inducing chemicals include leukotrienes, bradykinin, serotonin, histamine, potassium, protons, acetylcholine, substance P, and platelet-activating factor.
- The **spinothalamic pathway** is the main tract for pain transmission.
- Spinothalamic pathway is divided into:
  - Lateral fast signals.
    - Travel to the brainstem's thalamus and reticular area.
    - Help discriminate location, intensity, and duration of pain.
  - Medial slow/chronic pain.
    - Terminates in the spinal cord's lamina II and III.
    - A multisynaptic pathway with a large terminal distribution area.
- The thalamus is the key area for initial pain interpretation.
- Pain is divided into somatic pain or visceral pain.
- Visceral pain can be activated by:
  - Ischemia.
  - Chemical stimulation.
  - Spasm of hollow viscus.
  - Overdistention of hollow viscus.

CLINICAL CONSIDERATIONS IN PAIN MANAGEMENT

- Thorough assessment of medical condition is necessary for pain management.
- Pain affects a child's psychological, behavioral, physiologic, and emotional state.
- Only half of pediatric patients with significant pain receive analgesia.[2-8]
- Goal: To optimally and safely manage a patient's pain.
- Pediatric differences compared to adults include:
  - Cognitive abilities.
  - Developmental status.
  - Respiratory mechanics and airway anatomy.
  - Metabolism of drugs.

TABLE 18-1

Comparison of Different Neural Pain Fibers

	C Fibers	Aδ Fibers
Activation	80% of peripheral receptors Mechanical, thermal, and chemical	Primarily mechanical or thermal
Myelination	Nonmyelinated	Myelinated
Speed of Impulse Propagation	Slow: 0.5–2 m/sec	Fast: 5–30 m/sec
Diameter	<1.5 μm	1–5 μm

- Pain assessment should be:[9]
  - Individualized.
  - Comprehensive.
  - Measured.
  - Continuous.
  - Monitored.
  - Documented.
- Most reliable pain indicator is patient self-reporting.
- There are many different pain scales in use (Fig. 18-1).
- The American Academy of Pediatrics (AAP) and American Pain Society recommend observing behavior to complement self-reporting.
  - This is an acceptable alternative when valid self-reporting is unavailable.[11]

MODES OF PAIN RELIEF
- Two main pain relief strategies are nonpharmacologic and pharmacologic.[9,11]

Nonpharmacologic
- Cognitive: Music, imagery, positive reinforcement, hypnosis.
- Behavioral: Relaxation, biofeedback, breathing.
- Physical: Heat/cold application, massage, touch, TENS, acupuncture, immobilization.

Pharmacologic (Fig. 18-2, Tables 18-2 and 18-3)
- Have naloxone available in case of respiratory depression with opioids.
  - Dose: 0.1 mg/kg (maximum dose is 2 mg).
- Narcotic clearance is slower in neonates, and increases over the first 2 to 6 months.
- Dose accordingly.

DIFFERENT PAIN ASSESSMENT SCALES

Premature Infant Pain Profile (PIPP) (*Neonates*)
Children's Hospital for Eastern Ontario Pain Scale (CHEOPS) (*Birth to age 3 years*)
Oucher Scale (*Age 3-7 years*)
Faces pain scale – revised (*Age 5-12 years*)
Verbal rating scale (*Age over 7 years*)
Visual analog scale
Color scale
Faces
Body outline
Poker chip

FIGURE 18-1 ● Examples of pain assessment scales.[9,10]

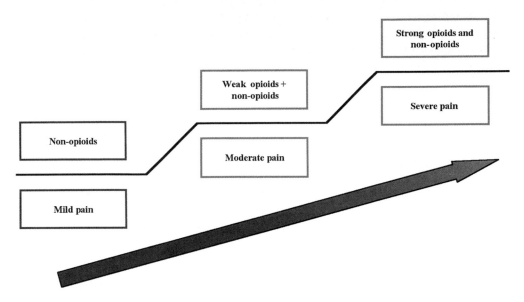

FIGURE 18-2 ● Pain relief ladder. (From Kowalczyk A, ed. *The 2004–2005 formulary of drugs. The Hospital for Sick Children, University of Toronto, 2004*, with permission.)

TABLE 18-2

Non-Opioid Analgesia[9,10,13]

Drug	Dosage	Route	Frequency	Max Dose
Acetaminophen	15 mg/kg	PO	4 hr	65 mg/kg or 4 g/day,
	30 mg/kg	PR	6 hr	whichever is less
Ibuprofen	10 mg/kg	PO	6 hr	40 mg/kg
Naproxen	5–10 mg/kg	PO	12 hr	1 g/day
Ketorolac	Load up to 0.5 mg/kg	IV/IM	6 hr	Maximum use of 30 mg/dose, only for 48 hours

TABLE 18-3

Opioid Analgesia[9,10,13]

Drug	Dosage	Route	Frequency	Max Dose
Codeine	0.5–1 mg/kg	PO	4 hr	3–6 mg/kg/day
Morphine	0.1–0.3 mg/kg	PO/PR	4 hr	
	0.05–0.1 mg/kg	IV	4 hr	
Fentanyl	0.5–1.0 µg/kg	IV	1 hr	

Local Anesthetics
- Local anesthetics used for laceration repair and regional analgesia.
- See Chapter 21 on Trauma Procedures for Regional Anesthesia Techniques.
- Toxicity related to:
  - Potency of local anesthetic.
  - Dose delivered.
  - Systemic absorption.
  - Protein binding.
  - Metabolism.
  - Excretion.
- Severe toxicity includes:
  - CNS.
    - Related to lipid solubility.
    - Acts by depression of inhibitory neurons.
    - Symptoms and signs are light-headedness, metallic taste, perioral paresthesias, drowsiness, seizure, and coma.
  - Cardiac toxicity.
    - Related to Na channel blockade.
    - Can have ventricular dysrhythmias, decreased myocardial contractility, and hypotension.
  - Allergic reaction.
    - Usually due to para-amino benzoic acid for esters.
    - Allergic reaction often from the preservative methylparaben.
    - True allergies are rare for amides (Table 18-4).

PROCEDURAL SEDATION
- Sedation is a continuum (Figs. 18-3 and 18-4).
- Sedation may cause loss of protective airway reflexes.
- Anyone administering sedation must be able to recognize and manage potential cardiorespiratory complications.
- Complication rate of 2.5% in an urban pediatric emergency department.
  - None required admission.[19]

TABLE 18-4

Local Anesthetic Properties[14]

AMIDES			
Drug	Latency	Duration	Dose
Bupivacaine	15–30 min	2.5–6 hr	2.5–3 mg/kg
Lidocaine	5–15 min	0.75–2 hr	4–5 mg/kg (7 mg/kg with epi)
Mepivacaine	5–15 min	1–1.25 hr	4–5 mg/kg (7 mg/kg with epi)
Prilocaine	15–25 min	0.75–2 hr	8 mg/kg

ESTERS			
Drug	Latency	Duration	Dose
Cocaine	–5min	20–30 min	3 mg/kg
Procaine	10–15 min	0.3–1 hr	12 mg/kg
Tetracaine	Up to 5min	1.5–3 hrs	3 mg/kg

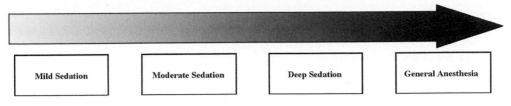

| Mild Sedation | Moderate Sedation | Deep Sedation | General Anesthesia |

FIGURE 18-3 ● Sedation as a continuum.

- Complications occur from:
  - Drug calculation error.
  - Drug–drug interactions.
  - Failure to recognize depth of sedation.
  - Inadequate resuscitation capabilities.
- *Procedural sedation* is a medically controlled state of depressed consciousness that:
  - Allows protective reflexes to be maintained.
  - Retains patient's ability to maintain a patent airway independently and continuously.
  - Permits appropriate patient response to physical stimulation or verbal command.
- Proper presedation assessment mandated by the American Society of Anesthesiologists (Figs. 18-5 and 18-6).[20]
- AAP guidelines for monitoring and managing pediatric patients during and after sedation.[21]
  - Thorough medical history to determine if patient is at risk for complications.
  - Careful physical exam, including airway assessment.
  - Informed parental consent.
  - Appropriate-sized equipment for the patient.

Mild sedation
- Responds to verbal command

Moderate sedation
- Intact protective reflexes
- Patent airway
- Appropriate response to physical stimulation or verbal command

Deep sedation
- Partial or complete loss of reflexes
- May not maintain airway reflexes
- Cannot respond to physical stimulation or command

General anesthesia
- Absence of airway reflex protection

FIGURE 18-4 ● Differences in sedation levels.[15-18]

PRESEDATION ASSESSMENT: HISTORY

- Informed consent from parent and assent from patient
- Focused history of current events
- Determination of ASA classification
- Prior anesthesia or sedation and any complications
- Current medications
- Drug allergies
- General medical problems
- Any pulmonary disease
    o Asthma
    o Pneumonia
    o URI
- Any cardiac problems
- History of neuromuscular disease

FIGURE 18-5 ● Presedation history assessment.[18,20,21]

- Specifically assign someone to monitor the patient's cardiorespiratory status, during and after the procedure.
  - Strict discharge criteria, with instructions on what to avoid and when to return.
- ASA guidelines for non-anesthesiologists.[20]
  - Remember that monitoring does *not* prevent complications.
  - Ensure that someone is watching the child for symptoms of apnea or difficulty breathing.
    - Level of consciousness.
- Sedation level based on verbal versus painful stimuli.
- If adverse drug responses are detected quickly, complications can be avoided.
- Pulmonary ventilation and oxygenation.
- Primary cause of morbidity and highest rate of complication is from respiratory depression.
- Early detection of hypoxemia through oximetry decreases likelihood of adverse effects.
- Monitoring hemodynamic parameters.
- Early detection of changes in blood pressure and heart rate can decrease risk of cardiovascular collapse.

Reversal Agents (Table 18-5)
- Naloxone
  - To reverse opioid-induced sedation or ventilatory depression.
  - Acute reversal can be associated with pain, hypertension, tachycardia, or pulmonary edema.
  - Multiple doses required if opioid half-life is longer than naloxone.

PRESEDATION ASSESSMENT: PHYSICAL EXAM

- Weight
- Baseline vital signs
- Cardiac and pulmonary examinations
- Upper airway assessment, with a Mallampati score (see anesthesia and airway section)
- Clarify last meal
    o Current recommendations at SickKids:
       2 hours for clear fluids
       4 hours for breast milk
       6 hours for cow's milk or formula
       8 hours for solids

FIGURE 18-6 ● Presedation physical exam and NPO status.[18,20–25]

TABLE 18-5

Medications Used for Conscious Sedation[9,15-17]

Drug	Dosing	Maximal Dose	Time to Onset (min)	Duration of Action (min)	Contraindications
SEDATIVE–HYPNOTICS					
Chloral hydrate[a]	PO: 25–50 mg/kg After 30 min may repeat 25–50 mg/kg	2 g or 100 mg/kg (whichever is less)	15–30	60–120	Avoid in cardiac, hepatic, renal patients Unpredictable effects
Midazolam[b,c]	IV: 0–5 yr: 0.05–0.1 mg/kg 6–12 yr: 0.025–0.05 mg/kg IM: 0.1–0.15 mg/kg PO: 0.5–0.75 mg/kg IN: 0.2–0.5 mg/kg PR: 0.25–0.5 mg/kg	0.6 mg/kg 0.4 mg/kg	2–3 10–20 15–30 10–15 10–30	45–60 60–120 60–90 60 60–90	
Pentobarbital[d]	IV: 1–6 mg/kg IM: 2–6 mg/kg PO/PR: <4 yr: 3–6 mg/kg >4 yr: 1.5–3 mg/kg	Increments of 1–2 mg/kg 100 mg 100 mg	3–5 10–15 15–60	15–45 60–120 60–240	Porphyria Can lead to paradoxical excitement
Thiopental	PR: 25 mg/kg		10–15	60	Respiratory depression Status asthmaticus Shock/cardiovascular collapse
Methohexital	PR: 25 mg/kg		10–15	60	Avoid in temporal-lobe epilepsy and porphyria
Propofol[e]	IV: 1 mg/kg, and titrate by increments of 0.05 mg/kg				Soy allergy May sting at site of injection Avoid prolonged infusion as it may result in lactic acidosis and death
Etomidate[f]	IV: 0.1–0.3 mg/kg				Adrenal suppresion
ANALGESIC AGENTS					
Fentanyl[g,h]	IV: 1 μg/kg	4 μg/kg	2–3	30–60	

(continued)

TABLE 18-5 (Continued)

Medications Used for Conscious Sedation[9,15-17]

Drug	Dosing	Maximal Dose	Time to Onset (min)	Duration of Action (min)	Contraindications
Ketamine[i]	IV: 1–1.5 mg/kg slowly over 1–2 min IM: 3–4 mg/kg	May repeat ½ dose every 10 min as required	1 3–5	60 90	Age <3 History of airway instability, tracheal surgery/stenosis Active pulmonary disease Head injury/CNS mass Glaucoma/eye injury Psychosis Porphyria Thyroid problems
Nitrous oxide	Mixture of minimum 40% oxygen; self-administered		<5	<5	Pregnancy Trapped gas pocket (bowel, inner ear, pneumothorax)
REVERSAL AGENTS					
Naloxone	IV/IM: 0.1 mg/kg/dose	Maximum of 2 mg/dose Can be repeated every 2 min PRN	IV: 2 IM: 10–15	20–40 60–90	
Flumazenil	IV: 0.02 mg/kg	1 mg	1–2	30–60	Patients on long-term benzodiazepines, cyclosporine, isoniazid, lithium, propoxyphene, theophylline, and TCA

aNo analgesia. Only single use in neonates.

bPreferred benzodiazepine agent due to shorter duration of action and multiple routes of administration. May produce paradoxical excitement, venous irritation, and respiratory depression.

cReversible with flumazenil.

dMay produce paradoxical excitement.

eWatch for respiratory depression and hypotension. Concern with propofol infusion syndrome in the pediatric population.

fCan cause adrenal suppression. Myoclonic jerks can also be observed.

gCan result in rigid chest wall syndrome. Treatment may require paralysis.

hReversible with naloxone.

iPreserves upper airway muscle tone and reflexes. Can result in laryngospasm. Watch for hallucinations/emergence reactions in patients >15, which can be blunted with midazolam; and increased secretions, which can be blunted with atropine or glycopyrolate; potentiates NMBs.

- Flumazenil
  - Antagonist of benzodiazepines.
  - Avoid in patients with known seizure disorder, chronic benzodiazepine use, or TCA overdose.
  - Multiple doses required if benzodiazepine half-life is longer than flumazenil.
- Do NOT use reversal agents to shorten duration of sedation.

CLINICAL PEARLS

DO
- Assess pain in all pediatric patients and treat accordingly.
- Realize that patient self-reporting is the most reliable means of assessing pain.
- Consider that narcotic clearance is slower in the first 6 months of life.
- Be aware that sedation should be performed by trained personnel who can manage the airway.
- Know the role of flumazenil and naloxone as reversal agents.

DON'T
- Sedate if not appropriately trained or lack necessary equipment.
- Oversedate patients into a general anesthetic.
- Rush into sedation. Always complete an appropriate assessment.

REFERENCES

1. Fink WA. The pathophysiology of acute pain. *Emerg Med Clin North Am* 2005;23(2):277–284.
2. Petrack E. Christopher N. Kriwinsky J. Pain management in the emergency department: patterns of analgesic utilization. *Pediatrics* 1997;99:711–714.
3. Simpson N, Finlay F. Acute pain management for children in A&E. *J Accid Emerg Med* 1997;14:58. Letter.
4. Friedland LR, Kulick RM. Emergency department analgesic use in pediatric trauma victims with fractures. *Ann Emerg Med* 1994;23:203–207.
5. Southall DP, Cronin BC, Hartmann H, et al. Invasive procedures in children receiving intensive care. *BMJ* 1993;306:1512–1513.
6. Schechter NL. The undertreatment of pain in children: an overview. *Pediatr Clin North Am* 1989;36: 781–794.
7. Maurice SC, O'Donnell JJ, Beattie TF. Emergency analgesia in the paediatric population. Part 1. Current practice and perspectives. *Emerg Med J* 2002;19:4–7.
8. Drendel AL, Brousseau DC, Gorelick MH. Pain assessment for pediatric patients in the emergency department. *Pediatrics* 2006;117:1511–1518.
9. Bauman BH, McManus JG. Pediatric pain management in the emergency department. *Emerg Med Clin North Am* 2005;23(2):393–414.
10. Cohen E, Zaarour C. Pain and sedation. In: Cheng A, Williams BA, Sivarajan BV, eds. *HSC handbook of pediatrics* Elsevier, Toronto; 2003.
11. Committee on psychosocial aspects of child and family health, American Academy of Pediatrics; task force on pain in infants, children, and adolescents, American Pain Society. The assessment and management of acute pain in infants, children, and adolescents. *Pediatrics* 2001;108:793–797.
12. Kowalczyk A, ed. *The 2004–2005 formulary of drugs.* The Hospital for Sick Children, University of Toronto, 2004.
13. Berde CB, Sethna NF. Analgesia for the treatment of pain in children. *N Engl J Med* 2002;347: 1094–1103.
14. Crystal CS, Blankenship RB. Local anesthetics and peripheral nerve blocks in the emergency department. *Emerg Med Clin North Am* 2005;23(2):477–502.
15. Shankar V, Deshpande JK. Procedural sedation in the pediatric patient. *Anesthesiol Clin North Am* 2005;23:635–654.
16. Rodriquez E, Jordan R. Contemporary trends in pediatric sedation and analgesia. *Emerg Med Clin North Am* 2002;20:199–222.
17. Krauss B, Green SM. Sedation and analgesia for procedures in children. *N Engl J Med* 2000;13:938–945.
18. American Academy of Pediatrics, committee on drugs and section on anesthesiology. Guidelines for the elective use of conscious sedation, deep sedation, and general anesthesia in pediatric patients. *Pediatrics* 1985;76:317–321.

19. Pena BM, Krauss B. Adverse events of procedural sedation and analgesia in a pediatric emergency department. *Ann Emerg Med* 1999;34:483–491.
20. Practice guidelines for sedation and analgesia by non-anesthesiologists: a report by the American Society of Anesthesiologists Task Force on Sedation and Analgesia by Non-Anesthesiologists. *Anesthesiology* 1996;84:459–471.
21. American Academy of Pediatrics, committee on drugs. Guidelines for monitoring and management of pediatric patients during and after sedation for diagnostic and therapeutic procedures. *Pediatrics* 1992;89:1110–1115.
22. Treston G. Prolonged pre-procedure fasting time is unnecessary when using titrated intravenous ketamine for pediatric procedural sedation. *Emerg Med Australasia* 2004;16:145–150.
23. Roback MG, Bajaj L, Wathen JE, et al. Preprocedural fasting and adverse events in procedural sedation and analgesia in a pediatric emergency department: are they related? *Ann Emerg Med* 2004;44: 454–459.
24. Kennedy RM, Luhmann JD. Pharmacological management of pain and anxiety during procedures in children. *Pediatr Drugs* 2001;3:337–354.
25. Agrawal D, Manzi SF, Gupta R, et al. Preprocedural fasting state and adverse events in children undergoing procedural sedation an analgesia in a pediatric emergency department. *Ann Emerg Med* 2003; 42:636–646.

CHAPTER 19

Nonaccidental Trauma

Michelle Shouldice, MD, FRCPC

EPIDEMIOLOGY
- A survey of over 10,000 Canadian adults indicated that 10% of adults experienced severe physical abuse during childhood.[1]
- Eleven percent of women and four percent of men reported a history of severe sexual abuse during childhood.[1]
- Rate of suspected cases reported to Children's Aid Societies (CAS) (child protection agencies) in Canada is just over 2%.[2]
  - Likely due to lack of recognition or under-reporting.
- In a retrospective review of children presenting to a pediatric emergency department who were referred to child protection agencies:[3]
  - The mean age was 6.4 years old.
  - The majority (55%) were referred for suspected physical abuse.
  - There were on average 4 to 5 previous emergency department visits.
  - The majority of reported cases did not have any physical findings (especially sexual abuse and neglect cases).
  - Of those with injuries, bruises were the most frequent injury reported.

HISTORY-TAKING
- Document source of history (parent, chart, CAS worker, etc.)
- Document thoroughly, in historian's own words, during the time history is taken.
- Give careful thought and consider consultation before directly questioning a young child if abuse is suspected.
  - Avoid extensive questioning, especially of young children.
  - When appropriate to question the child, ask only open-ended, non-leading, developmentally appropriate questions. For example, "Can you tell me how you hurt your leg?" **not** "Did your daddy hurt you?"
- Child's motor and language development.
- Injuries/possible physical abuse:
  - Thorough history of injury event, including location, time, who was present, detail of the injury event, symptoms in child, response of caregiver.
  - Previous injuries.
  - Family history as appropriate to the injury: Easy bruising, bleeding disorders, recurrent fractures, bone disorders.
- Possible sexual abuse/assault:
  - Determine whether child has active bleeding from the genital area and requires urgent assessment, and when the reported sexual contact occurred.
    - If no urgent need to assess/treat injuries, consult local child abuse expert PRIOR to beginning assessment.
    - If available, assessment by trained expert with medicolegal and child abuse experience is preferred.
  - For younger children, history from caregiver, preferably without the child present.
    - Reason for concern.

- History of vaginal bleeding or discharge.
- Other possible sources for bleeding: History of accidental injury, urinary symptoms, constipation, early signs of puberty, redness/irritation.
  - For older children and adolescents, history taken directly as discussed above:
    - History of events—time and date of assault, type of contact (skin, oral, genital, anal), pain, bleeding or discharge at the time of the assault or since, was a condom used, memory loss or confusion, possible consumption of mind-altering substances, other injuries.
    - Assailant's age, risk factors for sexually transmitted infections (STI) (multiple partners, previous sexual assault/incarceration, IV drug use, known previous or current STI).
    - History of previous sexual activity, last menstrual period, previous sexually transmitted infection, pregnancy.
    - Where adolescent lives, supports available. Are parents aware and discuss whether and how adolescents wish to inform parents.
    - Symptoms of fear, self-harm, suicidality.
    - Likelihood of forensic evidence available—has child bathed, showered, changed clothes, eaten, voided, defecated.
    - Discuss consent to inform police, complete a forensic evidence kit if appropriate (see below).

Red Flags in History for Nonaccidental Trauma
- History is inconsistent with mechanism or amount of force required to cause injury.
- History is inconsistent with the child's developmental level.
- History is inconsistent or changes.
- Delay in seeking medical attention without reasonable explanation.

PHYSICAL EXAMINATION
- Careful, thorough examination. Ensure all skin areas are seen, including ears, genitalia, buttocks, back.
- Clearly document any skin markings, preferably on a body diagram, and labeled with location, color, measured size, pattern.
  - Take photographs of all concerning skin injuries and store them in patient's record.
  - If photography is unavailable, CAS or police can organize photographs.
- Document growth parameters including head circumference.
- Assess fontanel and perform fundoscopic exam.
- Mouth: Look at upper lip frenulum, palate, and tongue frenulum.
- Abdominal exam: Tenderness, bruising.
- Palpate all body areas for pain, swelling, deformity, or callus.

Examination for Sexual Abuse Concerns:
- External genital examination only in prepubertal children, no internal vaginal examination or digital rectal examination (unless specific indication).
- Tanner stage of breast and pubic hair development.
- External genitalia—redness, bruising—document location, size, pattern, discharge, abrasions/lacerations.
- Labia should gently be retracted in a posterolateral direction to allow visualization of the hymen.
  - Carefully document redness, bruising, or injury (partial or complete transection) of the hymen.
  - Any abnormal hymenal findings should be reviewed with a clinician who has expertise and training in interpreting hymenal findings.
  - The source of any bleeding must be sought.
  - A gynecology consultation is required for ongoing internal bleeding to assess need for surgical intervention.
- External anal examination—document redness, bleeding, fissures, other acute injuries (lacerations).
  - A general surgery consultation is required for deep anal injuries or ongoing anal bleeding.

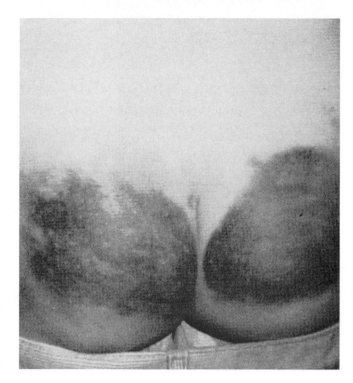

FIGURE 19-1 ● Buttock bruises. (From Ludwig S. Child abuse. In: Fleisher GR, Ludwig S, Baskin MN, eds. *Atlas of pediatric emergency medicine.* Philadelphia: Lippincott Williams & Wilkins; 2003: Figure 26.1D, with permission.)

Red Flags in Physical Examination for Nonaccidental Trauma

- Any bruising in a developmentally immobile (prior to cruising) child.
  - "Those who don't cruise rarely bruise."[4]
- Bruises of the cheeks, ears, or buttocks (Fig. 19-1).
- Patterned skin injuries (bruises or burns) (Fig. 19-2), including parallel linear bruises (Fig. 19-3), looped skin marks (Fig. 19-4), immersion-pattern scald burns (Fig.19-5).
- Torn upper lip or tongue frenulum in developmentally immobile child.
- Fracture in a developmentally immobile child without plausible explanation.
- Fractures of the ribs, (Fig. 19-6) limb bone metaphyses, scapula, vertebrae, sternum, long bones (Fig 19-7) without osteopenia/bone disorder.

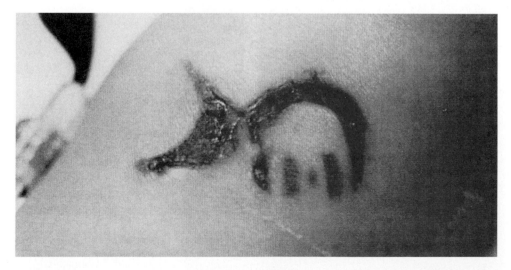

FIGURE 19-2 ● Cigarette lighter burn on a child. (From Ludwig S. Child abuse. In: Fleisher GR, Ludwig S, Baskin MN, eds. *Atlas of pediatric emergency medicine.* Philadelphia: Lippincott Williams & Wilkins; 2003: Figure 26.4, with permission.)

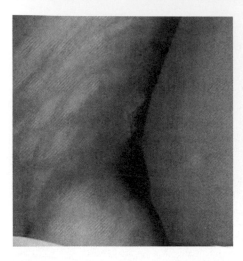

FIGURE 19-3 ● Linear marks. (From Ludwig S. Child abuse. In: Fleisher GR, Ludwig S, Baskin MN, eds. *Atlas of pediatric emergency medicine.* Philadelphia: Lippincott Williams & Wilkins; 2003: Figure 26.2A, with permission.)

- Severe life-threatening head injury from reported short (<5 feet/1.5 meter) fall. The exception to this is an epidural hematoma underlying a skull fracture, which can occur with a short fall and may be life-threatening.
- Multiple injuries, especially of different types and different ages.
- Sexual abuse:
  - Acute genital trauma without alternate explanation, particularly posterior hymenal injuries without history of accidental penetrating injury.
  - Sexually transmitted infection outside the perinatal transmission period and in the absence of a history of consensual sexual activity in an adolescent.

LABORATORY TESTING
- Children with suspicious bruising, intracranial hemorrhage, or retinal hemorrhage must have a CBC with platelet count, differential, and blood film, as well as INR and PTT to screen for coagulation disorders.

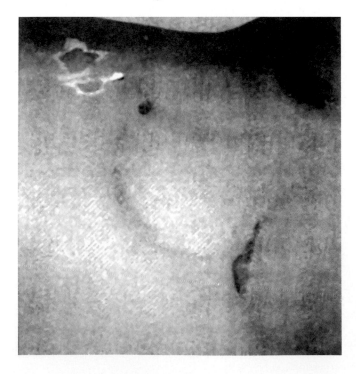

FIGURE 19-4 ● Loop-shaped marks. (From Ludwig S. Child abuse. In: Fleisher GR, Ludwig S, Baskin MN, eds. *Atlas of pediatric emergency medicine.* Philadelphia: Lippincott Williams & Wilkins; 2003: Figure 26.2B, with permission.)

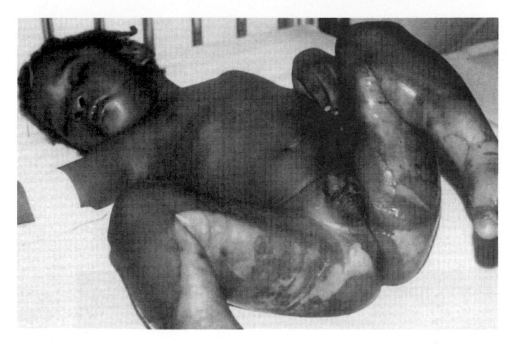

FIGURE 19-5 ● Immersion burns. (From Ludwig S. Child abuse. In: Fleisher GR, Ludwig S, Baskin MN, eds. *Atlas of pediatric emergency medicine.* Philadelphia: Lippincott Williams & Wilkins; 2003: Figure 26.3A, with permission.)

- Further coagulation testing may be indicated (discuss with child abuse or other expert).
- Children with suspicious fractures may require metabolic bone disease workup (discuss with child abuse or other expert).
- Children with seizures and intracranial hemorrhage should have metabolic screen, including blood gas, lactate, serum amino acids, urine organic acids.

Suspected Sexual Abuse
- Children/adolescents with suspected sexual abuse should have serology for hepatitis B and C, syphilis, and HIV.

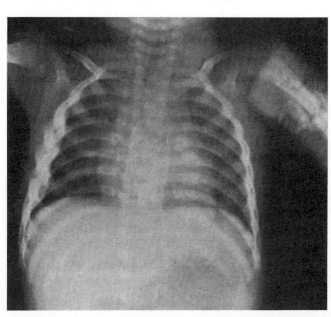

FIGURE 19-6 ● Multiple headline rib fractures and a humerus fracture. (From Ludwig S. Child abuse. In: Fleisher GR, Ludwig S, Baskin MN, eds. *Atlas of pediatric emergency medicine.* Philadelphia: Lippincott Williams & Wilkins; 2003: Figure 26.6B, with permission.)

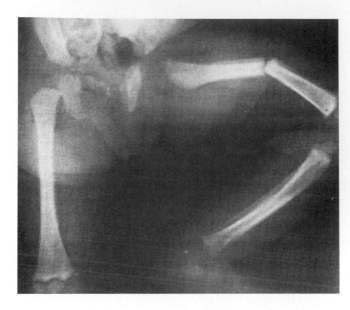

FIGURE 19-7 ● Femur Fracture. (From Ludwig S. Child abuse. In: Fleisher GR, Ludwig S, Baskin MN, eds. *Atlas of pediatric emergency medicine.* Philadelphia: Lippincott Williams & Wilkins; 2003: Figure 26.1C, with permission.)

- Children/adolescents with suspected sexual assault who had a period of memory loss/confusion or suspect a drug was administered to them should have blood and urine toxicology screens with specific request for Rohypnol/GHB/date rape drugs.

Testing for Sexually Transmitted Infections:
- Swabs for sexually transmitted infections are generally not indicated in acute sexual assault.
- Prepubertal children with vaginal discharge should have vaginal swabs for bacterial culture and *Chlamydia* culture.
  - Note that the hymen is very sensitive to touch in prepubertal children.
  - Small urethral swabs should be used and care taken to avoid contacting the hymen with the swab.
  - If culture is not available, nonculture tests (nucleic acid amplification tests) may be completed but a positive result must be confirmed with a second assay of a different type in this age group.
  - Adolescents with vaginal discharge should have a speculum examination with cervical swabs for bacterial culture and *Chlamydia* culture and a vaginal swab for *Trichomonas.*
  - Adolescents who have been previously sexually active should be referred for a nonurgent speculum examination, swabs, and a Pap test.

Sexual Assault Evidence Kit:
- A medicolegal (not medical) assessment conducted for the purposes of evidence collection for the police.
- Requires consent and cooperation from child/adolescent for completion, as well as active police involvement.
- Should be carefully considered—time consuming, invasive, yield varies. Collection of clothing, particularly underwear, has highest yield.
- Consider in prepubertal children reporting abuse/assault within the previous 24 hours, in adolescents reporting assault within the previous 72 hours.
- Instructions are clearly provided in the kit.
- You must stay with the kit at all times or lock it in a secure location until given to police.
- Document kit number and name/badge number of police officer along with date/time provided to police.

RADIOLOGIC EVALUATION

- All children under the age of 2 years or who are nonverbal or developmentally immobile must have a full skeletal survey (12+ views), **not** a babygram (1−2 views).[5]
  - Caregivers should be told that x-rays have been requested of all body areas to ensure there are no additional injuries **prior** to sending child to the x-ray department.
  - The skeletal survey should be completed before cast is applied.
  - The skeletal survey typically includes (all films done separately):[6]
    - AP and lateral skull.
    - AP and lateral complete spine.
    - AP and lateral chest for ribs.
    - AP pelvis.
    - AP both humeri.
    - AP both radius-ulna.
    - PA both hands and wrists.
    - AP both femora.
    - AP both tibia-fibula.
    - AP both feet.
- Children over the age of 2 years or who are ambulatory may require x-rays, although a full skeletal survey is typically **not** indicated.
  - This should be discussed with a child abuse expert.
- Children with suspected abdominal injuries (including those without symptoms/signs who have mild elevation of transaminases) must have an abdominal CT scan.
  - An abdominal ultrasound is not sufficiently sensitive for abdominal trauma.[7]
- All infants and children with suspected head injury must have a head CT with contrast and a dilated ophthalmic examination as soon as possible.
  - Retinal hemorrhages may resolve within days; therefore, the eye exam should be completed as soon as possible after the child is stabilized (Fig. 19–8).
  - Similarly, infants with fractures that are highly associated with abusive head trauma (skull fractures, rib fractures, and metaphyseal fractures of the limb bones) should have a CT scan and ophthalmologic examination.

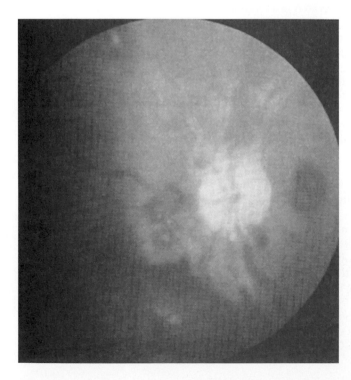

FIGURE 19-8 ● Retinal hemorrhage. (From Ludwig S. Child abuse. In: Fleisher GR, Ludwig S, Baskin MN, eds. *Atlas of pediatric emergency medicine.* Philadelphia: Lippincott Williams & Wilkins; 2003: Figure 26.11C, with permission.)

MANAGEMENT
General Considerations
- When abuse is suspected, tell caregivers about injuries but avoid specific discussion of mechanism.
- Use nonconfrontational, nonjudgmental language and approach with caregivers present.
  - For example, discuss "injuries" rather than "abuse," and avoid blame or accusation.
- As soon as abuse is suspected, a CAS or Child Protection Services (CPS) referral should be made.
  - In Ontario, this referral is mandated under the Child and Family Services Act (CFSA).[8]
  - A person suspecting abuse does not need to be certain of the diagnosis to make a referral, but must have reasonable grounds to suspect abuse or neglect.
  - The person with the most information about the concern must make the referral (e.g., if it is an injury, the physician must speak with the CAS and must not delegate this to a nurse or social worker).
  - The duty to report a concern of child maltreatment to the CAS/CPS overrides health care confidentiality, and information regarding the basis of the concern must be reported to the CAS.
  - If unsure whether CAS should be consulted or whether to be concerned, consult an expert such as the Suspected Child Abuse and Neglect (SCAN, child abuse) on-call clinician.
    - The SCAN program at SickKids provides 24-hour on call coverage for advice and recommendations for professionals in the hospital and the community. Similar child abuse programs are available in many parts of the country and North America.
  - In Ontario, CAS will contact police in cases of suspected child physical or sexual abuse, and the two agencies will conduct a joint investigation.

Injury Management
- Injuries should be managed as medically indicated.
- Head injuries: Infants and young children with inflicted traumatic brain injury who present with symptoms such as seizures, apnea, and altered level of consciousness frequently have significantly elevated intracranial pressure.
  - Early recognition and management is necessary to reduce secondary brain injury.
  - There is a significant mortality risk in these children.
  - See Chapter 5 on Head Trauma: Medical Management for details.

Acute Sexual Assault Management (Reported Assault Within 72 Hours)
- Offer emergency contraception (Choose one from below):
  - Plan B (levonorgestrel): 2 tablets immediately.
  - Ovral 2 tablets immediately, and repeat in 12 hours.
- Offer prophylaxis for sexually transmitted infections in nonpregnant, nonallergic patient.
  - Azithromycin:
    - <45 kg: 15 mg/kg PO in a single dose, max 1 g.
    - >45 kg: 1g PO in a single dose.
  - Cefixime:
    - <45 kg: 8 mg/kg PO in a single dose, max 400 mg.
    - >45 kg: 400 mg PO in a single dose.
- Ensure no allergies/contraindications and complete urine HCG in adolescents prior to administering these medications.
- Consider hepatitis B prophylaxis in nonimmune adolescents at high risk (high-risk assailant and exposure):
  - HBIG 0.06 mL/kg IM up to 14 days after exposure.
  - Begin hepatitis B vaccine series.
- Consider HIV prophylaxis. Consultation with a child abuse or infectious diseases expert recommended.

CLINICAL PEARLS

DO
- Have a high index of suspicion for child abuse in all injuries in nonambulatory children.
- Take a thorough injury history and do a thorough physical examination in all cases.
- Document clearly and completely.
- Perform skeletal survey in all cases of suspected physical abuse under 2 years old.
- Contact CAS/CPS immediately if you suspect child abuse.

DON'T
- Ask children leading questions about suspected abuse.
- Accuse parents of abusing their child.
- Delay! Contact CAS or child abuse expert immediately.

REFERENCES

1. MacMillan HL, Fleming JE, Trocmé N, et al. Prevalence of child physical and sexual abuse in the community. *JAMA* 1997;278:131–135.
2. Trocmé N, Wolfe D. *Canadian incidence study of reported child abuse and neglect: final report.* Ottawa: Minister of Public Works and Government Services; 2001.
3. Keshavarz R, Kawashima R, Low C. Child abuse and neglect presentations to a pediatric emergency department. *J Emerg Med* 2002;23:341–345.
4. Sugar N, Taylor J, Feldman K. Bruises in infants and toddlers. Those who don't cruise rarely bruise. *Arch Pediatr Adolesc Med* 1999;153:399–403.
5. American Academy of Pediatrics section on radiology. Diagnostic imaging of child abuse. *Pediatrics* 2000;105:1345–1348.
6. Ontario Hospital Association. *Identifying and managing child abuse and neglect. A manual for Ontario hospitals.* Ottawa: OHA; 2000.
7. Kleinman P. Visceral trauma. In: Kleinman P, ed. *Diagnostic imaging of child abuse.* St. Louis: Mosby; 1998.
8. Government of Ontario, Ministry of Community and Social Services. *Child and family services act.* 2001. Available at http://www.cfcs.gov.on.ca/mcss/splash.htm.

CHAPTER 20

Injury Prevention

Safe Kids Canada

EPIDEMIOLOGY

- In Canada, the leading cause of death for children is unintentional injury (Figs. 20-1 and 20-2).

Falls

- Babies fall off beds or out of cribs while playing, sleeping, or trying to get out of them.
  - Adult beds are involved in one-third of cases where a baby fell off a bed.[1]
  - Infant falls often result in head and neck injuries.[2]
  - Head injuries for infants can have lifelong implications on brain development.[1]
- Falls involving stairs and steps:
  - 63% of children injured were under age 5.
  - 23% were ages 5 to 9.
  - 14% were ages 10 to 14.[3]
- Playground falls:
  - 14% of children are hospitalized for head injuries.
  - 81% for broken bones to other parts of the body.
  - 5% for injuries such as dislocations and open wounds.[3]

Motor Vehicle Crashes

- The leading cause of injury-related death for Canadian children (Table 20-1).
- Can cause multiple serious injuries, such as spine and internal organ damage.
- Head injuries are a serious risk for children, especially when not restrained properly.[4,5]

Drowning

- Babies under age 1 are most likely to drown in the bathtub.[6]
- Toddlers ages 1 to 4 are most likely to drown* in home swimming pools followed by, large bodies of water such as rivers, ponds, and beach areas.[6]
  - Most toddler drownings occur when the child is walking or playing near water, not intending to swim, and often without an adult knowing the child is near the water.[6]
- In a 10-year review, the Canadian Red Cross found that 42% of drowning victims, ages 5 to 14, did not have adult supervision at the time.[6]

Burns

- 56% of hospitalizations for burns are caused by scald burns.
- Children under the age of 5 suffer 83% of all scald hospital admissions.[3]

Poisoning

- 64% of poisoning occurs in children ages 1 to 4.[3]
- Medication, both over-the-counter and prescription, is involved in 67% of all unintentional poisoning of children age 14 and under.[3]
- Other causes include household cleaners, alcohol, plants, fertilizers, pesticides, paint thinner, and antifreeze.[3]

TABLE 20-1

Annual Risk of Death and Injury for Canadian Children Under the Age of 14

Risk Factor	Number of Deaths per Year	Number of Hospitalizations per Year	Risk of Death	Risk of Serious Injury
Falls Related to Chairs, Beds, Stairs, and Steps		1,700		1 in 3,400
Playground Falls		2,500		1 in 2,300
Motor Vehicle Crashes	68	880	1 in 86,000	1 in 6,600
Cycling	20	1,800	1 in 333,000	1 in 3,300
Poisoning	7	1,700	1 in 820,000	1 in 3,400
Scalds and Burns	40	770	1 in 150,000	1 in 7,200
Drowning	58	140	1 in 100,000	1 in 47,600
Pedestrian	56	780	1 in 104,600	1 in 7,600
Choking, Strangulation, and Suffocation	44	380	1 in 132,800	1 in 15,400

(From Safe Kids Canada. *Child & Youth Unintentional Injury: 10 Years in Review, 1994–2003.* Toronto: Safe Kids Canada; 2006.)

Pedestrian

- Approximately 70% of deaths and 50% of serious injuries happen where there is no form of traffic control.[7]
- The child may have been trying to cross the street in the middle of the block, walking out from between parked cars, or crossing at an intersection without a stoplight.[7]

Choking, Strangulation, and Suffocation

- 80% of children treated for threats to breathing were under age 5.[3]
- Hospitalizations:
  - 94% choking on food or other objects.
  - 6% a mechanical cause (e.g., strangulation by blind cords).[3]
  - As of March 2006, 24 deaths and 21 near-miss incidents involving blinds or curtain cords and chains were reported.[3]

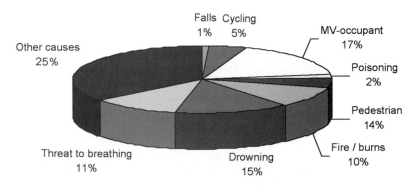

FIGURE 20-1 ● Major causes of unintentional injury deaths among Canadian children aged 0 to 14 years, 1994 to 2003. (Note: Death trends for 2003 were estimated from trends for the years 1994 to 2002. "Other causes" refers to types of injury such as sports-related deaths, firearms, or machinery. The death data are gathered in such a way that they often capture whether a child was struck by and struck against something, rather than the activity that the child was involved in at the time of injury. (From Statistics Canada, as used in Safe Kids Canada. *Child & Youth Unintentional Injury: 10 Years In Review, 1994–2003.* Toronto: Safe Kids Canada; 2006.)

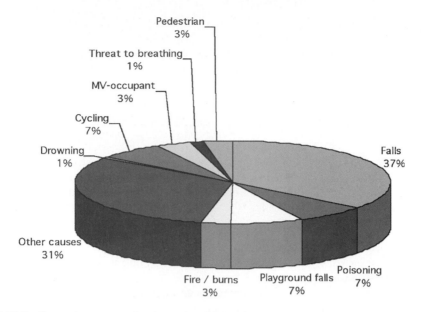

FIGURE 20-2 ● Major causes of unintentional injury hospitalization among Canadian children aged 0 to 14, 1994 to 2003. (From Canadian Institute for Health Information, as used in Safe Kids Canada. *Child & Youth Unintentional Injury: 10 Years in Review, 1994–2003.* Toronto: Safe Kids Canada; 2006.)

MANAGEMENT AND RISK REDUCTION STRATEGIES
- An estimated 90% of all injuries could be prevented.[8]
- Supervision and understanding child development are critical in keeping kids safe.
- Caregivers who receive counseling by front-line trauma workers have a safer home environment.[9]

Car Seats and Booster Seats
- Car seats, when used correctly:
  - Reduce the risk of death by:
    - 71% for infants.
    - 54% for children aged 1 to 4 years.[10]
  - Reduce the risk of hospitalization by 67% for children aged 4 and under.[11]
- Booster seats provide 59% more protection than seat belts alone.[5]
- Ensure parents understand the importance of correct restraint use for their children.
  - Most children between 4 and 9 are not correctly restrained by booster seats.[12]

ATVs
- Children under 16 should not operate ATVs.

Bike Helmets
- Wear a bike helmet correctly on every bike ride.
- A properly fitted helmet decreases the risk of serious head injury by up to 85%.[12]
- 4 out of 5 head injuries could be prevented if every cyclist wore a helmet.[13]
- Young cyclists ride at speeds averaging 11 to 16 km/hr.[14]
- The human skull is ~1 cm thick and can fracture at an impact of only 7 to 10 km/hr.[15]

Window Stops and Guards
- Children under 3 are most vulnerable to window falls.[16]
- Window screens are not a safety barrier. They cannot hold a child's weight.
- Use window guards or, stops to prevent the window opening more than 10 cm.

Playground Equipment

- Keep children under age 5 on equipment <1.5 m high
- Falls from heights >1.5 m double the risk of severe injury for children of all ages.[17]
- Appropriate playground surfacing can reduce injury severity compared to falls on a harder surface.[17,18]

Change Tables

- Always keep one hand on the child when using a change table.

Smoke Alarms

- Install smoke alarms on each level of the house, especially near sleeping areas.
  - There is a threefold increased risk of death in homes without smoke alarms.[17]
  - Most children who died in residential fires were in homes without smoke alarms or without working smoke alarms.[19]

Locks and Latches

- Keep all poisons locked out of reach.
  - Child-resistant packaging is required by law for certain medications and significantly reduces the chance of poisoning.[20]
  - Research shows that a small percentage of children may still be able to open the medication.[21] It must be kept locked up.

Carbon Monoxide Detectors

- Install on all levels of a home, particularly near sleeping areas.
- Ensure that fuel-burning appliances are in good working order.

Hot Water Temperature

- Reduce the tap water temperature to 49°C.
- Water temperature is typically 60°C, which can cause a third-degree burn on a child's sensitive skin in just 1 second.[22]
  - Tap water burns tend to be deep and cover a larger portion of the body.[23]

Gas Fireplaces

- Use gates to keep children away from gas fireplaces as they remain extremely hot even after being turned off.

Supervision Near Water

- Supervise young children by keeping them within arm's reach at all times when they are in or around water.

Life Jackets

- Use life jackets when young children are near or in water and on boats.

Private Swimming Pools

- Use four-sided fencing for private swimming pools.
- Proper fencing (1.2 m high, four-sided with a self-latching gate) could prevent 7 out of 10 drowning incidents in private swimming pools for children under age 5.[24]

Crossing the Street

- Do not let children under age 9 cross the road without an adult.[25]
  - Children under age 9:
    - Do not judge traffic safely.
    - Cannot determine how quickly a vehicle is moving.
    - Have undeveloped peripheral vision.
    - Believe that drivers will see them and stop when required.

Choking, Strangulation, and Suffocation

- Children under 4 should not have raw carrots, candies, popcorn, large pieces of hot dog, or access to small toys.

- Cut or tie up all blind and drapery cords.
- Children should sleep in their own crib, on their back, and with minimal, well-fitted bedding to reduce the risk of suffocation and SIDS.

Baby Walkers with Wheels
- Are banned in Canada.
- Serious injuries are three to five times more frequent in children who have fallen down stairs in baby walkers, compared to other types of falls.[26]

Baby Bath Seats
- Do not use baby bath seats.
- Canadian pediatricians reported 20 injuries and 12 near-miss drowning incidents involving baby bath seats between 2003 and 2005.[27]
- Health Canada issued a product advisory.
  - They received reports of 11 drowning deaths linked to infant bath seats and bath rings since 1991. Three of these deaths were in 2004 alone.[28]
  - Bath seats are mistakenly seen as a safe substitute for supervision, giving adults the misconception that they can do other activities while the child is in the tub.[29,30]

ADVOCACY
- Canada has seen reductions in injuries due, in part, to successful advocacy efforts to ban products and to introduce legislation.

Baby Walkers with Wheels
- In April 2004, Canada became the first country to ban the sale, importation, and advertisement of baby walkers.
- Prior to the ban, on average, each year in Canada Several hundred babies were injured, often head injuries, in baby walkers.

Helmet Legislation
- Some provinces in Canada have bike helmet legislation.
- A cross-Canada study demonstrated ~25% lower head injury rates among child and youth cyclists in provinces with helmet legislation, compared to provinces without legislation.
  - Over the 4 years studied, 687 hospitalizations for head injuries to child cyclists could have been prevented if every province had bicycle helmet legislation.[27]

Opportunities to Contribute
- Many organizations look to demonstrate strength through letter-writing campaigns to government, manufacturers, and media.
- Letters to the editor are effective in raising awareness around a specific issue or article featured in the newspaper.
- Be an expert—spokespeople for campaign and program launches give credibility to the message.
- Advocate for increases in prevention funding allocations and improved injury surveillance systems.

Hospital-Based Outreach Initiatives
- Many hospitals in Canada currently have programs addressing child and youth injury prevention.
- On-site child and youth injury prevention programs provide parents and caregivers with information, resources, and safety devices.
- Car seat loaner programs ensure children ride home safely after discharge.
- On-site bike helmet fittings teach children and caregivers the correct way to wear a helmet.

CANADIAN NATIONAL RESOURCES
Safe Kids Canada
- Works with community partners nationally in areas of research, education, and advocacy to prevent unintentional injuries to children and youth.
- Is uniquely positioned to be a partner in the knowledge translation process.
- Is able to take critical research findings and shape them into programs, messages, and advocacy initiatives to provide solutions to injury causes.

Canadian Hospitals Injury Reporting and Prevention Program (CHIRPP)
- CHIRPP is an emergency room surveillance system that tracks injuries seen in 10 pediatric hospitals and 5 general hospitals.
- The data collected provide good information on the details of the injury.
- CHIRPP coordinators report the data to a central location at Health Canada for compilation and analysis.
- CHIRPP is invaluable in identifying trends in child and youth injury patterns.

Canadian Pediatric Society
Resources for Health Care Professionals
- Position statements from the Canadian Paediatric Society (CPS) Injury Prevention Committee.
- The Canadian Pediatric Surveillance Program has undertaken several studies related to injury prevention, such as head injury secondary to suspected child maltreatment and lap-belt syndrome.
- The Caring for Kids website has a host of downloadable fact sheets on injury prevention to use in your practice or clinic.

Patient Education: Resources for Parents and Caregivers
- *Keeping Your Baby Safe:* A bilingual brochure that covers the basics of injury prevention for babies and young children, at home and in the car.
- Detailed brochures are available on topics such as playground safety, winter safety, safe sleep, and Halloween safety.

REFERENCES
1. Health Canada. For the safety of Canadian children and youth: from injury data to preventive measures. Ottawa: 1997;138.
2. Pickett W, Streight S, Simpson S. Injuries experienced by infant children: a population-based epidemiological analysis. *Pediatrics* 2003;111:365–370.
3. Safe Kids Canada. *Child & youth unintentional injury: 10 years in review, 1994–2003.* Toronto: Safe Kids Canada; 2006.
4. Muszynski C, Narayan Y, Pintar F, et al. Risk of pediatric head injury after motor vehicle accidents. *J Neurosurg (Pediatrics 4)* 2005;102:374–379.
5. Durbin D, Elliott M, Winston F. Belt-positioning booster seats and reduction in risk of injury among older children in vehicle crashes. *JAMA* 2003;289:2835–2840.
6. Canadian Red Cross. Drowning and other water-related injuries in Canada 1991–2000. 2006.
7. Transport Canada. Pedestrian fatalities and injuries 1988–1997. Fact sheet RS2001–401, February 2001. As cited in Safe Kids Canada. *Making it happen: pedestrian safety.* Toronto: Safe Kids Canada; 2004:9.
8. Cushman, R. Injury prevention: The time has come. *Canadian Medical Association Journal* 1995;152(1): 121–123.
9. Claudius IA, Nager AL. The utility of safety counseling in a pediatric emergency department. *Pediatrics* 2005;115;423–427.
10. National Highway Traffic Safety Administration. Research note: revised estimates of child restraint effectiveness. Washington, DC: U.S. Department of Transportation, National Highway Traffic Safety Administration; 1996. Report no. 96.855.
11. Kahane C. An evaluation of child passenger safety: the effectiveness and benefits of safety seats. Washington, DC: U.S. Department of Transportation. National Highway Traffic Safety Administration; 1986. Report no. 806 890.
12. Safe Kids Canada. *National child passenger safety survey results, 2004.* Toronto: Safe Kids Canada.
13. Thompson D, Rivara F, Thompson R. Helmets for preventing head and facial injuries in bicyclists. *Cochrane Database Syst Rev* 2001;4:1–37.

14. Thompson D, Rebolledo V, Thompson R, et al. Bike speed measurement in a recreational population: validity of self reported speed. *Inj Prev* 1997;3:43–45.
15. Canadian Bike Helmet Coalition. *How to organize a community project.* Canadian Bike Helmet Coalition; 1994.
16. Health Canada. Injuries associated with falls from windows. Canadian hospitals injury reporting and prevention program (CHIRPP), May 2000.
17. Macarthur C, Hu X, Wesson D, et al. Risk factors for severe injuries associated with falls from playground equipment. *Accid Anal Prev* 2000;32:377–382.
18. Chalmers D, Marshall S, Langley J, et al. Height and surfacing as risk factors for falls from playground equipment: a case control study. *Inj Prev* 1996;2:98–104.
19. Runyan C, Bangdiwala S, Linzer M, et al. Risk factors for fatal residential fires. *N Engl J Med* 1992;327:859–863.
20. Rodgers G. The effectiveness of child-resistant packaging for aspirin. *Arch Pediatr Adolesc Med* 2002; 156:929–933.
21. Chien C, Mariott K, Ashby K, et al. Unintentional ingestion of over the counter medications in children less than 5 years old. *J Paediatric Child Health* 2003;39:264–269.
22. Moritz A, Henriques F. Studies of thermal injury: the relative importance of time and surface temperature in the causation of cutaneous burns. *Am J Pathol* 1947;123:695–720.
23. Feldman K, Schalter R, Feldman J, McMillon M. Tap Water Scald Burns in Children. *Pediatrics* 1978; 62(1):1–7
24. Thompson D, Rivara F. Pool fencing for preventing drowning in children. *Cochrancer Review.* The Cochrane Library 3, 2004.
25. Malek M., Guyer B., Lescohier I. The Epidermiology and Prevention of Child Pedestrian Injury. *Accident Analysis and Prevention* 1990;22(4), 301–313.
26. Health Surveillance and Epidemiology Division, Public Health Agency of Canada. *Injuries associated with baby walkers.* Canadian Hospitals Injury Reporting and Prevention Program (CHIRPP).
27. Canadian Paediatric Surveillence Program. Infant bath seat survey: results and next steps. *Paediatr Child Health* 2005;10:27.
28. Health Canada. *Health Canada advises that a drowning hazard has been identified with respect to the use of infant bath seats and rings.* April 26, 2005.
29. Byard R, Donald T. Infant bath seats, drowning and near drowning. *J Paediatr Child Health* 2004; 40:305–307.
30. Macpherson A, To T, Macarthur C, et al. Impact of mandatory helmet legislation on bicycle-related head injures in children: a population-based study. *Pediatrics* 2002a;110:60.

CHAPTER 21

Trauma Procedures in the Emergency Department

Rahim Valani, MD, CCFP-EM, FRCPC, PG Dip Med Ed

INTRAOSSEOUS (IO) ACCESS[1–5] (FIG. 21-1)
- Immediate and urgent vascular access when intravenous (IV) access has failed.
- Can be used for any age.
- Safe to administer fluids, drugs, and blood products.
- IO needle can be left in place for up to 72 hours, but is generally not recommended.
- Used as a temporizing measure until peripheral venous access is obtained.

Indications
- Need for immediate access when IV access has failed.

Relative Contraindications
- Avoid IO in a fractured limb.
- Overlying infection.
- Previous attempt at the same site.
- Osteogenesis imperfecta or other medical conditions that are prone to fractures with minor trauma.

Complications
- Improper placement of needle into subcutaneous or subperiosteal tissue (extravasation of fluid) or poor landmarks.
- Bending of needle.
- Through and through penetration of bone.
- Infection—cellulitis, osteomyelitis.
- Compartment syndrome.
- Growth plate injuries.
- Local hematoma.

Procedure
- Use 14 to 20 G intraosseous needle with stylus.
- Prepare the area in a sterile fashion and infiltrate with local anesthetic.
- Landmark as illustrated for proximal tibial or distal femur placement (Fig. 21-1).
- Needle is inserted at 90 degrees to the bony surface.
- Avoid putting your other hand behind the limb where the IO needle is being inserted.
- Proper location will ensure that the needle is away from growth plate.
- Placement is confirmed when the cortex is infiltrated—you will feel a release (Fig. 21-2).
- You may aspirate marrow, but this is not always possible or necessary.
- Connect to IV tubing and infuse fluids.
- Watch for signs of fluid extravasation.

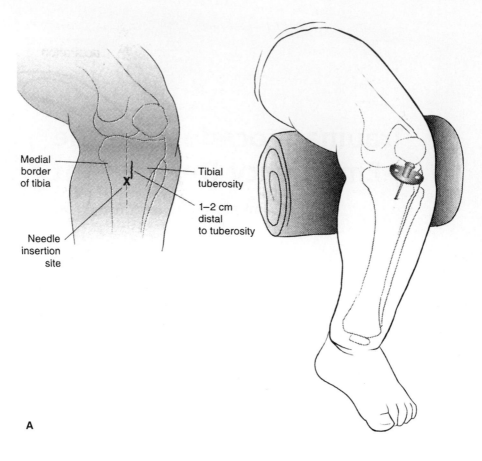

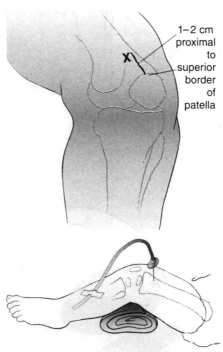

FIGURE 21-1 ● Landmarks for intraosseous infusion needle insertion. (From King C, Henretig FM. Intraosseous infusion. *Pocket atlas of pediatric emergency procedures.* Philadelphia: Lippincott Williams & Wilkins; 2000, Figs. 9.4 and 9.6, with permission.)

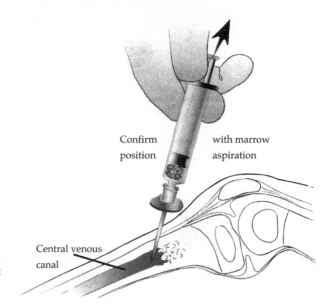

FIGURE 21-2 ● Insertion of intraosseous needle. (From King C, Henretig FM. Intraosseous infusion. *Pocket atlas of pediatric emergency procedures.* Philadelphia: Lippincott Williams & Wilkins; 2000, Fig. 9.2C, with permission.)

Confirm position with marrow aspiration

Central venous canal

CENTRAL LINE PLACEMENT[1-3,6,7]
- Sites for central venous line placement: femoral or subclavian (Table 21-1).

Indications
- Need for central venous pressure monitoring.
- Large volume infusions.
- Drug infusions requiring central access such as epinephrine and norepinephrine.
- Infusion of concentrated or peripherally sclerosing agents (>40 mEq/L of KCl, hypertonic saline).
- Emergency dialysis.

Contraindications
- Bleeding diathesis or coagulopathy.
- Distorted local anatomy.
- Proximal injury (e.g., avoid femoral line in pelvic fracture).
- Prior injury to the vesse.
- Complication rates of central line placements range from 0.3% to 18.8%.
- Ultrasound guided insertion is gaining popularity, and potentially may decrease complications.

Complications
- Bleeding.
- Thrombosis.
- Arterial puncture.
- Air embolism.
- Hemothorax.
- Pneumothorax.
- Systemic infection.
- Hematoma.
- Cellulitis.

TABLE 21-1

Sites for Central Venous Line Placement

Site	Advantages	Disadvantages
Femoral	Easy landmarks	Limits mobility of patient Femoral aneurysms Bowel or bladder injury
Subclavian	Can be performed during CPR or airway control	Pneumothorax Hemothorax Cannulation of subclavian artery Tracheal injury

Procedure
- See Figure 21-3 for landmarks.
- Prepare and drape the area in a sterile fashion.
- Consider using a "finder needle" to locate the vein.
- Infiltrate area with local anesthetic.

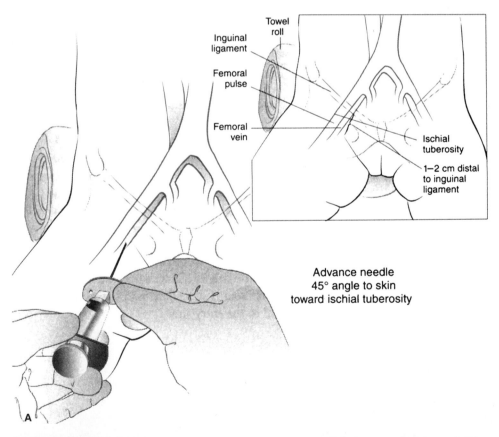

Towel roll
Inguinal ligament
Femoral pulse
Femoral vein
Ischial tuberosity
1–2 cm distal to inguinal ligament

Advance needle
45° angle to skin
toward ischial tuberosity

A

FIGURE 21-3 ●   Landmarks for central line placement. **A.** Femoral site. **B.** Internal Jugular Site **C.** Subclavian Vein (From King C, Henretig FM. Central Venous Access. *Pocket atlas of pediatric emergency procedures.* Philadelphia: Lippincott Williams & Wilkins; 2000, Figs. 7.2, 7.3, and 7.4, with permission.)

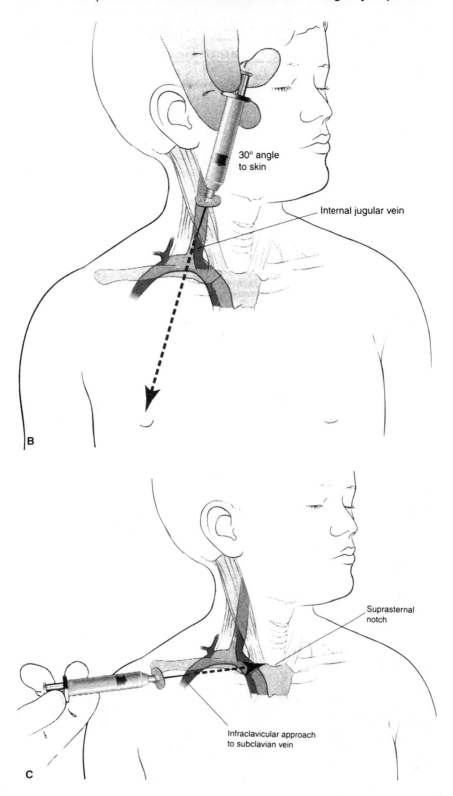

FIGURE 21-3 ● *(Continued)*

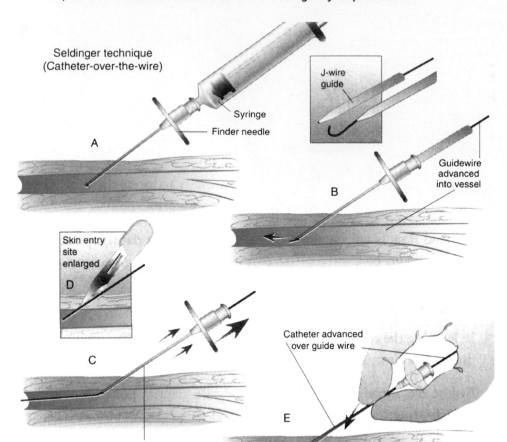

FIGURE 21-4 ● Seldinger technique for insertion of central venous line over guidewire. (From King C, Henretig FM. Central venous access. *Pocket atlas of pediatric emergency procedures.* Philadelphia: Lippincott Williams & Wilkins; 2000, Fig. 7.1, with permission.)

- Seldinger technique (Fig. 21-4):
  - Use a 5-mL syringe connected to the entry needle.
  - Use specified landmarks for the central vein being cannulated (Fig. 21-3).
  - Insert needle while continuously drawing back. A rapid draw suggests the vessel is accessed.
- Can confirm venous placement versus arterial with:
  - Rapid blood gas analysis.
  - Lack of pulsatile flow.
  - Transduce with short segment of IV tubing.
  - Color of blood is not a reliable marker.
- Once vessel is accessed, remove syringe while stabilizing needle and insert guidewire. It should thread in easily.
- If guidewire not threading easily, reconnect syringe and ensure the needle tip is positioned in the vessel.
- Remove needle while leaving guide wire in place.
- *DO NOT LET GO OF THE GUIDEWIRE!*
- Place selected catheter over guidewire, and remove guidewire.
- Secure central line.
- Obtain chest x-ray for subclavian line to ensure no pneumothorax, correct placement, and location of catheter tip.

ARTERIAL LINE PLACEMENT[1–3]
- Various kits are available that aid in the Seldinger technique.
- Potential sites include:
  - Radial (most common site).
  - Ulnar.
  - Posterior tibial.
  - Femoral.

Indications
- Continuous monitoring of hemodynamic parameters (blood pressure and heart rate).
- Frequent need for blood sampling and arterial gas sampling.

Contraindications
- Hand—absence of collateral circulation. All other sites, absence of pulse.
  - Can cause compromise of circulation and distal ischemia.
- Prior surgery over the site.
- Bleeding diathesis.

Complications
- Arterial spasm.
- Poor waveform.
- Ischemic limb/digits.
- Aneurysm.
- Infection.

Procedure
- Palpate artery over area of maximal impulse.
- Prep the area in a sterile fashion.
- Insert the needle at a 10- to 20-degree angle to the skin surface.
- Blood will appear in the catheter hub when the artery is punctured.
- Advance the catheter slowly until the angle to the skin surface is 10 degrees.
- Advance the catheter over needle into the artery.
- Remove the needle while compressing the artery proximal to the tip of the catheter.
- Connect the catheter to the arterial line system.
  - Zero the system.
  - Assess the waveform.
  - Secure the catheter.
  - Use heparinized solution only.

TUBE THORACOSTOMY (CHEST TUBE)[1–3,8–11]
- Common procedure performed for blunt or penetrating thoracic trauma.
- Purpose is to drain air or blood from the pleural space.
- In trauma, the open procedure with a larger chest tube size is preferable.
- For small, spontaneous pneumothoraces, a percutaneous kit can be utilized.

Indications
- Drainage of contents from the pleural space:
  - Air (pneumothorax)—tension, open, or simple.
  - Blood (hemothorax).
  - Chyle.
  - Esophageal contents.
- Prevention of tension pneumothorax in ventilated patient with rib fractures.
- Traumatic arrest—requires bilateral tube thoracostomy.
- Suspected chest injury prior to transfer to definitive trauma center.

Contraindications
- Uncontrolled bleeding diathesis/coagulopathy.
- Infection over the site.

TABLE 21-2

Typical Chest Tube Sizes

Patient	Size
Teen male or adult	28–32F
Teen female or adult	28F
Child	18F
Newborn	12–14F

Complications
- Complication rate estimated at 2% to 10%, the majority being minor.
- Injuries to the heart, lung, hilum, great vessels, and liver have all been documented.
- Avoid trocar sets as they have an increased incidence of such injury.

Chest Tube Sizes (Table 21-2)
- Rough guide: 4 times the size of the endotracheal tube.

Procedure
- Sterile preparation of the appropriate hemithorax.
- Insert tube between the anterior and midaxillary line along the fourth or fifth inter-costal space (Fig. 21-5).
- Ensure adequate sedation and analgesia if patient is alert (see Chapter 18 on Pain Management for details).

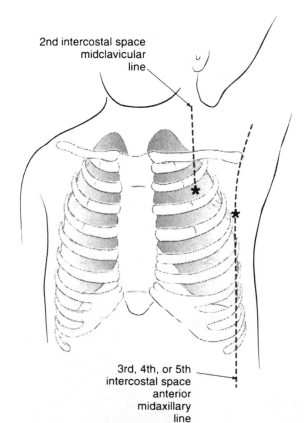

2nd intercostal space
midclavicular
line

3rd, 4th, or 5th
intercostal space
anterior
midaxillary
line

FIGURE 21-5 ● Landmarks for insertion of chest tube. (From King C, Henretig FM. Tube thoracostomy and needle decompression of the chest. *Pocket atlas of pediatric emergency procedures.* Philadelphia: Lippincott Williams & Wilkins; 2000, Fig. 15.1, with permission.)

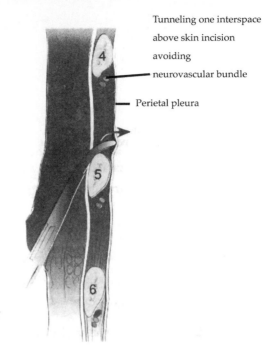

Tunneling one interspace
above skin incision
avoiding
neurovascular bundle

Perietal pleura

FIGURE 21-6 ● Landmarks for insertion of chest tube. (From King C, Henretig FM. Tube thoracostomy and needle decompression of the chest. *Pocket atlas of pediatric emergency procedures.* Philadelphia: Lippincott Williams & Wilkins; 2000, Fig. 15.6B, with permission.)

- Infiltrate local anesthetic along the area of incision and deep into the pleural space.
- Incise the upper border of the rib below the intercostal space being used (avoid the neurovascular bundle).
- A 2-cm incision will suffice for most teens and young adults.
- Bluntly dissect (Kelly clamp) through the muscle layers to the pleural space (Fig. 21-6).

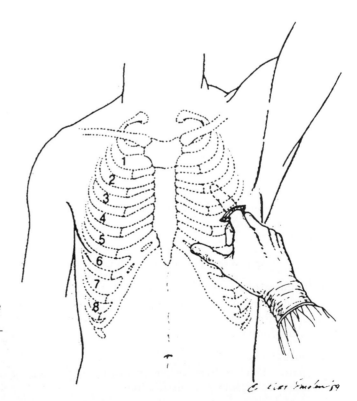

FIGURE 21-7 ● Sweep your finger into the cavity to ensure you feel lung parenchyma. (From Feliciano DV. Tube thoracostomy. In: Benumof JL, ed. *Clinical procedures in anesthesia and intensive care.* Philadelphia: Lippincott; 1992, Fig. 15.3, with permission.)

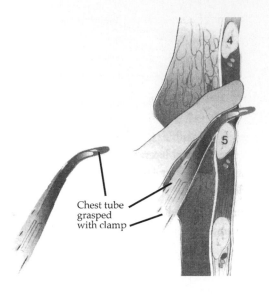

Chest tube grasped with clamp

FIGURE 21-8 ● Insertion of chest tube with Kelly. (From King C, Henretig FM. Tube thoracostomy and needle decompression of the chest. *Pocket atlas of pediatric emergency procedures.* Philadelphia: Lippincott Williams & Wilkins; 2000, Fig. 15.6E and F, with permission.)

- Use a curved Kelly to pierce the pleural space, and extend the opening.
- Feel for lung or soft tissues using your finger (sweep inside the pleural cavity) (Fig. 21-7).
- Insert appropriate chest tube, using the curved Kelly as a guide.
- Direct the chest tube posteriorly within the thorax (Fig. 21-8).
- Secure chest tube in place with a stitch.
- Connect chest tube to an underwater seal and suction.
- Obtain chest x-ray to check position and result of chest tube insertion.

NEEDLE CRICOTHYROIDOTOMY[1–3,12–14]
- Performed only in emergent situation when attempts to secure the airway have failed.
- Incidence of surgical airway procedures in the ED is decreasing with increased competency of ED physicians in airway management.
- Incidence of emergency cricothyroidotomies for blunt or penetrating injuries is 0.5%.
- Only a temporizing measure to oxygenate but not ventilate the patient.
- Simplest technique that can be used by ED physicians until backup from ENT and anesthesia becomes available.
  - Used for children under the age of 12.
  - Can be used to oxygenate for up to 45 minutes.
  - Limiting factor is hypercapnia.

Indications
- The need for a definitive airway is necessary, and other means have failed.
- Severe maxillofacial injury.
- Fractured larynx.
- Oral burns.
- Severe bruxism or inability to open the mouth due to other conditions.
- Laryngeal spasm from allergic reaction.

Contraindications
- More conventional means of securing the airway are possible.
- Tracheal transection with retraction of the distal end.
- Fractured larynx.

Procedure
- Prepare a 12 G or 14 G needle over catheter connected to a 5-mL syringe.
- Prepare the neck in a sterile fashion.

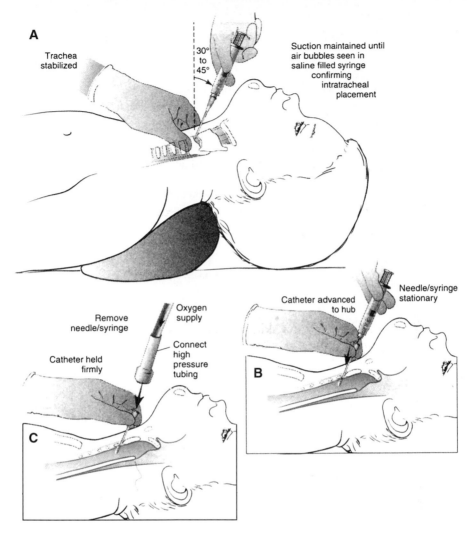

FIGURE 21-9 ● Performing a needle cricothyroidotomy. (From King C, Henretig FM. Obtaining a percutaneous or surgical airway. *Pocket atlas of pediatric emergency procedures.* Philadelphia: Lippincott Williams & Wilkins; 2000, Figs. 6.3A to C, with permission.)

- Identify the cricothyroid membrane, between the thyroid and cricoid cartilage.
- Stabilize the trachea, and puncture the cricothyroid membrane in the midline, directing it 45 degrees inferiorly, and withdrawing on the syringe at the same time (Fig. 21-9).
- Air is aspirated when the needle tip enters the trachea.
- Remove the syringe and needle while advancing the catheter.
- Attach oxygen tubing to the end of the catheter.
- Methods of oxygenation include:
  - Transtracheal jet ventilation (need specialized equipment).
  - Attaching a syringe hub to the catheter, and then placing an ETT into the syringe and continuing to bag through it.

Complications
- Bleeding.
- Puncture of the esophagus.
- Hypercarbia from prolonged use.

- Emphysema.
- Creation of a false lumen.
- Cellulitis.

NEEDLE PERICARDIOCENTESIS[1-3]

- Blood in the pericardial sac decreases the compliance of the heart.
- Recognize the clinical signs of tamponade.
  - Beck triad of hypotension, distended neck veins, and muffled heart sounds.
  - The full triad is not always present.
- Suspect tamponade in any patient who has sustained an injury to the cardiac box.
- The procedure has a high false-positive (intracardiac puncture) and false-negative (clotted blood) rate.
- Can present as pulseless electrical activity (PEA); therefore can be a lifesaving procedure.
- Only a temporizing measure until a formal pericardial window can be established.
- Hemodynamically stable patients should have drainage performed under echocardiographic guidance.

Indications

- Diagnostic and therapeutic intervention for PEA or clinical cardiac tamponade.

Contraindications

- Hemodynamically stable patient should undergo echo-guided aspiration.

Procedure (Fig. 21-10)

- Place patient in reverse Trendelenburg position if possible.
- Prepare the lower sternum and epigastrium in a sterile fashion.
- Attach a 10-mL syringe to an 18 G or 20 G spinal needle.
- Insert inferior and to the left of the xiphoid, aiming toward the left shoulder.
- Advance the needle while withdrawing on syringe.
- Continue until aspiration of blood seen OR evidence of ECG changes.
- If patient's clinical status improves, prepare for a formal pericardial window.

Proper angle and path of needle to pericardium

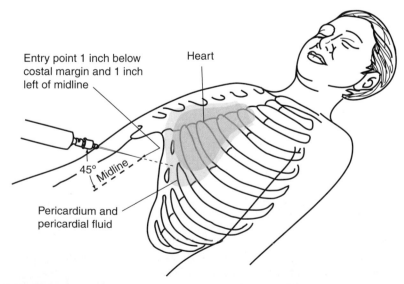

FIGURE 21-10 ● Pericardiocentesis. Aim the needle towards the left shoulder. (From Feliciano DV. Tube thoracostomy. In: Benumof JL, ed. *Clinical procedures in anesthesia and intensive care.* Philadelphia: Lippincott; 1992, Fig. 15.3, with permission.)

Complications
- Arrhythmias.
- Ventricular wall perforation.
- Laceration of coronary artery.
- Procedure can cause tamponade.
- Pulmonary edema.
- Pneumothorax.

ED THORACOTOMY[1–3,15–22]
- Can be a lifesaving procedure.
- Should only be performed by properly trained individuals.
- Survival after ED thoracotomy varies from 18% to 33% for penetrating injury, and up to 2.5% for blunt injury.
- Isolated cardiac stab wounds causing tamponade have the highest rate of survival, approaching 70%.
- Successful outcome is possible if the patient has tamponade and the definitive intervention is performed within 10 minutes of loss of cardiac output.
- Consider the following to decide whether or not the thoracotomy is necessary:
  - Mechanism of injury (blunt versus penetrating).
  - Vital signs present in the ED.
- Goals of the thoracotomy are to:
  - Relieve cardiac tamponade that is causing the compromise.
  - Manage cardiac or great vessel bleeding.
  - Perform open cardiac massage.
  - Limit subdiaphragmatic bleeding via aortic cross-clamping.

Indications
- Penetrating injury with prior witnessed cardiac activity.
- Penetrating injury with persistent and unresponsive hypotension (SBP <70).

Contraindications
- Blunt injury with no witnessed cardiac activity in ED.
- Multiple blunt trauma.
- Severe head injury.
- Loss of cardiac output for more than 10 minutes.
- Lack of expertise.

Procedure: Clam Shell Technique (Fig. 21-11)
- Procedure should only be performed if appropriate training and surgical presence.
- Access to the chest should take no more than 1 to 2 minutes.
- Easier to perform and provides better access and visualization compared to traditional left anterior approach.
- Prepare the area rapidly with antiseptic solution.
- Make bilateral thoracostomy incisions to relieve any tension. If output resumes, you can stop at this point.
- Connect the two sites to form a complete incision.
- Use the Gigli saw or heavy scissors to cut through the sternum.
- Lift the anterior chest wall to obtain the best view of the thoracic cavity (either with clamps or having assistants lift the chest wall).

Tamponade
- Open the pericardium longitudinally to avoid damage to the phrenic nerve.
- Evacuate blood and/or clots from the cavity (Fig. 21-12).

Cardiac Wounds (Fig. 21-13)
- Direct finger pressure over the wound (especially if <1 cm).

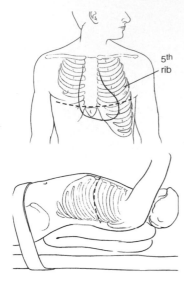

FIGURE 21-11 ● Incision landmarks for a clamshell thoracotomy.

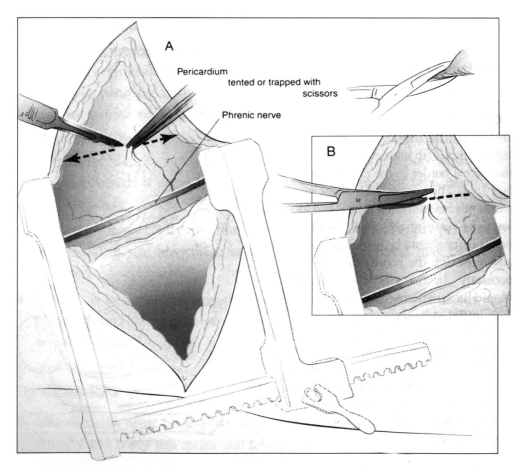

FIGURE 21-12 ● Relief of tamponade. Tent the pericardium with a pair of forceps and cut along the midline. Avoid lateral aspects due to the phrenic nerve. (From King C, Henretig FM. Emergency thoracotomy. *Pocket atlas of pediatric emergency procedures.* Philadelphia: Lippincott Williams & Wilkins; 2000, Fig. 16.3A and B, with permission.)

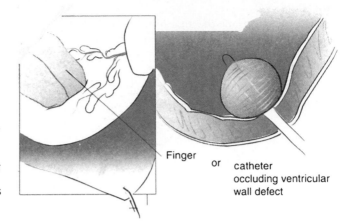

FIGURE 21-13 ● Ventricular wall defect occluded with finger or Foley catheter. (From King C, Henretig FM. Emergency thoracotomy. *Pocket atlas of pediatric emergency procedures.* Philadelphia: Lippincott Williams & Wilkins; 2000, Fig. 16.4, with permission.)

Finger   or   catheter occluding ventricular wall defect

- Larger wounds should be sutured if possible, or temporized by inserting and inflating a Foley catheter.
- Always examine the posterior cardiac region to ensure no other wounds are present.

Aortic Cross–Clamping
- The purpose is to redirect blood flow to the coronary and cerebral vascular beds.
- Can limit hemorrhage in the abdomen and pelvis.
- Clamp at the area of the diaphragm.
- If clamp time should not be longer than 30 minutes.
- Once perfusion is restored, the patient should be moved to the operating room for exploration and definitive treatment.

REGIONAL ANESTHESIA[1–3]
- Local anesthesia to provide a regional block of nerve distribution to facilitate procedures such as suturing.
- Can reduce the amount of local anesthetic used by blocking the nerve proximally and gaining a large anesthetic field distally.
- See Chapter 18 on Pain Management for local anesthetic types, dosages, and duration of action.

Indications
- Anesthesia for surgical procedures that can be done without a general anesthetic.
- Wound repair over a large area innervated by a few proximal nerves.
- Specific regions:
  - Complex hand wounds.
  - Multiple facial lacerations on ipsilateral side.

Contraindications
- Avoid use of epinephrine in end-arteriole systems (fingers, nose, penis, toes, pinna of the ear).
- Local injury at site of infusion.
- Distorted anatomy.

Complications
- Intravascular injection.
- Nerve injury.
- Hematoma.

Procedure
- Prepare and drape the area of injection.
- Use a 25 G needle for infiltration, and inject slowly to decrease discomfort.
- If paresthesias are noted by patient, stop and withdraw a few millimetres and continue to infiltrate.
- The goal is to bathe the nerve in the anesthetic, not inject it.

Locations and Nerve Distribution
Hand
- Anatomy of hand with nerve distribution (Fig. 21-14).

Median Nerve (Fig. 21-15)
- Median nerve runs in the carpal tunnel along with nine other tendons.
- Inject at the flexor crease of the wrist, slightly radial to palmaris longus.

Ulnar Nerve (Fig. 21-16)
- Ulnar nerve hides under the flexor carpi ulnaris about 1 cm deep.
- Inject under the flexor carpi ulnaris, tangential to the hand surface (lateral approach).

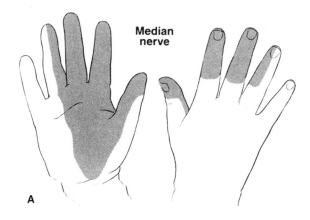

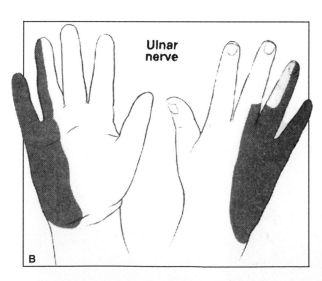

FIGURE 21-14 • Nerve distribution in the hand. **A.** Median nerve. **B.** Ulnar nerve. **C.** Radial nerve. (From King C, Henretig FM. Regional anesthesia. *Pocket atlas of pediatric emergency procedures.* Philadelphia: Lippincott Williams & Wilkins; 2000, Figs. 17.1B, 17.2B, and 17.3B, with permission.)

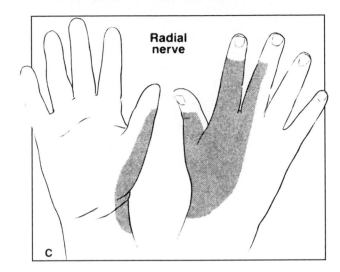

FIGURE 21-14 ● *(Continued)*

Radial Nerve (Fig. 21-17)
- Radial nerve fans out at the dorsum of the hand at the region of the snuffbox.
- Inject distal to radial styloid, and fan out to infiltrate all branches.

Face
- Anatomy of head with nerve distribution (Fig. 21-18).

Infraorbital Nerve Block (Fig. 21-19)
- The nerve exits the infraorbital foramen, about 1 to 2 cm below the inferior orbital rim.
- Intraoral injection better tolerated.
- Consider oral topical anesthetic.
- Retract the lip, and use the maxillary canine/premolar as a landmark. Inject superior to this to the level of the nerve (slightly below the infraorbital foramen).
- Avoid injecting into the foramen.

Mental Block (Fig. 21-20)
- The nerve exits at the mental foramen, about 0.5 to 1 cm inferior and anterior to the inferior premolar.
- Consider topical local anesthetic.
- Inject inferiorly to the level of the nerve.

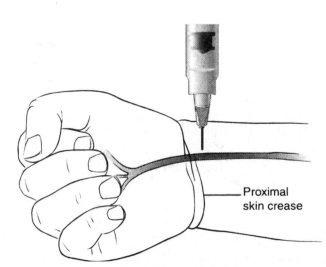

FIGURE 21-15 ● Wrist block of the median nerve. (From King C, Henretig FM. Regional anesthesia. *Pocket atlas of pediatric emergency procedures.* Philadelphia: Lippincott Williams & Wilkins; 2000, Fig. 17.1C, with permission.)

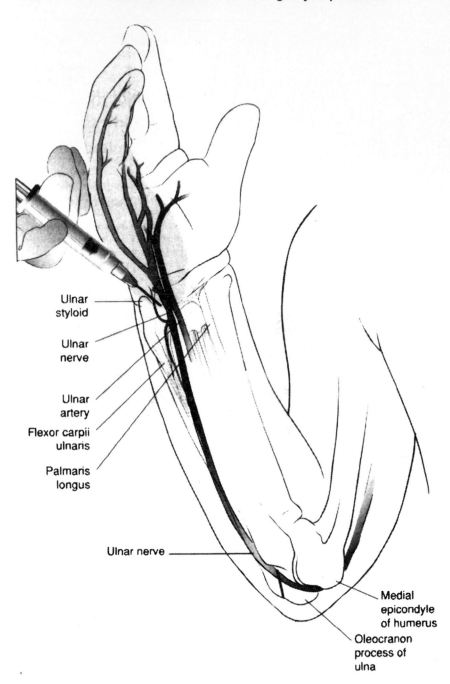

Ulnar
styloid

Ulnar
nerve

Ulnar
artery

Flexor carpii
ulnaris

Palmaris
longus

Ulnar nerve

Medial
epicondyle
of humerus

Oleocranon
process of
ulna

FIGURE 21-16 ● Wrist block of the ulnar nerve. (From King C, Henretig FM. Regional anesthesia. *Pocket atlas of pediatric emergency procedures.* Philadelphia: Lippincott Williams & Wilkins; 2000, Fig. 17.2A, with permission.)

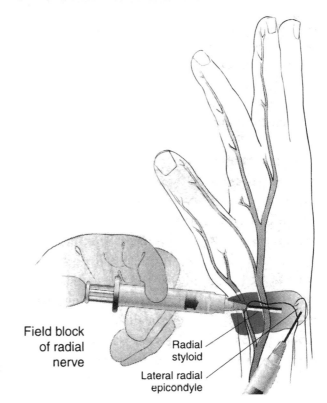

FIGURE 21-17 ● Wrist block of the radial nerve. (From King C, Henretig FM. Regional anesthesia. *Pocket atlas of pediatric emergency procedures.* Philadelphia: Lippincott Williams & Wilkins; 2000, Fig. 17.3C, with permission.)

Field block of radial nerve

Radial styloid

Lateral radial epicondyle

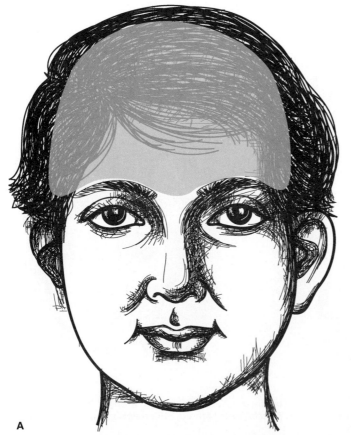

FIGURE 21-18 ● Sensory nerve distribution of the face. **A.** Supraorbital nerve. **B.** Infraorbital nerve. **C.** Mental nerve. (From Simon RR, Brenner BE. Anesthesia and regional blocks. *Emergency procedures & techniques.* 4th ed. Philadelphia: Lippincott Williams & Wilkins; 2002, with permission.)

A

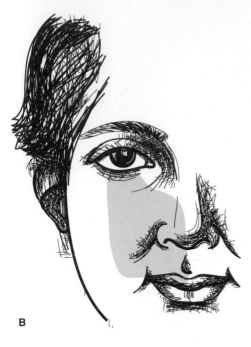

B

C

FIGURE 21-18 ● *(Continued)*

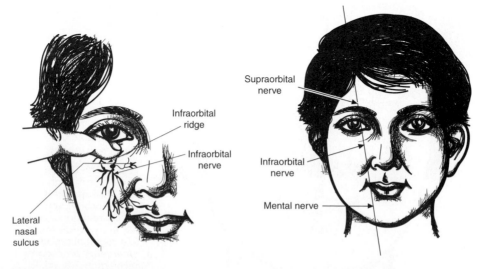

Supraorbital
nerve

Infraorbital
ridge

Infraorbital
nerve

Infraorbital
nerve

Mental nerve

Lateral
nasal
sulcus

FIGURE 21-19 ● Infraorbital nerve block landmarks. (From Simon RR, Brenner BE. Anesthesia and regional blocks. *Emergency procedures & techniques.* 4th ed. Philadelphia: Lippincott Williams & Wilkins; 2002, with permission.)

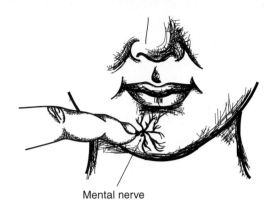

Mental nerve

FIGURE 21-20 ● Mental nerve block landmarks. (From Simon RR, Brenner BE. Anesthesia and regional blocks. *Emergency procedures & techniques.* 4th ed. Philadelphia: Lippincott Williams & Wilkins; 2002, with permission.)

REFERENCES

1. Baxter BT, Moore EE, Moore JB, et al. Emergency department thoracotomy following injury: critical determinants of patient salvage. *World J. Surg* 1988;12:671–675.
2. Beaver BL, Columbani PM, Buck JR, et al. Efficacy of emergency room thoracotomy in pediatric trauma. *J Pediatric Surg* 1987;22:19–23.
3. Biffl WL, Moore, EE, Harken AH. Emergency department thoracotomy. In: Mattox KL, Moore EE, Feliciano DV, eds. *Trauma.* McGraw Hill, New York; 2000.
4. Branney SW, Moore EE, Feldhaus KM, et al. Critical analysis of two decades of experience with postinjury emergency department thoracotomy in a regional trauma center. *J Trauma* 1998;45:87–94.
5. Rothenberg SS, Moore EE, Moore FA, et al. Emergency department thoracotomy in children—a critical analysis. *J Trauma* 1989;29:1322–1325.
6. Karmy-Jones R, Jurkovich GJ, Nathens AB, et al. Timing of urgent thoracotomy for hemorrhage after trauma: a multicenter study. *Arch Surg* 2001;136:513–518.
7. Rhee PM, Acosta J, Bridgeman A, et al. Survival after emergency department thoracotomy: review of published data from the past 25 years. *J Am Coll Surg* 2000;190:288–298.
8. Wise D, Davies G, Coats T, et al. Emergency thoracotomy: how to do it. *Emerg Med J* 2005;22:22–24.
9. King C, Henretig FM. *Pocket atlas of pediatric emergency procedures.* Philadelphia: Lippincott Williams & Wilkins; 2000.
10. Simon R, Brenner B. *Emergency procedures and techniques.* Philadelphia: Lippincott Williams & Wilkins; 2002.
11. Robers JR, Hedges JR. *Clinical procedures in emergency medicine.* 4th ed. Philadelphia: Saunders; 2004.
12. Mattox KL, Allen MK. Systematic approach to pneumothorax, haemothorax, pneumomediastinum and subcutaneous emphysema. *Injury* 1986;17:309–312. Symposium paper.
13. Etoch SW, Bar-Natan MF, Miller FB, et al. Tube thoracostomy. Factors relating to complications. *Arch Surg* 1995;130:521–525.
14. Milikan JS, Moore EE, Steiner E, et al. Complications of tube thoracostomy for acute trauma. *Am J Surgery* 1980;140:738–741.
15. Bailey RC. Complications of tube thoracostomy in trauma. *J Accid Emerg Med* 2000;17:111–114.
16. Abboud PC, Kendall JL. Ultrasound guidance for vascular access. *Emerg Med Clin North Am* 2004;22:749–773.
17. Dearlove OR. NICE guidelines for central venous catheterization in children. *Br J Anaesth* 2005;94:136–137.
18. Iserson KV, Criss E. Intraosseous infusions: a usable technique. *Am J Emerg Med* 1986;4:540–542.
19. Kruse JA, Vyskocil JJ, Haupt MT. Intraosseous infusions: a flexible option for the adult or child with delayed, difficult, or impossible conventional vascular access. *Crit Care Med* 1994;22:728–729.
20. Granholm T, Framer DL. The surgical airway. *Respir Clin North Am* 2001;7:13–23.
21. Schroeder AA. Cricothyroidotomy: when, why and why not? *Am J Otolaryngol* 2000;21:195–201.
22. Rehm CG, Wanek SM, Gagnon EB, et al. Cricothyroidotomy for elective airway management in critically ill trauma patients with technically challenging neck anatomy. *Crit Care* 2002;6:531–535.

CHAPTER 22

Transport of the Pediatric Trauma Patient

Adam Cheng, MD, FRCPC (Ped EM), FAAP

BACKGROUND
- Critically ill children have better outcomes when treated in pediatric trauma centers and tertiary pediatric intensive care units.[1]
- Pediatric intensive care unit centralization has increased the need for interhospital pediatric transports.
- Specialized pediatric retrieval teams have been developed in many countries to undertake the stabilization and safe transfer of critically ill children.
- Pediatric trauma patients are best cared for in centers that are prepared to treat sustained injuries.[1]

COMPOSITION OF PEDIATRIC TRANSPORT TEAMS
- Team may include critical care paramedics, nurses, respiratory therapists, or physicians.
- Recommend at least 2 patient care providers per transport, with 3 care providers for more critically ill children.[2]
- Aim to match team members' skills to patient needs.
- Incidence of complications is decreased with dedicated, specialized transport teams.[2]

PREPARING FOR TRANSPORT: EQUIPMENT AND MODE OF TRANSPORT
Equipment
- See Table 22-1 for list of equipment required to transport a critically ill child.
- Optimally small, lightweight, and sturdy.
- Regularly check and service all transport equipment.
- Bring extra batteries/power source for all equipment.
- Replenish used medications and supplies after each transport.

Mode of Transport
- Determined by several factors:
  - Urgency of case.
  - Distance.
  - Traffic conditions.
  - Weather.
  - Availability of air/land transport.
- Equipment availability may vary by mode of transport.
  - Check beforehand and bring additional supplies.
- Voltage capacity in different settings may vary. Having additional battery packs may be useful but cumbersome.
- See Table 22-2 for Selected Modes of Transport.

TABLE 22-1

Equipment Required When Transporting a Critically Ill Child

Monitors	Heart rate/rhythm
	Blood pressure
	Pulse oximetry
	End-tidal CO_2
	Temperature
	Blood glucose
	Extra batteries
Infusion Pumps	Multiple infusion pumps
	Pressure infuser
	Extra extension tubing, stopcocks, T-connectors
	Various IV fluids
	Extra batteries
Resuscitation Equipment	Airway equipment
	Suction equipment
	Central lines
	Chest tubes
	Intravenous and intraosseous needles
	Proper-sized resuscitation board/stretcher
Drugs and Fluids	Resuscitation drugs
	Infusion drugs
	Sedative/paralytic drugs
	Antibiotics
	Intravenous fluids/blood if necessary
Portable Oxygen Supply	Oxygen: Ensure adequate amount for transport
Ventilator	Appropriate ventilator for desired mode
	Appropriately sized circuit (neonate vs. child vs. adult)
Document Folder	Patient chart
	Transport record
	Information for parents
	Telephone numbers
Clothing	Personal protective clothing: Gowns, gloves, and masks
	Warm clothes
	Change of clothes (for long transports)
	Appropriate footwear
Communication	Portable phone
	Extra batteries
Personal Care	Food and beverage for longer transports
	Personal hygiene items for potential overnight transports

PREPARING FOR TRANSPORT: PRIOR TO LEAVING THE SENDING FACILITY
General Principles
- Do no harm:[1]
  - Avoid undue delay.
    - Especially if patient requires specialized tertiary care.
  - Ensure safety of transport.
- Timely, optimization of patient condition prior to transport.
- Aim to provide care equivalent to sending hospital's capabilities.
- Follow an organized, structured approach to assessing patient.
- Ensure patient has received a full primary and secondary survey.
  - See Chapter 2 on Primary and Secondary Survey for details.
- Communicate with receiving hospital prior to departure.
- Anticipate patient care needs during transport.

TABLE 22-2

Selected Modes of Transport[3]

Road/Land Ambulance	**Advantages** Rapid mobilization Large working area Ability to stop for procedures **Disadvantages** Slow transit time Bumpy ride, motion sickness
Helicopter/Rotor-Wing	**Advantages** Rapid mobilization if service available Fast Can land directly at facility/scene **Disadvantages** Limited work area Noisy Vibration with turbulence Operation limited by weather Pressure considerations
Fixed-Wing Aircraft	**Advantages** Long distances traveled in short times **Disadvantages** Noisy Vibration with turbulence Operation limited by weather Requires additional legs of patient transport (to/from airport or hospital) Pressure considerations

Airway

- Ensure airway is patent and protected.
- Assess risk of losing airway on transport.
  - Consider need for intubation prior to departure.
  - See Chapter 3 on Airway Management for details on RSI.
- If patient is intubated, mechanical ventilation is preferred over hand-bagging.
- Confirm ETT placement prior to departure:
  - End-tidal CO_2 detection and continuous monitoring.
  - Chest x-ray.
- Secure position of ETT.
- Consider predeparture blood gas to ensure adequate oxygenation and ventilation.
- Ensure suction is working:
  - All patients, whether intubated or not, may require suctioning.
- Protect cervical spine if indicated:
  - C-spine collar.
  - Secure head to spine board using blocks/sandbags and tapes.

Breathing

- Provide supplemental oxygen and consider altitude.
- Monitor oxygen saturation and end-tidal CO_2 continuously.
- Ensure adequate oxygen supply for duration of transport.
- Ensure head-injured patients are adequately oxygenated to prevent secondary brain injury.

- Consider need for tube thoracostomy prior to transport.
  - Insert if clinical signs of chest trauma and respiratory distress.[1]
  - Bring appropriate size of chest tubes if risk of pneumothorax is high.
    - Sending hospital may not have all pediatric sizes.
- Flight strategies for dealing with potential expansion of free air:
  - Pressurize cabin to sea level.
  - Limit flight altitude.

Circulation

- Ensure adequate or ongoing fluid resuscitation of patient.
- Control external hemorrhage by direct pressure, staples, or sutures.
- Consider ongoing fluid losses in fluid calculations.
- Secure two large-bore IVs for transport.
- For fluid-refractory shock:
  - Prepare appropriate inotrope infusions prior to departure.
  - Bring necessary blood products if clinically indicated.
  - Ensure sufficient intravenous fluids for duration of transport.
- Secure and protect all intravenous and central lines.
  - Ensure patency and evaluate for kinking or blockage of tubing.
- Obtain intraosseous (IO) access if unable to procure intravenous access.
  - Secure IO with tape and gauze to prevent dislodgement.

Monitoring and Tubes

- Ensure all monitors in good, working order.
- Use frequent cycling, external blood pressure monitoring en route.
- Continuous end-tidal CO_2 monitoring of all intubated patients.
- Foley catheter to monitor urine output and decompress bladder.
- Nasogastric tube as needed to decompress stomach.

Analgesia, Sedation, and Drugs

- See Chapter 18 on Pain Management for details.
- Assess patient need for analgesia, sedation, and neuromuscular blockade.
- Ensure proper and sufficient medications are available en route.
- Consider continuous infusions of sedatives/analgesics, rather than intermittent boluses, especially for longer transports.
- See Table 22-3 for list of critical care transport drugs.

TABLE 22-3

Drugs List for Pediatric Critical Care Transport

Antibiotics	Ampicillin, cefazolin, cefotaxime, cetriaxone, clindamycin, gentamicin, vancomycin
Anticonvulsants	Lorazepam, midazolam, phenobarbital, phenytoin
Cardiac Drugs	Adenosine, amiodarone, atropine, calcium gluconate, digoxin, dobutamine, dopamine, epinephrine, isoproterenol, lidocaine, nifedipine, nitroprusside, propanolol, prostaglandin, vasopressin
Fluids and Blood Products	Albumin, dextrose 10%, dextrose 50%, dextrose 5% normal saline, normal saline, 3% saline, sterile water
Sedatives, Analgesics, and Paralytics	Etomidate, fentanyl, ketamine, morphine, pancuronium, propofol, rocuronium, succinylcholine, thiopental, vecuronium
Other Medications	Dexamethasone, diphenhydramine, furosemide, glucagon, heparin, hydrocortisone, insulin, mannitol, methylprednisolone, naloxone, neostigmine, potassium chloride, salbutamol, racemic epinephrine, sodium bicarbonate

Orthopedic Injuries
- See Chapter 12 on Orthopedic Injuries for details.
- Stabilize any potential fractures prior to transport (e.g., pelvis, femur).
- Monitor for signs of hypovolemic shock for long bone and pelvic fractures.
- Prevent neurovascular compromise by reassessing any known injuries.

Burns
- See Chapter 14 on Thermal Injuries for details.
- Protect airway as needed prior to transport.
- Ensure ongoing, adequate fluid resuscitation.
- Calculate ongoing fluid requirements prior to departing sending facility.
- Cover, cleanse, and dress wounds.

Documentation and Communication
- Ensure appropriate handover from sending facility.
- Bring all documentation and x-rays.
- Provide information to the parents:
  - Update on child's condition.
  - Directions to receiving hospital.
  - Contact telephone number of receiving hospital.
  - Instruct family not to follow ambulance at high speed.
- At receiving facility: Provide appropriate patient handover.

TRANSPORT BY AIR: SPECIAL CONSIDERATIONS
- Patient evaluation and stabilization are affected by certain flight-imposed stresses.[4]

Boyle's Law
- Gas expands as cabin altitude rises and as barometric pressure falls.
- Pneumothoraces should be drained prior to air transport.
  - Vent chest tubes into a Heimlich (flap) valve for portability.
- Fill endotracheal cuffs and Foley balloons with water/saline instead of air.
- Monitor for increased intracranial pressure in head-injured patients.
- Place a nasogastric tube to decompress stomach and prevent gastric distention.

Increased Oxygen Requirements
- Oxygen requirements increase with altitude.
- Provide supplemental oxygen for patients.
- Patients requiring 100% oxygen on the ground may need a change in ventilatory support to tolerate transport at altitude.
- Saturations may be lower at altitude; therefore the benefits/risks of air transport need to be considered.

Noise
- Difficult to communicate and causes fatigue.
- Auscultation is difficult (breath sounds, heart sounds, or blood pressure).

Temperature
- Decreases with increasing altitude.
- Monitor patient temperature, particularly infants (use isolette).
- Ensure patient is appropriately covered and draped.
- Foil blankets aid in retaining thermal heat.
- Bring extra clothes for transport team members.

Turbulence and Vibration
- Depends on prevalent weather conditions: Worse when air is warm.
- Abrupt changes in altitude or aircraft position may cause motion sickness.
- Secure patient with belts, blankets, and restraints (if necessary).
- Ensure all equipment is secured.

Dehydration
- Lack of moisture at high altitudes.
- Maintain adequate hydration for patient and team members.

Acceleration/Deceleration in Fixed-Wing Aircraft
- Rear-load (head facing rear of aircraft) hemodynamically compromised patients to prevent compromise in cerebral perfusion during takeoff.
- Front-load (head facing front of aircraft) head-injured patients to prevent increases in intracranial pressure during takeoff.

ADVERSE EVENTS DURING TRANSPORT
- Adverse events occur commonly (up to 50%).[5,6]
- Incidence of adverse events proportional to severity of patient's illness.
- Type of adverse events:
  - Alteration in vital signs: Hypothermia/hyperthermia, hypertension/hypotension, bradycardia/tachycardia.
  - Equipment related: Accidental extubation, oxygen supply loss, ventilator malfunction, loss of IV catheter infusing vasoactive drugs.
  - Other: Drug error, respiratory arrest, cardiac arrest, death.
- Minimize adverse events:
  - Provide adequate resuscitation prior to transfer.
  - Provide appropriate monitoring during transfer.
  - Anticipate potential problems during transfer.
  - Team composition and equipment should reflect pretransport severity of illness and anticipated duration of transport.

CLINICAL PEARLS

DO
- Draw up appropriate medications and fluids before departing sending facility.
- Adequately fluid-resuscitate patient prior to transport.
- Maintain open lines of communication with receiving facility.

DON'T
- Send a team unprepared to deal with the patient's severity of illness.
- Delay transport if patient needs definitive care at tertiary care hospital.
- Leave sending facility before ensuring airway is patent and secure.

REFERENCES
1. Graneto JW, Soglin DF. Transport and stabilization of the pediatric trauma patient. *Pediatr Clin North Am* 1993;40:365–378.
2. Woodward GA, Insoft RM, Pearson-Shaver AL, et al. The state of pediatric interfacility transport: consensus of the second national pediatric and neonatal interfacility transport medicine leadership conference. *Pediatr Emerg Care* 2002;18:38–43.
3. Macrae DJ. Paediatric intensive care transport. *Arch Dis Child* 1994;71:175–178.
4. Brink LW, Neuman B, Wynn J. Air transport. *Pediatr Clin North Am* 1993;40:439–455.
5. Wallen E, Venkataraman ST, Grosso MJ, et al. Intrahospital transport of critically ill pediatric patients. *Crit Care Med* 1995;23:1588–1595.
6. Barry PW, Ralston C. Adverse events occurring during interhospital transfer of the critically ill. *Arch Dis Child* 1994;71:8–11.

Index

Page numbers followed by *f* or *t* indicate figures or tables, respectively.